FOREIGN PRACTICES

McGill-Queen's/Associated Medical Services Studies in the History of Medicine, Health, and Society

Series editors: J.T.H. Connor and Erika Dyck

This series presents books in the history of medicine, health studies, and social policy, exploring interactions between the institutions, ideas, and practices of medicine and those of society as a whole. To begin to understand these complex relationships and their history is a vital step to ensuring the protection of a fundamental human right: the right to health. Volumes in this series have received financial support to assist publication from Associated Medical Services, Inc. (AMS), a Canadian charitable organization with an impressive history as a catalyst for change in Canadian healthcare. For eighty years, AMS has had a profound impact through its support of the history of medicine and the education of healthcare professionals, and by making strategic investments to address critical issues in our healthcare system. AMS has funded eight chairs in the history of medicine across Canada, is a primary sponsor of many of the country's history of medicine and nursing organizations, and offers fellowships and grants through the AMS History of Medicine and Healthcare Program (www.amshealthcare.ca).

FOREIGN
PRACTICES

Immigrant Doctors and the
History of Canadian Medicare

SASHA MULLALLY AND DAVID WRIGHT

MCGILL-QUEEN'S UNIVERSITY PRESS
Montreal & Kingston • London • Chicago

© McGill-Queen's University Press 2020

ISBN 978-0-2280-0371-7 (cloth)
ISBN 978-0-2280-0372-4 (paper)
ISBN 978-0-2280-0492-9 (ePDF)

Legal deposit fourth quarter 2020
Bibliothèque nationale du Québec

Printed in Canada on acid-free paper that is 100% ancient forest free
(100% post-consumer recycled), processed chlorine free

This book has been published with the help of a grant from the Canadian
Federation for the Humanities and Social Sciences, through the Awards to
Scholarly Publications Program, using funds provided by the Social
Sciences and Humanities Research Council of Canada.

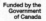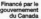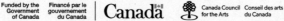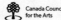

We acknowledge the support of the Canada Council for the Arts.

Nous remercions le Conseil des arts du Canada de son soutien.

Library and Archives Canada Cataloguing in Publication

Title: Foreign practices : immigrant doctors and the history of Canadian
    medicare / Sasha Mullally and David Wright.
Names: Mullally, Sasha, author. | Wright, David, 1965- author.
Series: McGill-Queen's/Associated Medical Services (Hannah Institute)
    studies in the history of medicine, health, and society ; 55.
Description: Series statement: McGill-Queen's/Associated Medical Services
    studies in the history of medicine, health, and society ; 55 | Includes
    bibliographical references and index.
Identifiers: Canadiana (print) 20200299662 | Canadiana (ebook)
    2020029976X | ISBN 9780228003717 (cloth) | ISBN 9780228003724 (paper) |
    ISBN 9780228004929 (ePDF)
Subjects: LCSH: Physicians, Foreign—Canada—History—20th century. |
    LCSH: Physicians—Canada—History—20th century. | LCSH: Immi-
    grants—Canada—History—20th century. | LCSH: Medical care—
    Canada—History—20th century.
Classification: LCC R697.F6 M85 2020 | DDC 610.97109/045—dc23

To Mona and Andrew

Contents

Tables and Figures

FIGURES

Acknowledgments

This book began life almost twenty years ago, arising from a conversation held over coffee between the two authors at an annual conference of the Canadian Society for the History of Medicine. It has since been nurtured and supported by various institutions and funding agencies, as an idea became a pilot project, and the pilot project evolved into a multiyear collaborative initiative, leading to articles and book chapters, and ultimately this monograph. Needless to say, over such a long period of gestation, we have many institutions and people to thank. We would like to acknowledge our respective institutions over the last two decades – University of Alberta, St Mary's University, and the University of New Brunswick (Mullally) as well as McMaster University and McGill University (Wright) – for their generous support of time and research facilities. David Wright's position at McMaster was supported by an endowment (Hannah Chair endowment) from Associated Medical Services (AMS), Toronto. AMS also generously funded a seed grant involving both of the authors in 2008 and, later, a conference held at McGill University in 2012. The Social Sciences and Humanities Research Council of Canada has contributed support through a Research Development Initiative grant (2007), through a conference workshop (2012), and ultimately, in conjunction with the Canada Research Chairs (CRC) program (2012–19), the Tier 1 CRC in the History of Health Policy at McGill University.

At McGill University, David has received generous assistance from the Institute for Health and Social Policy (IHSP), a jointly funded research institute between the Faculty of Medicine and the Faculty of Arts, McGill University. The IHSP has provided a vibrant intellectual home as well as crucial infrastructure for research and workshops, and hosted Sasha as visiting professor during her 2015 sabbatical as the first chapters for this book were drafted. Her work was also supported by McGill's Osler Library, which awarded her an Edward H. Bensley Travel Grant in 2015 to access medical directories and biographical materials. The institute also provided training for interns who have worked on various aspects of this project; they include Emma Avery, John Clarke, Saskia de Vries, Elliot Huzman, Robyn Lee, Andrew Madeiros, Abbey Mahon, Farwa Malik, and Haley Welch. In addition, we were both fortunate to hire, some for short periods of time, others for longer, a series of research assistants who contributed to the project in a myriad of ways. Johanna Bleecker, Katherine Macdonald, and Emma Avery conducted GIS research and mapping; John Clarke and Taylor Dysart inputted data on the American-trained and Newfoundland-based foreign doctors, respectively, as part of miniprojects. Alexandra Ketchum contributed research and insights on the role of American "draft doctors" who moved north during the Vietnam War. Gregory Marks revolutionized the data gathering from the contemporary directories of the Canadian and American medical associations, with his own flair for adapting freeware. Barry MacKenzie, Cody Hamilton, Sharon Black, and Renée Saucier transcribed oral interviews over several years. Renée Saucier worked assiduously, for several years, on many different aspects of the book, in particular research into the Indian response to the medical brain drain, background pieces on rural medicine, as well as preproduction fact checking and permissions for images. Her influence appears throughout almost every aspect of the book.

We would also like to thank the many colleagues and graduate students whose intellectual suggestions and research shaped the contours of our own book and contributed to scholarly articles over the past ten years: Annmarie Adams, John Armstrong, Sanjoy Bhattacharya, Laura Bisaillon, Linda Bryder, Lisa Chilton, Jim Connor, Colleen Cordukes, Nathan Flis, Martin Gorsky, Mona Gupta, Laura Madokoro, Gregory Marchildon, Sean Mills, Laurence Monnais, James Moran, Jan Raska, and Mat Savelli. Papers were test-driven in various locales around the world, including annual conferences of the Canadian Society for the History of Medicine (Edmonton, Montreal, Toronto, Vancouver), the American Association for the History of Medicine (Montreal, Minneapolis, Nashville), the Canadian Association for the History of Nursing (Toronto), as well as seminars and colloquia as far afield as Auckland (New Zealand), Stockholm, and

Gothenburg (Sweden), Memorial University (Newfoundland), Dalhousie and St Mary's University (Nova Scotia), University of Warwick (Great Britain), University of Oxford (Great Britain), Durban (South Africa), Charlottetown (Prince Edward Island), and Hong Kong. Many thanks for those who assisted in the organization of these papers and invited lectures, including Sanjoy Bhattacharya, Kelvin Chan, Erica Charters, Cathy Coleborne, Mark Harrison, Howard Jones, Solveig Jülich, Susan Lamb, Hilary Marland, James Moran, Jock Murray, Shannon Murray, Anders Ottosson, Julie Parle, Howard Phillips, Maria Sjöberg, and Peter Twohig. Visiting fellowships and lectureships were funded and organized by the University of Warwick (Great Britain) and Otago University (New Zealand). We thank individuals involved in the immigration process, who proved invaluable to our understanding of the assessment of new immigrants in the 1960s and 1970s, including Gerry Maffre and members of the Canadian Immigration History Society network as well as Michael McCormick of the Department of Citizenship and Immigration.

Parts of this book appeared in earlier versions in articles and book chapters. We are grateful to the University of Toronto Press for material that appeared in the *Journal of Canadian Studies* and in the edited volume *Doctors Without Borders*, to Oxford University Press for material that appeared in the *Journal of the History of Medicine and Allied Sciences*, and to the University of Pittsburgh Press, for material that appeared in a book edited by Patrick Manning and Mat Savelli entitled *Global Transformations in the Life Sciences, 1945–80*. We also thank the individuals and institutions who have granted us permission to feature images from their collections, including Gary L Saunders, Dr Richard Swinson, Dr Denis Danemen, the estate of Dr George Dewar, the University of Calgary Archives, Pier 21, the World Health Organization, the archives and special collections of the University of Manitoba, the Osler Library, the university archives and special collections of the University of Saskatchewan, the Toronto Public Library, the McCord Museum, and Archives du Centre International de Documentation et d'Information Haitienne, Caribéenne et Afro-Canadienne (Montreal), Bibliothèque et Archives nationales du Québec, and Library and Archives Canada.

Finally, we must also acknowledge the advice, support, and encouragement of our editor Kyla Madden and her excellent team at McGill-Queen's University Press who guided this book to publication. Noeline

Bridge crafted an excellent index. We also want to thank the foreign-trained doctors who generously donated their time for interviews and whose life stories helped shape our narrative. Some thirty provided interviews both in person and over the telephone, others shared stories over email and in letters, while still other life stories were captured in published memoirs and in the many medical journals we culled for stories of emigration, immigration, relocation, and settlement. Their collective stories are both the inspiration and the lifeblood of the book that follows.

FOREIGN PRACTICES

Introduction

In 1969, Jagdish Gupta, a forty-two-year-old Indian ophthalmologist, arrived in Sydney, Nova Scotia, to near universal relief. The local inhabitants, it was to become apparent, were seriously short of doctors and had been forced to travel hundreds of miles, often suffering and in poor health, for specialist treatment. The only two ophthalmic surgeons on the island of Cape Breton had recently retired, leaving the medical community with the prospect of sending all urgent cases to Halifax, more than 400 kilometres away. Dr Gupta had never seen Sydney before. A visit to Halifax had led to an offer to relocate to one of Dalhousie's teaching hospitals, and letters exchanged with medical institutions in Toronto had also elicited potential positions but with the proviso that he undertake a year's retraining. However, the head of St Rita's hospital in the small mining and steel town of Sydney, on Cape Breton Island's northeast coast, offered him an immediate permanent position with no local medical competition. The hospital administrator convinced his peers at the College of Physicians and Surgeons of Nova Scotia not to impose any recertification requirements. The Punjabi surgeon accepted the offer and returned to India to close down his Delhi practice. Because of inaccurate Indian documentation, he listed Canada Day – 1 July – on his formal immigration application for landed immigrant status.[1]

Gupta seemed, at first, like an ambitious surgeon who was bound to make a go of it in his home country. In 1946, he attended Lahore medical school, a "scholarship Hindu" at a predominantly Muslim institution, full of promise and ambition. But he was forced to complete his medical studies in the so-called camp sites of Panjab University after the Partition of British India tore his native Punjab apart the next year. Ultimately

Gupta completed his undergraduate medical education and a further master of surgery at Lucknow. Over his student life, he endured a brief incarceration by the British colonial authorities for participation in political rallies, but he nonetheless did not let this stop him from being drawn to the opportunities that the British Commonwealth might offer him. He subsequently accepted a postgraduate scholarship to pursue his fellowship training in England. From 1956 to 1959, along with a growing cohort of Indian doctors in Britain,[2] he trained as an ophthalmologist in some of the most famous London teaching hospitals – Great Ormond Street and Bartholomew's – before taking his first staff position as a house officer in the Sheffield Eye Hospital.

Typical of many of his classmates at the time, he had no firm plans to remain in Britain. Indeed, he returned to the Indian subcontinent once his training in Britain was complete in 1959, securing a comfortable position in a new teaching hospital in New Delhi. There, he married a graduate student studying political science, and together they began a life with many of the trappings of middle-class Indian professionals. They benefitted from the comfort of a generous house with servants, and Gupta enjoyed the prestige of being a British-trained medical doctor in the postpartition Indian capital. Yet, as with many of his classmates who had studied abroad, the experience of life in Britain had shifted the landscape of his professional identity. In 1968 a letter from one of his former roommates in England alerted him to a program in the province of Nova Scotia, Canada, which was apparently licensing English-speaking Commonwealth doctors who had (British) General Medical Council specialist qualifications. He visited the Canadian consulate in Delhi, and within a year he had packed his bags to inquire further. After signing his contract, his wife, eight months pregnant, and his five-year-old son would arrive in late September of 1969, only weeks before the first Cape Breton snowstorm of the year.[3]

For the next twelve years, Dr Gupta would be the only practising ophthalmologist on the island of Cape Breton – he was, in effect, permanently on call for the 40,000 residents for more than a decade. Providing clinical services in his fourth language (in addition to his native Punjabi, he spoke Urdu and Hindi), he set up practice in Sydney and also tutored himself in basic French medical terminology to better serve the occasional unilingual Acadian patient arriving from Cheticamp or one of the western Cape Breton outports. However, he would not constitute the first, or the

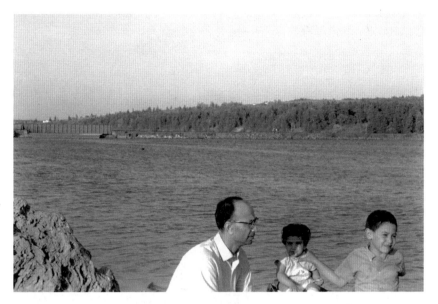

Figure I.1 Dr Jagdish Gupta in Cape Breton
A Punjabi-born surgeon who specialized in ophthalmology in the British teaching hospitals in the 1950s, Dr Gupta returned to postpartition India, only to remigrate to Cape Breton in the late 1960s. By the time of the Immigration Act of 1976, there would be almost 500 doctors who completed their undergraduate medical degrees in India who were listed as practicing in Canada under the newly inauguarated system of Medicare. The family photo in Cape Breton was taken with his two children, who would both become doctors.

last, South Asian practitioner in this remote part of Atlantic Canada. He was preceded by Mohan Virick, a Burmese-trained general practitioner,[4] and followed, in the subsequent seven years, by Drs Naqvi, Gursahani, Bhattacharjee, Chokshi, Singh, Mian, Chauhan, Chaturvedi, Khalsa, Khalifa, Patel, Rajani, Kooka, Qureshi, and several other foreign-trained physicians and their families in the Sydney and nearby Glace Bay municipalities. By the early 1970s, a sizeable minority of all the practicing physicians in the two principal cities of Sydney and Glace Bay were foreign-trained doctors and half of these foreign medical graduates were South Asian practitioners ministering to the ill-health, occupational accidents, and mental disorders of this economically impoverished, but culturally dynamic, Scottish Canadian community.

Taken as a microhistory of immigration in the 1960s, the South Asian medical community of Cape Breton would constitute an unusual and intriguing case study of Canadian social history at the time of the nation's centenary. However, it represents so much more. The Sydney and Glace Bay doctors form part of a much larger transnational event in the history of medicine – a relocation of hundreds of thousands of physicians, surgeons, nurses, dentists, lab technicians and allied health practitioners during the 1960s and 1970s. The transformation of immigration policies – not just in Canada but across the global north – facilitated a surge in medical migration that included huge international diasporas of South Asian, British, Taiwanese, South African, Haitian, and Irish doctors, to name only a few of the principal nationalities represented in this heterogeneous group. These intertwined medical diasporas would transform the health care systems of their adopted nations and, indirectly, raise profound questions about global health inequities. The timing of their arrival was equally important for Canada, for they would settle at the very moment of the inception of its most revered social policy of twentieth century – the inauguration of Medicare.

MEDICARE AND MIGRATION

Universal health insurance, or Medicare as it is known in Canada, occupies a central place in the self-identity of Canadians, who tend to express patriotism through a peculiar type of welfare-state nationalism. Indeed, when the Canadian Broadcasting Corporation ran a national contest to identify the "Greatest Canadian of All Time," few were surprised when the "father" of Medicare – Tommy Douglas – won by a large margin.[5] Douglas has become an iconic figure in Canadian political history, widely regarded as the leader of the first socialist government in North America. The Saskatchewan premier and his Cooperative Commonwealth Federation (CCF) government implemented a prototype of what would evolve into the national health care insurance program.[6] Douglas's vision, his own poverty-to-power biography, as well as his charismatic personality cast a long shadow on the history of Canadian medicine in this period.[7] It is hard to disaggregate his own contributions to Medicare with the narrative of the Canadian political left and the national New Democratic Party (of which he was the first national leader). He also encapsulated the pride that Saskatchewan, for long a have-not province, felt in "leading the way."[8] Yet, even in the dramatized CBC documentary of his life, a biopic entitled *Prairie Giant*, Douglas's efforts to implement free, state-funded health care in Saskatchewan were successful only when the provincial government flew in foreign doctors to staff the system. Although the audiences get only one brief glimpse of these ambiguously dark-complexioned physicians, airlifted from Britain by charter plane, they represent a turning point in the conflict narrative, providing the crux of the CCF government's efforts to break the back of a provincial doctors' strike, where medical practitioners feared for their future under a new regime of "socialized medicine."[9]

As with the narrative construction of *Prairie Giant*, Canadians' collective welfare-state nationalism has always privileged the role of the prairie preacher and only hinted at other parallel, and equally compelling, story lines. Focusing overwhelmingly on Douglas and the fight against entrenched medical interests, however, obscures other aspects of the construction of national health insurance in this country, of which the immigration of foreign-trained doctors to populate the Canadian health care system was but one of many fascinating and underappreciated elements. This one-sidedness in the historical record can be seen in the policy histories that have dominated the historical record on the implementation of Medicare. Several authors, the most prominent of which was Malcolm Taylor, focussed on the challenges of implementing such a pan-Canadian policy within a confederation in which health care was enshrined as a constitutional provincial responsibility.[10] Similarly, David Naylor authored an excellent book on the dynamics between the provincial medical associations and various proposals, leading up to the Medical Care Act of 1966, to implement hospital and medical insurance systems. He explored the troubled history between the state (defined both as the provincial and federal state), the medical profession, and the political fortunes of various parties.[11] Within this political science and public policy framework, historians have also documented the rise of prepayment schemes that emerged in different provinces, reflecting each province's different policy approach.[12] Other studies have analyzed the initial and ongoing problems associated with both funding and administering the new system by poorer

provinces in Canada.[13] Some of this regional scholarship has been collected
in a book edited by Greg Marchildon, a volume of essays that also includes
illuminating reflections by some of the principal actors.[14] From time to
time, political scientists have also tried to broaden our understanding of
the emergence of Medicare in Canada by introducing a comparative developmental perspective. For example, Antonia Maioni explored the long-
debated question as to how and why Canada and the United States took
divergent paths with regard to universal health insurance in the post-
WWII era.[15] More recently, Esyllt Jones has examined the influence of international leftist movements and the interwar circulation of ideas on
"socialist medicine," situating Canada within a larger transnational movement of ideas.[16]

Within this body of literature, it must be said that social history perspectives have not figured prominently. Constellations of medical practitioners tended to be assessed narrowly in terms of how they lined up
for, or against, universal health insurance proposals. The principal plotline
revolves around the battle – between politicians and medical organization
– for the hearts and minds of the public on a social policy seen as a litmus
test of social justice and professional freedom. However, there are some
exceptions to this general rule. A small number of nursing historians, for
example, have utilized the methods of labour history and critical race theory to explore the ways in which postwar health care expansion must be
understood within broader transnational themes. As Karen Flynn has
pointed out, over the course of the late 1950s and early 1960s Canada and
many other countries began to expand their quotas on nonwhite countries specifically to recruit health care personnel.[17] In Canada, these
measures took the form of "exceptional" entry for Afro-Caribbean nurses,
whose prospective employers could demonstrate that there were no
native-born Canadians who were able to fill these essential positions.[18]
Flynn's work has nuanced our understanding of health care diasporas as
well as to sensitize Canadians to the interplay between race, immigration,
and health care personnel.[19]

Oral history has figured prominently in several books that have inspired our own work and mixed methodology. Catherine Choy's *Empire
of Care*[20] used participant interviews to analyze the vast diaspora of

Filipina nurses and caregivers, as part of the now well-known phenomenon of the exportation of health and social care workers and the remittance of billions of dollars to the Philippine economy. Emma Jones and Stephanie Snow have explored the professional challenges of "black and ethnic minority" medical practitioners in the post-WWII Manchester area in their brief book *Against the Odds*.[21] Through the skilful deployment of the memories of medical practitioners, they document how "Asian" (that is, South Asian in North American parlance) doctors were directed into underserviced areas and specialties. This latter theme was taken up by Raghuram and Bornat who, through extensive participant testimonies, have demonstrated how Indian doctors were crucial to the creation, and evolution, of geriatrics in Britain. In these British publications, foreign doctors performed the "dirty work" of the NHS – the jobs and locations that were unwanted by British-born medical practitioners. Ultimately, Julian Simpson and his colleagues used oral history to write migrants into the history of the National Health Service, something Simpson has achieved in his recent work on South Asian doctors and the evolution of general practice under the NHS.[22]

As our book will demonstrate, the immigration and remigration of physicians in the twentieth century was simultaneously a Canadian and a transnational[23] story. Unsurprisingly then, there are scholars in other national contexts who have approached similar themes of immigration and medical history as it affected their home countries. John Armstrong, for example, conducted an exhaustive quantitative study of medical obituaries, in order to understand the history of medical migration (primarily for postgraduate education) of New Zealand medical graduates.[24] Fallon Mody has recently published several articles on British medical graduates in mid-twentieth-century New South Wales, focusing in particular on the history of women doctors.[25] Anna Greenwood has analyzed the central role of Indian-trained doctors in Kenya and the circulation of ideas and practitioners between East Africa and the Indian subcontinent.[26] There have also been studies of the systematic "exportation" of physicians, particularly from Ireland[27] and Cuba.[28] Our book, therefore, should be seen as contributing a Canadian perspective to a much wider and interconnected story in transnational history.

PRINCIPAL THEMES

This book examines the immigration of foreign-trained doctors to Canada during the establishment and early years of Medicare. To understand the intersection of these two historical events, we pose the following questions: What were the characteristics of medical practitioners who would settle in Canada in the post-WWII era? Where and in what specialties did they practice? Did they put down roots permanently or remain mobile, moving within Canada? Do major differences appear in the professional experiences of the "national" groups, such as the Indian, South African, British, Haitian, Irish, and American doctors? How does this picture compare to the United States, which was a net recipient nation, or to Britain, a nation that was, like Canada, both a major "recipient" and "donor" of physicians to the global health care marketplace over this period? Ultimately, we address the impact foreign-trained physicians had on the delivery of health care in Canada, since introducing universal health insurance in a country where an estimated 40 per cent of individuals had no or inadequate medical coverage was a considerable gamble.

Three dominant themes have informed our analytic perspective. First, we survey the immigration and settlement of physicians and surgeons[29] between 1957 and 1984. This period witnessed the arrival of thousands of foreign-trained doctors who would, by the end of our period of study, comprise about one third of the entire Canadian workforce of doctors. The beginning and end dates represent two landmark moments in the construction and consolidation of universal health insurance – 1957 saw the passage of the Hospital Insurance and Diagnostic Services Act (which guaranteed federal cofunding of hospital care and hospital-based diagnostics); 1984 marked the royal assent to the Canada Health Act, which updated the 1966 Medical Care Act and has constituted the framework of Medicare in Canada for the past four decades. The same time period includes three of the most important moments in Canadian immigration history: the 1962 Fairclough Directive, ostensibly eliminating race and religion as criteria for selecting new immigrants; the 1967 Immigration (Appeals Board) Act, which introduced the merit-based "points system" that favoured highly educated professionals; and the 1976 Immigration Act, which incorporated these changes but also began to de-emphasize medical trainees at a time when the 1970s economy was in stagnation and provinces increasingly felt they had too many doctors.

In the quarter of a century following the 1957 Hospital Insurance and Diagnostic Services Act, more than 15,000 foreign-trained doctors entered the country, the overwhelming majority of whom were foreign-born.[30] We aim to document the pathways of the international medical graduate (IMG) immigration to Canada over this period, situating migration patterns to, and within, Canada in policy and professional discourses emergent in Canada at the time. We interrogate the complex reasons why migrant physicians with non-Canadian credentials chose Canada over a range of other national options, what guided their careers after they arrived, and bureaucratic structures that enabled (or inhibited) their migration and settlement. We conceive of these doctors as elite migrant groups, who, to borrow the words of the migration historian, Dirk Hoerder, operated within "distinct cultural subsystems" that were inflected by cultural and linguistic affinities.[31] These affinities include shared colonial institutional legacies, which, as we shall show, is a key reason why the Commonwealth network of countries provided a path from regions such as South Asia and South Africa to Canada. By looking at pathways, but recognizing and documenting roadblocks and diversions, this book is concerned with charting the routes by which doctors moved across national borders and then chose particular communities from the many options that presented across the continental landscape.

We aim to write a national history of the interplay of Medicare and the immigration of foreign-trained doctors, but it is a history in which certain regions and sectors were more implicated than others. We have focused our inquiry on three interrelated areas of health service delivery where we believe the impact has been very strong. These include (1) the provision of medical care in marginalized, rural, and remote communities in Canada; (2) the context of new forms of collaborative practices, including private or incorporated group practices and the consumer and union-directed community health centres persistent into midcentury; and (3) the dramatic expansion of health education (particularly in the form of new medical schools) in Canada. By doing so, we will be able to examine the ways in which foreign-trained doctors fit into and exerted an influence on the economic and corporate structures of medicine that were in flux over the 1960s and 1970s.

These metaquestions emerge from concerns with health policy, but as we discuss in the section on methodology and sources, they will be answered by the dynamic interplay and creative consideration of the "big picture" and the individual experience. At first, a consideration of international medical migration seems to be a topic best answered from a macroperspective. Certainly, writers of the later 1970s increasingly embraced a "push-pull" model of migration that emphasized the ways in which individual decisions are affected by conditions in donor and destination countries/regions. In the end, however, as Rosemary Stevens observed in her contemporary study of "Alien Doctors" in the United States, "[a]ll these assumptions are mechanistic; they assume that the immigrants are relatively passive participants in the process of migration, affected by national considerations beyond their control."[32] We will pay close attention to migrant physicians' careers, the obligations and privileges that went along with their professional status and work, and their broader role as citizens and community members. These are expressed in local, regional, and sometimes national and even international terms. While "manpower" trends so discussed in contemporary policy documents are valuable in themselves, they are rendered more meaningful when considered against institutional and governmental policies, and the individual cultural, economic, and political factors that guided decision making and shaped experiences over the arc of discrete lives and careers.

As the research perspective moves back and forth between macro- and microanalyses, the broader questions listed above have fascinating specific iterations that we will address as a matter of course. This is because the Medicare generation of foreign-trained doctors have rich storied lives that lie at the intersection of the history of medicine, history of public policy, and immigration history. Asking questions about cohort, mobility, service impact, and community relations will touch on the broader themes inherent in the phenomenon often coined, in more popular terms, as the "brain drain." As well, our focus on the impact on several service areas prompts us to keep an eye on the more general role they played in the evolution of public policy in Canada. Ultimately, the book situates the evolution of universal health insurance in Canada within the context of the complicated postwar phenomenon of globalization. Medicare may have been subsequently embraced as a principal component of national pride – of Canadianism – but it owes significant personnel and intellectual roots elsewhere.[33]

METHODS AND SOURCES

Ever since the organization (and occupational closure) of the formal medical profession in the nineteenth century, all medical practitioners in Canada have been required by law to be licensed and formally registered. This procedure was paramount for providing, to the public, a mechanism for ensuring that the qualifications of a doctor were legitimate and appropriate to their scope of practice. In post-Confederation Canada, this process of professional self-regulation was delegated to arm's-length provincial organizations referred to as the College of Physicians and Surgeons.[34] Part of that regulation included annual public disclosure of the qualifications, names, and addresses of all licensed practitioners. Over time, the Canadian Medical Association aggregated the provincial lists of licensed practitioners into a larger, printed tome known as the *Canadian Medical Directory* (CMD), the first of which appeared in 1955.[35] By the late 1950s, the CMD included more than 400 pages with listings of more than 20,000 doctors. There were three principal sections of the CMD. The largest (the "white pages") included an alphabetical listing of all licensed practitioners in the country for that year. Individual entries of doctors included last name and initials, address of practice, place of undergraduate medical education, year of graduation, and (often) professional affiliations that indicated diplomas and further medical specialization. White page entries also included interns, residents, retired doctors, doctors on leave (or away), and doctors working for the armed services.[36] For most of the period under study, the CMD was distributed in print form across the country; it was not available in digital form but would be organized as a database when it was subcontracted to the Southam Media Group (and known, throughout the 1970s and 1980s, as the Southam Medical Database).[37]

The second part of the CMD (the "blue pages") was grouped by province and subdivided by county or municipality. These entries listed only names of the practitioners and the population of the county or municipality. The blue pages excluded residents, interns, and doctors working for the armed services. Keeping in mind this minor difference from the white page entries, doctors' names for particular communities can be cross-referenced with the larger individual physician list, permitting an analysis of the composition of the physician workforce at the local level.

Finally, as a reference work, the CMD also included a third principal section – the so-called "buff pages" – with the addresses and officers of the
provincial colleges, the medical schools of Canada, and their principal
administrators as well as a listing of the major medical and psychiatric
institutions and their chief medical officers. The buff pages also included
those omitted from the white and blue pages, including some doctors attached to the armed services as well as those who graduated from medical
school after the deadline for moving to production of the CMD (usually
around September). During the summer months of any particular year,
a group of university students were employed to sort through the entire
directory, make changes (or additions), and contact doctors to confirm
the accuracy of their individual entries.

The printed versions of the CMD thus acted as an annual census of all
licensed medical practitioners in the country and, like traditional censuses, can be used for historical research. Through a complicated and
time-consuming process, all of the entries of the 1961, 1966, 1971, and 1976
editions of the CMD were scanned and entered into four spreadsheets and
then "sifted" into discrete columns pertaining to name, place of practice,
place of undergraduate medical education, and year of undergraduate
medical education. The 132,000 entries were then "cleaned" (by reviewing
them individually for errors) and coded for province of practice, country
of undergraduate medical education, and for whether the practitioner
self-identified as no longer or not currently practicing (due to retirement
or "being abroad"). Once completed, the databases permitted the reconstruction of particular cohorts, which included doctors trained in what
contemporaries called the "mother" countries (Britain and Ireland),
countries of growing significance in medical migration (such as India and
Pakistan), as well as medical practitioners escaping from countries in considerable domestic turmoil in the 1960s (for example, Haiti, South Africa,
Czechoslovakia, and Taiwan).

The resultant spreadsheets of 1961, 1966, 1971, and 1976 give a snapshot
of the size, composition, and geographical distribution of physicians at
particular moments in time. No source is perfect, and case studies of particular communities suggest that the principal drawback of the CMD was
one of underreporting, perhaps by about 5 per cent. Further, the frequent
use of initials renders the changing composition of female and male doctors much more difficult than one would have originally anticipated. Yet

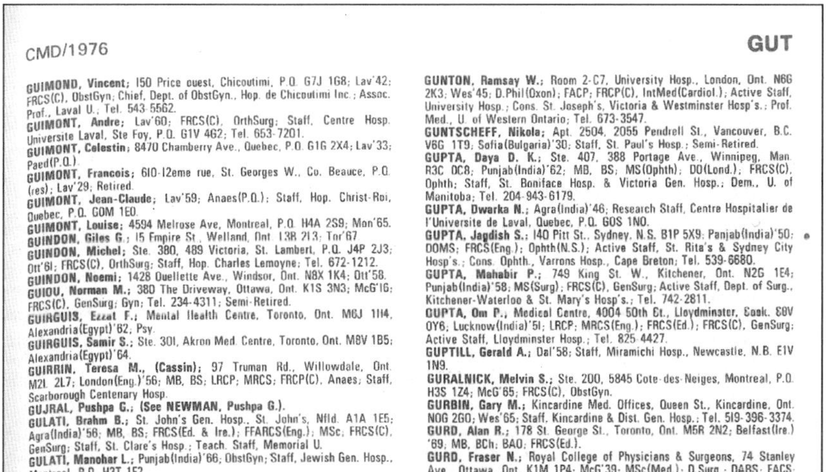

CMD/1976   **GUT**

GUIMOND, Vincent; 150 Price ouest, Chicoutimi, P.Q. G7J 1G8; Lav'42; FRCS(C), ObstGyn, Chief, Dept. of ObstGyn., Hop. de Chicoutimi Inc.; Assoc. Prof., Laval U., Tel. 543-5562.
GUIMONT, Andre; Lav'60; FRCS(C), OrthSurg: Staff, Centre Hosp. Universite Laval, Ste Foy, P.Q. G1V 4G2; Tel. 653-7201.
GUIMONT, Celestin; 8470 Chamberry Ave., Quebec, P.Q. G1G 2X4; Lav'33; Paed(P.Q.)
GUIMONT, Francois; 610-12eme rue, St. Georges W., Co. Beauce, P.Q. (res); Lav'29; Retired.
GUIMONT, Jean-Claude; Lav'59; Anaes(P.Q.); Staff, Hop. Christ-Roi, Quebec, P.Q. GOM 1E0.
GUIMONT, Louise; 4594 Melrose Ave, Montreal, P.Q. H4A 2S9; Mon'65.
GUINDON, Giles G.; 15 Empire St., Welland, Ont. 13R 2L3; Tor'67
GUINDON, Michel; Ste. 380, 489 Victoria, St. Lambert, P.Q. J4P 2J3; Ott'61; FRCS(C), OrthSurg: Staff, Hop. Charles Lemoyne; Tel. 672-1212.
GUINDON, Noemi; 1428 Ouellette Ave., Windsor, Ont. N8X 1K4; Ott'58.
GUIDOU, Norman M.; 380 The Driveway, Ottawa, Ont. K1S 3N3; McG'16; FRCS(C), GenSurg; Gyn; Tel. 234-4311; Semi-Retired.
GUIRGUIS, Ezzat F.; Mental Health Centre, Toronto, Ont. M6J 1H4, Alexandria(Egypt)'62; Psy.
GUIRGUIS, Samir S.; Ste. 301, Akron Med Centre, Toronto, Ont. M8V 1B5; Alexandria(Egypt)'64.
GUIRRIN, Teresa M., (Cassin); 97 Truman Rd., Willowdale, Ont M2L 2L7; London(Eng.)'56; MB, BS; LRCP; MRCS; FRCP(C), Anaes; Staff, Scarborough Centenary Hosp.
GUJRAL, Pushpa C., (See NEWMAN, Pushpa G.).
GULATI, Brahm B.; St. John's Gen. Hosp., St. John's, Nfld. A1A 1E5; Agra(India)'56; MB, BS; FRCS(Ed. & Ire.); FFARCS(Eng.); MSc; FRCS(C); GenSurg; Staff, St. Clare's Hosp.; Teach. Staff, Memorial U.
GULATI, Manohar L.; Punjab(India)'66; ObstGyn; Staff, Jewish Gen. Hosp., Montreal, P.Q. H3T 1E2.
GULENS, Voldemars; Box 39 Dashwood, Ont NOM 1N0, Riga(Latvia)'37...

GUNTON, Ramsay W.; Room 2-C7, University Hosp., London, Ont. N6G 2K3; Wes'45; D.Phil(Oxon); FACP; FRCP(C), IntMed(Cardiol.); Active Staff, University Hosp.; Cons. St. Joseph's, Victoria & Westminster Hosp's.; Prof. Med., U. of Western Ontario; Tel. 673-3547.
GUNTSCHEFF, Nikola; Apt. 2504, 2055 Pendrell St., Vancouver, B.C. V6G 1T9; Sofia(Bulgaria)'30; Staff, St. Paul's Hosp.; Semi-Retired.
GUPTA, Daya D. K.; Ste. 407, 388 Portage Ave., Winnipeg, Man. R3C 0C8; Punjab(India)'62; MB, BS; MS(Ophth); DO(Lond.); FRCS(C), Ophth; Staff, St. Boniface Hosp. & Victoria Gen. Hosp.; Dem., U. of Manitoba; Tel. 204-943-6179.
GUPTA, Dwarka N.; Agra(India)'46; Research Staff, Centre Hospitalier de l'Universite de Laval, Quebec, P.Q. GOS 1N0.
GUPTA, Jagdish S.; 140 Pitt St., Sydney, N.S. B1P 5X9; Panjab(India)'50; DOMS; FRCS(Eng.); Ophth(N.S.); Active Staff, St. Rita's & Sydney City Hosp's.; Cons. Ophth., Varrons Hosp., Cape Breton; Tel. 539-6680.
GUPTA, Mahabir P.; 749 King St. W., Kitchener, Ont. N2G 1E4; Punjab(India)'58, MS(Surg); FRCS(C), GenSurg; Active Staff, Dept. of Surg., Kitchener-Waterloo & St. Mary's Hosp's.; Tel. 742-2811.
GUPTA, Om P.; Medical Centre, 4004 50th St., Lloydminster, Sask. S8V 0Y6; Lucknow(India)'51; LRCP; MRCS(Eng.); FRCS(Ed.); FRCS(C), GenSurg; Active Staff, Lloydminster Hosp.; Tel. 825-4427.
GUPTILL, Gerald A.; Dal'58; Staff, Miramichi Hosp., Newcastle, N.B. E1V 1N9.
GURALNICK, Melvin S.; Ste. 200, 5845 Cote-des-Neiges, Montreal, P.Q. H3S 1Z4; McG'65; ObstGyn.
GURBIN, Gary M.; Kincardine Med. Offices, Queen St., Kincardine, Ont. N0G 2G0; Wes'65; Staff, Kincardine & Dist. Gen. Hosp.; Tel. 519-396-3374.
GURD, Alan R.; 178 St. George St., Toronto, Ont. M5R 2N2; Belfast(Ire.)'89, MB, BCh; BAO; FRCS(Ed.).
GURD, Fraser N.; Royal College of Physicians & Surgeons, 74 Stanley Ave., Ottawa, Ont. K1M 1P4; McG'39; MSc(Med.); D.Surg.; DABS; FACS; FRCS(C), GenSurg; Assoc. Sec. RCPS; Cons. Staff, Montreal Gen. Hosp...

Figure I.2 *Canadian Medical Directory*'s white pages, 1976
The *Canadian Medical Directory* was established in 1955 as a compendium of all licensed medical practitioners in the country. This directory of several hundred pages was an administrative resource for every medical office, providing an easy means of contacting practitioners for consultation. By 1976, there would be 36,000 doctors listed in the *Canadian Medical Directory*, of whom some 12,000 were graduates of medical schools outside the country. A 1976 extract above, including Dr Gupta.

despite these issues, the CMD permits, in theory at least, a broad-ranging quasi-prosopographical approach – that is, the reconstruction of the life careers of cohorts of individuals (in this case, doctors) through a database analysis of historical records extant in different jurisdictions. One can determine, for example, where these physicians were trained, approximately when they arrived in Canada, where they were practicing, in what specialty, and, by linking different editions of the CMD over time, where they were relatively stationary or mobile. They can also be combined with other qualitative and quantitative sources, as diverse as obituaries to institutional sources in their home countries (such as medical school graduation lists or equivalent public lists of licensed physicians), though given the fact that there were thousands of foreign-trained doctors arriving from scores of countries under the period under study, time limited such transnational reconstructions to a select few.

The CMD, as a historical source, can be supplemented and validated by other sources, including the annual returns of the federal Department of Immigration and Citizenship (which changed its name over the period under question). Appended to each annual report were tables of landed immigrants for that calendar year, broken down by a number of variables, including "intended occupation." Within intended occupation there was a section on health care occupations, which listed "physician or surgeon" as a discrete entry (as well as "dentists," "veterinarians," "osteopaths and chiropractors," "health diagnostic technicians," "nurses," "therapists," "pharmacists," and "optometrists"). These annual returns provide a time series of medical immigration to Canada over decades, where one can also disaggregate the inflow of doctors by "nationality."[38] In addition, the Canadian Medical Association, through its journal (the *Canadian Medical Association Journal*), regularly conducted its own research into the physician supply and distribution, publishing articles on a number of issues relevant to this book including the problem of medical practitioners in underserviced areas, the looming national doctor shortage in the 1960s, as well as the growing presence of immigrant doctors. There was also a journal of the Association of Canadian Medical Colleges – the ACMD *Forum* – that expressed the particular concerns of medical training institutions. The provincial medical associations – such as the Nova Scotia Medical Association or the Manitoba Medical Association – presented these (and other) quantitative findings to various provincial or national inquiries, not the least of which was the Royal Commission on Health Services (Hall Commission), which held hearings across the country in 1961 and 1962 (see below).[39] The accuracy of these findings can be matched against research from source countries. For example, one can compare the number of British-trained physicians entering Canada with estimates made by British medical and parliamentary reports on the brain drain of physicians to Canada and the United States or, by contrast, contemporary Indian Medical Association reports on the number of Indian doctors practicing or studying abroad.

The current iteration of the CMD – now run by a private company called Scott's Medical Database – provides a digitized version of the CMD, though the composition of entries has not changed significantly from the 1950s. It is now largely used for commercial purposes, providing digital addresses to other companies selling medical supplies. What they permit, for the historian, is the easy identification of foreign-trained doctors, still practicing or semiretired, who were first licensed in Canada during our period of study. With Research Ethics Board approval, we used the Scott's Medical Database to identify and recruit oral history interviews for our period under study (1957 to 1984). As our research questions evolved, we placed greater emphasis on clusters of foreign-trained doctors from particular countries of origin highlighted in chapters five and six. In total we interviewed thirty foreign-trained doctors.[40]

Oral testimonies of doctors who were trained abroad but would ultimately settle in Canada, can also be found in diverse research projects, from hospital histories, to histories of medical schools, to projects funded on important Canadian medical pioneers, to sites dedicated to specific "national" or "ethnic" groups. Organizations and institutions involved in the history of immigration (such as Pier 21 in Halifax) also have rich oral history collections. For some of these, the interviews of doctors arose coincidental to the larger research themes, such as the history of particular national groups, specific medical specialties, individual medical schools or hospitals. Further, over the last decade we have also collected written accounts from IMGs who came to Canada as an ongoing part of our research. These personal accounts are published either in memoir form or have been written up as a "reminiscences" and published in a magazine, a medical journal, or online. Some appear as published or unpublished autobiographies. While qualitatively different from the oral histories, these memoirs in their short and longer forms provide points of comparison and contrast to the oral histories we collected. Sometimes written as a first-hand, first-person account, other times written as an end-of-career reflection, sometimes printed in local newspapers or on-line, other times published in monograph form, this wide-ranging literature all falls under the loose category of life writing. These accounts humanize the sometimes mundane and occasionally dramatic life stories of this remarkable transnational event.

STRUCTURE OF CHAPTERS

The chapters of this book are organized in a chronological manner, weaving the findings from our statistical analyses, the exploration of the contemporary immigration and health policy documents, and our examination of oral histories and life stories into a new historical perspective on the establishment of Medicare. Chapter 1 begins by examining medical practice and physician migration to Canada leading up to and immediately after the Second World War. It outlines the tensions between the provincial regulation of medical practice and accreditation, the federal responsibility for immigration processing, and the globalizing trends of highly skilled migrants that were emerging at the time. As the chapter demonstrates, foreign-trained doctors were far from a rare phenomenon in 1950s Canada, with some 300–400 arriving every year. However, these medical practitioners were mostly British-born and British-trained doctors leaving the National Health Service, with a smaller number of Irish-trained medical practitioners, some of whom may well have been born in parts of Canada with no medical school (such as New Brunswick) and therefore left for undergraduate medical training. Immigration to Canada, framed by the 1952 Immigration Act, emphasized the acceptance of new Canadians who could easily assimilate into Canadian culture, society, and economy. British and Irish, and to a lesser extent American, doctors were therefore an easy fit. However, basic demographic and economic pressures necessitated a rethinking of the unofficial whites-only policy, as hospitals and local health authorities began to press for doctors and nurses from nontraditional countries to be granted landed immigrant status under the "exceptionality" clause of the immigration regulations.

The longstanding colonial connection of Canadian, British, and Commonwealth medicine provided the pathway through which later waves of British (and non-British) medical practitioners would enter the country. In many respects, Britain became a transfer terminal through which thousands of foreign-trained doctors would pass, en route to Canada. Chapter 2 examines the shortcomings of the British National Health Service (NHS) in the 1950s, which precipitated several interrelated phenomena – not only the outmigration of British (and Irish) physicians to Canada (as documented in chapter 1) but also the assimilation of English-speaking medical graduates from the former colonies (Indians, Kenyans, South Africans, New Zealanders) into the lower-ranking positions in British hospitals. By the end of the 1950s, as many as 50 per cent of house officers were not British-born, something that was an emerging political headache for the British government which refused to accept that the influx of foreign doctors constituted a negative commentary on the health of the NHS itself.

By the early 1960s, Britain responded to growing anxieties about race, language, and culture in the National Health Service (and British society in general) by instituting greater restrictions on immigration to Britain. Hundreds of non-British practitioners, sensing a growing resentment to their presence by health authorities, certain politicians, and some patients chose either to return home or to seek employment elsewhere. Having received their postgraduate qualifications in Britain, many would continue their transnational migration by resettling in Canada.

The timing of the arrival of hundreds of foreign-trained doctors proved crucial. The 1950s witnessed important experimentations in health insurance in the province of Saskatchewan (and in more limited form elsewhere) that would form the basis of the first step towards a national health insurance system. Chapter 3 will revisit the Saskatchewan Hospitalization Act of 1946[41] and the principle of hospitalization insurance that would prove to be popular and ultimately adopted at the federal level one decade later. The federal legislation of 1957, entitled the Hospital Insurance and Diagnostic Services Act (HIDS), committed Ottawa to cofund specific hospitalization stays and (within-hospital) diagnostic services provided by provincial health insurance systems. In a protocol to be followed in the future, the federal government promised to reimburse the provinces at the end of the year (a health transfer) 50 per cent of the costs of hospital stays and diagnostic tests. Some provinces quickly passed legislation enabling the federal funding, others (like Quebec) at first refused.[42] Nevertheless, the advent of "free" hospitalization triggered a surge in the use of hospitals, one that necessitated more and more health care personnel. By 1960 it was clear that the policy of free hospitalization was both popular and deeply unworkable given a health human resource infrastructure that had barely changed for a generation. It became apparent to medical leaders and politicians alike that there were not enough medical staff to support the new system. A national discourse around doctor and nurse "shortages" began to emerge at the same time as the doctors in Saskatchewan pushed back against the prospect of socialized medicine, engaging in a brief, but famous, strike in July of 1962.

The challenges of the health care system were one aspect that forced politicians to rethink whom they let into the country and for what societal objectives. With the arrival of the Diefenbaker government in 1958, a new culture and perspective emerged in Ottawa, which was encouraged to rethink the evaluation and processing of landed immigrant applicants. This new orientation arose in part from Diefenbaker's desire to pass a Bill of Rights in the country, which he did in 1960. The Bill of Rights articulated the idea of nondiscrimination within the civil service and, in exhortatory manner, within Canadian society more generally. Ellen Fairclough, an MP from Hamilton, Ontario and the first woman federal cabinet minister in Canadian history, was tasked with shepherding a number of changes that would, in theory at least, also eliminate race as a criterion in the evaluation of immigration candidates. Her ministerial initiatives began in 1962 and would be continued under Pearson's government, when the Liberals returned to power the next year. Chapter 4 examines this crucial period of the early 1960s when not just Canada but also the United States and other Western countries, refocused their immigration policies on attracting "highly skilled manpower" regardless of colour or creed. In Canada, an amendment Act passed in the very year of Canada's centenary would provide the basis of immigration (the points system) for the last third of the twentieth century. It would dramatically change the face of the country.

The very year of the centenary celebrations, 1967, marked the convergence of several important events that are important to this book. It witnessed the new "points system" for immigration, followed just months after the passing of the Medical Care Act of 1966, and also the disbursement of almost half of a billion dollars of (yet more) federal funding for new medical training facilities across the country. For the next six years, while medical, nursing, and dental schools from St John's to Calgary were being built, staffed, and welcoming their first students, Canada admitted more foreign-trained doctors (and nurses) than it graduated domestically. It was a situation without parallel in modern Canadian history. Chapter 5 examines the contours of the admission of the thousands of IMGs as they entered the country, looking in particular at four illustrative countries of origin: Czechoslovakia, Egypt, Taiwan, and Pakistan. The peak of medical immigration occurred in 1972, not coincidentally the very year that the last province passed enabling legislation for universal health insurance. It was also the year that Canada celebrated its 10,000,000th immigrant – none other than a foreign-trained doctor.

By the 1970s, the brain drain of doctors and nurses would become a polarizing debate within global health policy circles. American and European scholars also took interest, as the migration of doctors and nurses began to capture the attention of labour economists and sociologists. Between 1967 and 1978, a number of monographs appeared, exploring the growing phenomenon of "alien doctors" in the United States. These authors observed the demographic pressures of the baby boom and the expansion of health services in the United States that were made possible by an ever-increasing number of international medical graduates.[43] As the transnational nature of physician migration became apparent, some researchers refocused on the global picture, unnerved by the movement of medical practitioners from "developing" to "developed" countries.[44] By the early 1970s there were several multinational studies, some sponsored by the Rockefeller Foundation, others by the World Health Organization, that examined the transnational flow of professionals.[45] The significance of this transnational phenomenon also reached the World Health Organization, which commissioned Alfonso Mejía to research and report back on transnational migration of health care personnel.[46] Although by the time of the publication of the last of his studies – *Physician and Nurse Migration* (1979) – most wealthy countries had begun to restrict the licensing of foreign-trained health care practitioners. Chapter 6 traces the emergence of a global health care debate over the ethics of physician migration, examining the situation of two politically polarized countries of origin: Haiti and South Africa.

In a country as geographically diverse as Canada, the impact of foreign-trained doctors was far from homogenous. Contemporary commentators reflected on the maldistribution of medical resources throughout Canada, often referring to "rural and remote" areas as if this was some catchall category. Chapter 7 surveys the use of foreign-trained physicians to service diverse nonmetropolitan communities across the country, blending policy analyses with on-the-ground accounts of service challenges. Drawing on submissions to the Hall Commission, it was clear that there were many sectors of medical care that were in desperate shortage of personnel – including Indian Health Services and the large provincially run psychiatric facilities across the country. By contrast, the dramatic increase in physician immigration was leading to a growing consensus about the problem of "overdoctoring" in certain segments of the country. Medical economists began to claim that "nobody loves an immigrant physician."[47]

But some certainly did, and over this period a number of foreign-trained doctors were actively recruited to group practices throughout Canada. Chapter 8 examines their experiences, comparing the distribution of foreign-trained physicians in more established industrial towns alongside the newer resource towns in Canada's "new north," where mining and other extractive industries created communities and helped power the economy of midcentury Canada. These were communities that experimented with new health service models. The Community Health Centre in Sault St Marie was one group practice that recruited heavily, but often unsuccessfully, from the ranks of what were increasingly called international medical graduates (IMGs). Looking at the group practice experience from such physicians' perspectives reveals some of the medical cultures that disrupted the smooth functioning of the innovative health service system, unique to the Sault. On the other hand, the case study of Thompson, the "muskeg metropolis" of Manitoba's emerging nickel belt, became perhaps one of the most international nonmetropolitan medical communities in Canada at that time. The impact that medical immigration and Medicare had on the otherwise tightly controlled group practices of the northern city illuminate the profound shifts in medical economics between 1965 and 1975 and underscore the ways that quick local incentivization could work on the ground to draw prospective foreign-trained physicians to such regions.

Resource towns notwithstanding, some provincial ministers of health began complaining that they had *too many* doctors by the 1970s and blamed, in part, the intra-Canadian movement of foreign-trained doctors for worsening their situation. In reality, the combination of the previous generation of accelerated medical immigration, the completion of new medical schools, as well as the economic downturn from 1973 onwards, all shifted the culture around the desirability of yet more foreign-trained doctors in the Canadian health care system. Chapter 9 engages with the changes in policy that emerge in the mid-1970s, by which time the acute phase of the doctor shortage has passed. Indeed, by 1974–75, many provincial ministers of health met with their federal counterparts in order to convince federal immigration officials to no longer prioritize immigrant doctors under the points system. Meanwhile, the growing disquiet over what some claimed was unrestrained (general) immigration led to a consolidation of immigration regulations enshrined in the 1976 Immigration

Act. From 1976 onwards, doctors would begin to enter the country in significantly reduced numbers (dropping by two-thirds in the first year alone). If they did receive landed immigrant status, they found it harder and harder to secure a license to practice. The focus of health policy was less and less about recruiting foreign-trained medical practitioners than forcing the reduced number still entering the country into underserviced areas. As a consequence, the early 1980s witnessed a range of novel practices – from provisional licenses to differential remuneration schemes – in order to correct the maldistribution (rather than overall shortage) of physicians in the country. While foreign-trained doctors continued to be recruited for niche university-related research positions, many others found themselves practicing, in the words of one interviewee, "in the middle of nowhere."[48]

By the end of the twentieth century, the brain drain of doctors and nurses had emerged as a polarizing debate within global health circles. It attracted commentary at all levels, as countries such as South Africa strained under the double constraints of the loss of health care practitioners and devastating epidemics. For more than a generation, countries like Canada had strategically used their immigration regulations to underpin the expansion and staffing of their health services. In our Conclusion we bring a historical perspective to this vexing issue of global health inequalities and the rights of migrants. We also introduce the thoughts of some of our physician interviewees on their own reflections on transnational physician migration. This final chapter concludes with observations about how the story of physician immigration to Canada at midcentury holds lessons for contemporary policymakers and our understanding of Medicare as a cardinal moment in the nation building of Canada.

Chapter One

Medical Practice in Postwar Canada

INTRODUCTION

Late in life, the New Brunswick medical practitioner Arthur Leatherbarrow recalled a blinding blizzard, which took place one night during an emergency obstetrical call early in his career. The weather, narrow roads, and heavy snowfall provided significant obstacles to the ten-mile journey ahead. "However, I got a man with two horses and a sleigh, and we started out," he remembered vividly. "We left Hampton [New Brunswick] at six o'clock in the evening, and by eleven o'clock that night we had covered the first six miles. By then our horses were played out." Rousing a local man, who went off to get help, Leatherbarrow was surprised when the stranger returned from a logging camp with not only a horse but "a big pung [sleigh], and twenty-three men with shovels." Over the last four miles, the doctor rode just behind the men who shovelled in front of him as he lumbered forward, arriving at 4 a.m. to deliver the baby while the men piled into the small kitchen to warm up and wait out the night. Leatherbarrow remained at the farm into the following afternoon to make sure mother, baby, and household were stable. He then returned home, twenty-four hours on the clock after he received the initial call.[1]

Leatherbarrow's reminiscences of life as a country doctor could be read as a lively narrative of personal adventure and the undeniable sense of community in rural Canada in the early twentieth century. However, one noteworthy element of Leatherbarrow's biography is that he was not Canadian at all but rather an Irishman, who had sought refuge from his own country's turmoil, gambling his fortune on his medical degree and his sheer determination to succeed in a foreign land. Graduating from medical school at Queen's University, Belfast, in 1916, Leatherbarrow left for Canada later that same year, following a long-trodden passage of Irish medical émigrés.[2] His was a bold but not uncommon gambit: an immigrant fleeing unrest in his home country. The doctor left just before the escalation of the Civil War and Partition in the 1920s.[3]

Notwithstanding wintry deliveries in the countryside of New Brunswick, Leatherbarrow's integration into professional life in his new homeland appears, in retrospect, to have been relatively smooth. According to professional records, he passed the examination of the Council of Physicians and Surgeons of New Brunswick shortly after he arrived and set up a general practice in Hampton, forty kilometres northeast of Saint John. There, the young Irish doctor married Annie DeMille, a woman from a prominent local family, and became, over time, a well-known and well-respected rural practitioner.[4] Over the course of his career, he augmented his thriving general practice with public duties, serving as New Brunswick's executive member of the Department of Obstetrics under the Canadian Medical Association, as provincial coroner in the 1930s, and as medical staff of the Department of Pensions and National Health (DPNH) during the war years.[5] At the war's close, he worked in the service of the Department of Veteran's Affairs, retiring in 1950.[6] All evidence points to a prosperous career as a local family doctor, successful in his professional life, with a large family, and the respect of his peers and community. Indeed, the community recognized his contributions by naming the local primary school after him.[7]

This chapter takes the Irish immigrant doctor's life story as a point of departure to examine the intersection of medical immigration and clinical practice in Canada in the early twentieth century. Leatherbarrow was amongst hundreds of Irish- and British-trained doctors who arrived in Canada a century ago. As this chapter will demonstrate, about 50 per cent of newly licensed doctors hailed from or received their training in the British Isles. In some respects, their arrival may well have been considered unremarkable, in light of the wave of migration from Britain and Ireland before and after the Second World War. We will demonstrate, however, that this general pattern of medical migration from the British Isles disguised something more structural – the growing need for highly skilled immigrants in the Canadian economy and society that would reach a crisis by the 1950s.

Seen in its most general terms, Canada could boast one of the most robust physician per population ratios in the Western world by the end of the Second World War, with just under 1,000 residents per physician.

Nonetheless, there were signs that the older system of medical education would still be insufficient to service Canada's postwar economic growth, the baby boom, and changing demands of technological medicine. Not only the population but the infrastructures – including health infra-structures – to service growing urban and suburban communities, would expand dramatically. For health care, this was especially so with the ex-pansion of prepayment schemes for personal and family care and event-ually the advent of universal hospital insurance. Early experiments with state-run hospital systems and community care, such as those in the largely rural provinces of Saskatchewan and Newfoundland described later in this book, illustrated how individual doctors, like Leatherbarrow, were unable to meet community needs as health care expanded in the postwar years. Indeed, the Irish general practitioner would, in many ways, be the last of his kind of medical immigrant, as the crisis in rural medicine reconfigured medical practice in Canada and led to innovations that would forever change both Canadian health care and immigration.

MEDICAL EDUCATION IN CANADA

British- and Irish-trained doctors were integral to the very establishment of Canadian medical education in the nineteenth century. The first medical school in Canada, at McGill University, was itself populated by Scottish-born and Scottish-trained surgeons and physicians; Royal Victoria Hospi-tal, looming imposingly above the city of Montreal, was an architectural testament to this Celtic-Canadian connection.[8] The University of Toronto, after confusing stages of affiliated proprietary schools in the middle of the nineteenth century, also relied heavily on British-born practitioners as it consolidated medical education in the "Queen's City" by the 1880s.[9] Around the time of Confederation, these two universities had embraced the new medical doctorate, or MD, as the gold standard for medical education. New medical journals – such as the *Dominion Medical Journal* and the *Canadian Lancet* – reflected the professionalization of medicine in the expanding confederation of Canadian provinces.[10] British North America witnessed a steady stream of British-trained doctors who were received more openly than their American-trained counterparts.[11]

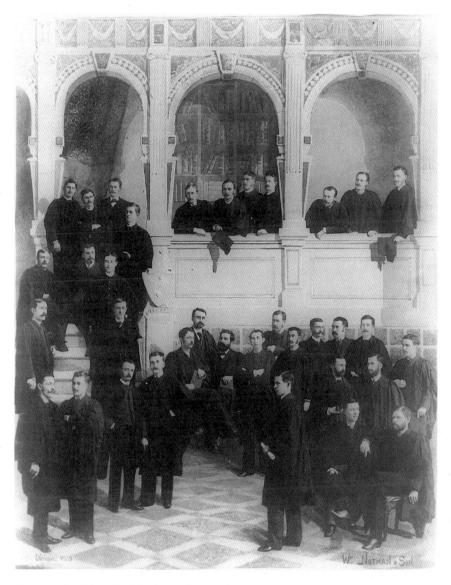

Figure 1.1 McGill medical faculty graduating class, 1883.
McGill was the oldest and most prestigious of the medical faculties in Canada, counting
Dr William Osler and Sir Thomas Roddick as two of its most notable professors. This composite photograph reflects the self-representation and ideal of medical schools in Canada
as refined environments of learning in the Scottish tradition. It also represents how McGill
maintained a training environment that was exclusively male.

Medical education also began to flourish outside of the two principal cities of central Canada. Dalhousie University, building on the Halifax Medical College, acted as a *de facto* training ground for young men of the Maritimes, being the only medical school in that region of the country until the last third of the twentieth century. With the booming population of Ontario, medical schools were also founded at Queen's University (Kingston) in the 1850s and the University of Western Ontario (London) in the 1880s. As the Prairies and Northwest became settled with Europeans, partial undergraduate medical degree training became available. The Manitoba Medical College, founded in 1883, merged with the University of Manitoba in 1918. The University of Alberta and the University of Saskatchewan (Saskatoon) also offered two-year programs by the early 1920s. Students who began their MD degrees in these prairie universities were required to move and complete their studies elsewhere. Université Laval, in Quebec City, constituted the only permanent[12] French-language medical school in the Dominion, though it would seed a "branch" university in Montreal that would evolve into the Université de Montréal by the interwar period. Until that time Francophones had to either travel to Quebec City or France, or adapt to the English-language instruction and traditions of McGill. Shortly after World War II, the University of Ottawa Faculty of Medicine was founded and graduated its first class in 1951. The University of British Columbia's medical school completed the transnational network in 1950.[13]

By the dawn of the 1950s, there were twelve medical schools in Canada (see figure 1.2) providing medical education in the country for Canadian-born medical students and, in the case of McGill University and the University of Toronto, a small but significant cohort from the United States and the British Caribbean.[14] The expansion of the domestic Canadian medical school system did not, however, signal an end of colonial medical ties. It was not uncommon for medical students in Canada, upon graduation, to travel to Britain for postgraduate diplomas, attracted by a certain allure of the famous teaching hospitals in London, Glasgow, and Edinburgh. Moreover, some Canadian-born or Newfoundland-born medical students elected, for a variety of personal reasons, to relocate to Britain and Ireland for their undergraduate medical education before returning home. Their travels reflected a circulation of English-speaking doctors throughout the British Commonwealth. The system of reciprocity between Britain's General Medical Council (GMC) and its colonial and Commonwealth equivalent governing bodies ensured that those graduating with medical credentials from universities in Britain, Ireland, and other parts of Canada would receive a relatively easy passage to medical practice throughout the British Empire and, later, Commonwealth.[15] Whether it be for medical missionary work, for the adventure of exploring more remote parts of the world, or for sheer professional calculation, English-speaking doctors were mobile in the early twentieth century.

The Canadian medical schools were openly discriminatory and restrictive in their admission of students. McGill University excluded women until 1922, almost exactly a century after its precursor – the Montreal Medical Institute – was founded.[16] Women did have a brief window of opportunity in the 1890s to attend the short-lived medical school at Bishops University, in Lennoxville (Quebec), before it was folded into McGill University's medical school in 1905. During the First World War, McGill-affiliated hospitals restricted the clinical training of its small annual cohort of black Caribbean students, whereas Queen's University expelled its own black trainees, deciding to abandon the admission of black students to the University until well after WWII.[17] McGill University and the University of Manitoba systematically limited the number of Jewish students.[18] By contrast, the University of Toronto graduated ever-increasing numbers of Jewish doctors from its MD program in the interwar period (approximately 10–25 per cent of any given cohort),[19] but the city's medical elite made it almost impossible for these graduates to secure internships in the affiliated teaching hospitals.[20] Women fared slightly better in Toronto than in Montreal, being admitted into a separate but affiliated Women's Medical College from the 1880s, which was then amalgamated into the "regular" medical school in the academic year 1905–06. Women graduates in Toronto then at least had Women's College Hospital as a refuge from an often-hostile medical hierarchy. Queen's University briefly experimented with coeducation in the early 1880s but abandoned the initiative altogether until the 1940s.[21] The newer medical schools proved to be somewhat more receptive to women graduates. Dalhousie University, for example, was coeducational by 1888, and the University of Western Ontario began accepting women students in 1919, even if the numbers of women medical students remained small. Given this context, it is unsurprising that the 1951 Canadian census lists only 10 per cent of the physician workforce as female,[22] and these women doctors were often channelled (or self-selected) into particular types of practice that were considered to be acceptable pursuits for their sex: paediatrics, general practice, school medical officers, pathology, and basic laboratory science.

Arising from this network of Canadian medical schools, the Dominion of Canada witnessed a steady domestic supply of Canadian-trained medical graduates by the beginning of the twentieth century, approximately 800 per year (though perhaps as many as one hundred of these were Americans who returned south of the border).[23] In addition, reciprocity between Canadian provinces facilitated the dispersion of Canadian-born and Canadian-trained medical practitioners. Graduates from the two largest medical schools – McGill University and the University of Toronto – could be found in disparate regions throughout the country. Meanwhile, many of the Maritime provinces continued to supplement Canadian-trained physicians with graduates of medical schools in the British Isles. Nova Scotia, for example, had a long history, extending back to the nineteenth century, of accepting Scottish medical credentials due to cultural affinities and the predominance of the University of Edinburgh as a respected and sought-after medical school for most of the period.[24] And as the Leatherbarrow vignette illustrates, Irish-trained doctors dotted the landscape of the Maritimes in the interwar period.

The circulation of medical practitioners across provincial and national borders was not, however, without its tensions. Over the course of the nineteenth century, when the professionalization of medicine was an ongoing project, the credentialing of foreign-trained doctors was a recurring point of debate. Politicians were eager to ensure the presence of adequate numbers of medical practitioners in their communities. Medical societies and provincial associations, by contrast, were anxious to protect the livelihood of individual practitioners against potential oversupply. The proliferation of American medical schools, and a certain anti-American bias, often resulted in a restriction of access for American-trained practitioners who wanted to practice north of the border.[25] This prejudice was reinforced by the Flexner Report of 1910, a North American survey of the state of medical education, which revealed many of the educational shortcomings of the largely unregulated American proprietary medical schools.[26] Even the principle of reciprocity and registration between Britain's GMC and the Commonwealth led to skirmishes, particularly in the interwar period, as "White Dominions" began to assert their independence and the economic downturn of the 1930s fuelled protectionist and anti-immigrant sentiments. For example, half of Canadian provinces revoked or restricted reciprocity in the interwar period only to reinstate it due to the exigencies of medical relocation during the Second World War.[27]

The regulation of licensed medical practitioners in Canada was made more contentious by the ambiguous relationship between the federal government and provincial governments in the area of medical practice. The horse trading that resulted in the Canadian Confederation in 1867 revolved around the cardinal issues of minority language and religious education, as well as taxation powers. "Health care" was a secondary issue and would not have had meaning as a term in the 1860s; rather, the British North America Act (1867) assigned the administration and regulation of medical and quasi-medical institutions – "hospitals, asylums, charities and eleemosynary [charitable] institutions" – to the provinces under Section 92. Moreover, public health initiatives (such as vaccination and sanitary reform) that were ongoing at the time of the constitutional negotiations (the 1860s) were also implicit in the duties assigned to the provinces, since they were organized at the municipal level. To confuse jurisdictional matters, however, the federal government retained responsibility for immigration, which also included the medical inspection (and if necessary rejection) of new arrivals, as well as the right to enact emergency border measures related to immigration and trade, such as quarantine.[28] Indeed, it was in response to the flu pandemic of 1918 that the federal government established its own Department of Health. Finally, the federal government also assumed responsibility over medical and nursing care of "Indians" [First Nations], an issue further clarified in the Indian Act of 1876 and which continued until after World War II.[29]

This awkward division of responsibilities played itself out in overlapping federal and provincial bodies regulating medical practitioners. Provincial legislation regarding medical and midwifery practice dates back to colonial times (in the case of Quebec, the 1780s). Some colonies, such as Nova Scotia, passed medical acts in the first half of the nineteenth century, providing some degree of professional closure and self-governance, even if the legislation was resisted and distrusted by a sceptical public who were wary of government-sponsored monopolies.[30] At the time of Confederation, the provinces maintained their right to control the licensing of medical practitioners. However, the need to have some sort of national standard led the federal government of Canada to create the Medical Council of Canada in 1912. The requirement to become a Licentiate of the Medical Council of Canada (LMCC), through the LMCC examination, ensured a national standard over the quality of practitioners in Canada. Over time, the LMCC became the unofficial "final exam" of Canadian medical graduates (regardless of province) as well as the go-to examination for foreign-trained doctors whose credentials were considered to be either incomplete or requiring further validation.[31]

The actual licensing of individual practitioners remained the prerogative of provincial bodies most often called, at the provincial level, the College of Physicians and Surgeons. In practice, these colleges established committees whose principal responsibility was to vet and deliberate upon out-of-province (including foreign) applicants. For Canadian-born and Canadian-trained medical practitioners who had completed their MD and passed their LMCC exams, this was a relatively straightforward process of compiling the necessary paperwork and perhaps requiring, at most, a one-year internship under supervision. In cases of those trained abroad, even Canadian-born graduates who had travelled to Britain and Ireland for education, the vetting took longer and sometimes obliged the candidate to sit the LMCC examination. Unsurprisingly, the vetting process and preferences varied between provinces, reflective of different medical cultures and their need for different types of practitioners, not the least of which was a desire or intention of newcomers to practice in underserviced areas or sectors, such as rural and remote parts of a province, or in institutions chronically lacking medical personnel, such as provincial mental hospitals.

Medical education during the interwar period, it should be emphasized, was overwhelmingly undergraduate medical education leading to the doctor of medicine (MD) degree. Although individuals might well "specialize" in particular areas after graduation, the formal three- to five-year postgraduate residency system was not then universally embraced. Rather, there existed a patchwork of graduate diplomas (both in Canada and in the British Isles) for those who wished to further their training or begin research careers. Summer- or year-long postgraduate diploma courses in surgery, paediatrics, and psychiatry, for example, became increasingly popular in Canada by the 1930s and 1940s. Meanwhile, it was also common for medical graduates with the means to travel to Britain or Europe for a

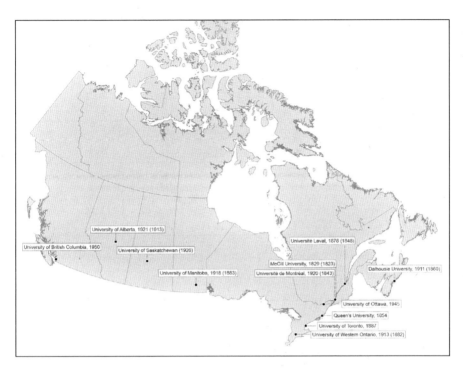

Figure 1.2 Map of Canadian medical schools, 1950
By 1950, Canada boasted twelve medical schools. The dates in parentheses represent
the founding date of schools that became affiliated with the respective universities over
time. This map excludes some proprietary medical schools that came and went in the
nineteenth century.

year to two. This reliance on Britain and Europe for graduate training, although not uncommon among former British colonies, increasingly irked
some senior members of the Canadian medical establishment. The famous
Montreal neurosurgeon Wilder Penfield, for instance, called for enhanced
support of specialist training and medical research as a necessary part of
a new commitment of the Canadian government to postwar medical
training. "For generations," he observed in the middle of the Second World
War, "young Canadians have gone, hat in hand, to the universities of Europe for graduate training ... the time has come for us to pay our way and
to support those institutions of higher learning here to which the students
of the world will want to come."[32] It was an appeal that would find fertile
ground in a new program – the federal health grants (1948) – that would

be part of the new surge of spending during postwar reconstruction. As Britain and Europe struggled to recover from the devastation of the Second World War, the directionality of graduate medical education began to reverse itself. As we shall see, British and European medical trainees increasingly came to North America to hone their clinical skills.

IMMIGRATION AFTER THE SECOND WORLD WAR

By all accounts, the Canadian economy flourished in the quarter century after the conclusion of the Second World War. A period of economic and demographic expansion unfolded in the immediate postwar years and continued, with temporary pauses, until the economic crises of the early 1970s. Canada would emerge as the second wealthiest country in the world by the late 1950s. Significant American investment in the extraction and refining of natural resources was accompanied by a dramtic growth in manufacturing, fuelled by strict tariffs on value-added goods. Canada's gross national product rose dramatically from $5.7 billion in 1939 to $36 billion in 1962, a six-fold increase in less than a decade and a half. At the same time, unemployment was low for much of the 1950s. Flush with cash, successive federal governments embraced the so-called "liberal consensus," investing millions of public dollars in physical infrastructure and new social welfare programs, from the family benefit to unemployment insurance. Indeed, it was during this period that the basic elements of the Canadian welfare state were established. Canadians themselves were keen to purchase goods, having endured the austerity of the Depression and war effort, thus giving the economy an additional boost from consumer spending. The postwar boom also included larger families as a reflection of national prosperity. Between 1941 and 1962, Canada's population rose from 11.5 million to 18.5 million, as the long-term decline in fertility experienced an unusual twenty-year reversal.

Postwar Canadian expansion reflected and was fuelled both by domestic growth and renewed immigration. Over the previous century the colonies, and later provinces, that would form the Dominion of Canada witnessed several surges of immigration – such as the two decades during Wilfrid Laurier's reign – often followed by relative periods of retrenchment, such as the closed-door policy of the Depression years.[33] Immigration to Canada, of course, was a searing political topic that touched upon the fault lines of religion, language, and ethnicity. As pressure mounted for Canada to accept thousands of displaced persons from postwar Europe, Prime Minister Mackenzie King attempted to walk a fine line, supporting immigration in general but only those immigrants, he emphasized, who could be easily "absorbed."[34] King was wary of any significant and sudden change in policy, particularly how it would be received in Quebec. "It is not a 'fundamental human right' of any alien to enter Canada," he reassured the House of Commons. "It is a privilege."[35]

Despite public pronouncements, the crisis of refugees in Europe forced the government to respond with a modernization of its immigration bureaucracy. In 1950, the federal government of Canada created a new Department of Citizenship and Immigration. Until that time the immigration branch was housed, tellingly, as a backwater of the federal government infrastructure as a part of the Department of Mines and Resources. That same year, empowered by a broader and more independent mandate, the Department of Citizenship and Immigration expanded the admissible classes of European immigrants to include "any healthy applicant of good character who has skills needed in Canada and who could readily integrate into Canadian society."[36] In effect this opened the door to European nationalities, such as tens of thousands of southern Europeans – Greeks, Italians, and Portuguese – as well as northern Europeans – such as Germans and the Dutch.[37] These new regulations also widened the admissible classes of what were termed "Asiatics"; the following year agreements were signed with Commonwealth governments of India, Pakistan, and Ceylon (Sri Lanka), whereby Canada agreed to accept limited numbers of immigrants from the Indian subcontinent.[38] Many restrictions remained, and such barriers tell us a great deal about the persistence of racial ideologies embedded within Canadian immigration policy and Canadian society. As Patricia Roy observed, the 1947 repeal of the Chinese Immigration Act (which banned East Asian immigration to Canada) proved to be not much more than a token gesture, as orders in council still limited Chinese immigration to wives and children of those already citizens.[39]

Administrative changes in how Canada accepted newcomers were consolidated in the Immigration Act of 1952. The act reiterated a preference for immigrants from traditional countries – those from the British Isles, France, and, somewhat begrudgingly, a wider array of southern and eastern European nations. It also contained a curious list of exclusions, including a prohibition on those deemed to be a medical burden ("epileptics," "the insane," and "imbeciles") that dated from the nineteenth century, supplemented by exclusions of "homosexuals" and those guilty of "moral turpitude." However, the operation of the new act was overtaken by international events, such as the Hungarian Revolution of 1956, which witnessed thousands of political refugees enter in the country by order-in-council. Annual intakes fluctuated wildly, reaching a peak in 1957. That year alone 280,000 individuals immigrated to Canada.

As with any major piece of legislation, the impact of the Immigration Act of 1952 was guided by structural constraints as well as individual prejudices. Applying to immigrate to Canada was a complicated and confusing process, one that depended upon the accessibility of Canadian consulates and embassies, and the guidance of immigration officers both at home and abroad. The 1952 Immigration Act gave the minister (and immigration officials and agents abroad) significant powers of interpretation; it also empowered the civil service, through discretionary interpretations of the act, to limit admission of people for a wide array of reasons. These, most immigration historians agree, were designed to, or resulted in, keeping out nonwhite immigrants.[40] For instance, while immigrants from Europe and the Americas could sponsor relatives, other nationalities could not because of fears that a dramatic influx of relatives from places like India would otherwise result. As Valerie Knowles has argued, immigration policies of this era continued to defend "Canada's right to discriminate, stating that the racial and national balance of immigration would be regulated so as not to alter the fundamental character of the Canadian population."[41]

It is in this 1950s context that health care practitioners – doctors, nurses, dentists, medical technicians – came to occupy a central place in the regulation and admission of new immigrants. Canada witnessed a steady immigration of British and Irish doctors and nurses who, like Leatherbarrow, arrived in the early decades of the twentieth century to take up positions in various Canadian provinces. But by the 1950s Canada relied, informally, on one-third of all newly licensed doctors coming from abroad. As the next chapter will demonstrate, there were certainly no small numbers of British-born and Irish-born doctors who, disillusioned with the National

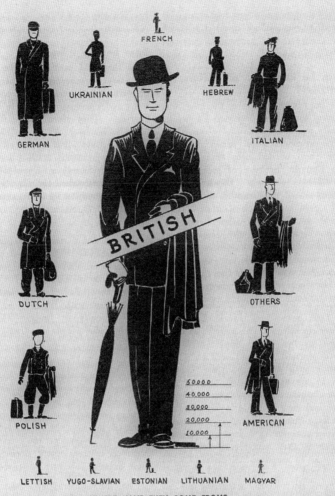

FRENCH

UKRAINIAN

HEBREW

GERMAN

ITALIAN

BRITISH

DUTCH

OTHERS

50,000
40,000
30,000
20,000
10,000

POLISH

AMERICAN

LETTISH   YUGO-SLAVIAN   ESTONIAN   LITHUANIAN   MAGYAR

WHERE HAVE THEY COME FROM?

The "ethnic origin" of newcomers to Canada, 1946-1951, is indicated by the graph above, not the country from which emigration actually took place. "Ethnic origin" is determined by the Department of Immigration on the basis of the father's language, except in the case of the United States and British Isles. "British" includes Scotch, Welsh and Irish.

Figure 1.3 Pictogram of immigration to Canada, 1953
The Immigration Act of 1952 prioritized candidates from the British Isles. However, slowly, this approach was augmented, in the 1950s, by immigration from a wider range of European countries, as depicted in this pictogram that attempts to convey the arrival of professional male immigrants by stereotyping their dress and configuring their size to their relative importance in immigration statistics. The norm continued to be white European immigrants as the most likely to successfully adapt to Canadian society.

Health Service, were willing to take a chance on a medical living in Canada. Speaking to the 1951 annual meeting of the Canadian Medical Association in Halifax, St John's physician Leonard Miller described the endemic problems with physician recruitment and retention in his home province of Newfoundland: "Up to the present Newfoundland has not been able to produce and hold from its native sons a sufficient number of doctors to look after the needs of the population."[42] Though he attributed this problem to the difficulties inherent in the north Atlantic coastal environment – most community physicians attended to populations of 3,000 residents or more – the solution was to recruit and encourage foreign-trained physicians. "Through the years," Miller noted, "we have welcomed medical graduates from the mainland of Canada and from England, Scotland, and Ireland. Today, our medical register shows a high percentage of graduates from across the seas including local men, and others who have made our province their permanent home."[43]

Miller's observations were confined to Newfoundland; however, he may well have been commenting on various rural and remote parts of the country, from Northern Ontario to the rural and dispersed communities of the Prairies. Indeed, in the years immediately after the Second World War Canadian bureaucrats observed that there was a pool of refugee doctors who might be able to help with underserviced areas and began discussions with the Canadian Medical Association over plans to welcome them *en masse*. Apparently, since the beginning of the war, sixty physicians had already been admitted to Canada with refugee status. The Canadian Medical Association (CMA) remained skittish about the wholesale licensing of refugee physicians detained in displaced persons camps after the war, even were they to come to service areas without any medical practitioners. "The answer to the lack of medical care in the rural communities does not lie in forcing, co-opting or importing a doctor and setting him down there," a CMA statement on "the refugee doctor" warned in 1947. Staking out a convenient moral high ground, the CMA authors argued that other parts of the world "needed" such physicians more than Canada and thus concluded that "we would have no more right to bring doctors from Europe than we would have to ask Europe to send us food parcels."[44]

The problem of providing doctors in rural and remote areas was not, however, something the CMA could put off forever. It was a significant problem and one that provincial governments were already addressing.

In Albert Leatherbarrow's adopted province of New Brunswick, the increasing number of applications for practice stymied the local medical council, the body that granted licenses on behalf of the College of Physicians and Surgeons. In 1951, they reported a spike in the number of registered physicians in the province, mainly because "the number of applications of immigrant doctors from continental Europe for enabling certificates [to sit registration exams] was increasing." The council took a dim view of such applicants, whom they suspected "never thought of practicing in New Brunswick, but were attempting to use the NB Medical Council as a backdoor to practice in the more industrialized parts of Canada." In response, the provincial body had formalized several regulations. Many of these were standard criteria for practice, including graduation from "a medical school approved by the Council" and having at least two years of premedical studies or basic science before applying. These were standard criteria, but, in addition to training, the council required the applicant be Canadian born, "born in the British Isles," or have "acquired Canadian citizenship" before applying. This last requirement elicited considerable discussion at the annual meeting in 1953, where the clause caused several members to critique the decisions of the council and "take exception" to the citizenship requirement. After lengthy debate, members of the society present at the meeting recommended that the council wait and reconsider the problem posed by the influx of foreign-trained physicians, and the citizenship requirement was ostensibly dropped.[45]

The actions in New Brunswick, however, were not isolated. Three years earlier, Ontario had adopted a citizenship requirement, likely because it was home to the very "industrialized parts of the country" to which provinces like New Brunswick were losing their new physicians. The public relations problem this posed did not escape the notice of James Burns McGeachy, a frequent lay columnist in the *Canadian Medical Association Journal* during the 1950s. In 1956 he warned Canadian doctors that, due to the very serious physician shortages in parts of Ontario outlined by William Victor Johnson almost a decade previous, such dubious restrictions on medical licensing posed a political challenge for the profession. "The projected rule about naturalization," he wrote, "cannot be defended at all except on the ground that it will help maintain this scarcity and guarantee to the doctors the extra income."[46] Giving in to any "protectionist spirit" when setting licensing requirements for immigrant physicians was anathema to the larger professional ethic of service. He concluded, "It appears to me that the doctors should think twice, in the general interest, before they make it tougher than it is at present for a foreign doctor to establish himself and make himself useful in this country."[47]

Protectionism could take many forms, and it seems clear from the professional discourse of the era that the national organization should set the terms for licensing. At the contentious New Brunswick meeting one year earlier, members observed how "the matter is receiving continued study by the Medical Councils of Canada; and opinion among the several provinces has not reached a point where general agreement is yet possible."[48] Eventually, the LMCC requirement was decoupled from the citizenship requirement, and the regulations of Canadian licensing bodies, like the national immigration regulations, adopted policies that more equitably assessed skills, education, and training credentials separately from the issue of nationality. But the separate discussions about the citizenship requirements in provinces like New Brunswick and Ontario in the 1950s call into question what kind of barriers to practice local Colleges of Physicians and Surgeons would erect to limit the participation of foreign-trained physicians to their jurisdiction. There are only occasional and scattered references to some in the national and regional medical journals of the day; as chapters 7 and 8 detail, local regulatory regimes at the provincial and hospital administrative levels could operate to delimit options for physicians with foreign credentials. The provincial debates captured here reveal concerns and prejudices about immigrant physicians' opportunism, their mobility among Canadian jurisdictions, as well as how physician shortages in some areas made the idea of professional "protectionism" volatile for physician organizations in 1950s Canada.

THE CHALLENGES OF RURAL MEDICAL PRACTICE

The crisis in rural medicine was felt most acutely in provinces such as Saskatchewan and Newfoundland where dispersed populations and relatively low household incomes posed challenges to the viability of private practices. Both provinces created unique systems to respond to the urgent need for medical care. The better known of the two emerged in Saskatchewan, which, following the election of North America's first socialist government, the Co-operative Commonwealth Federation (CCF) under T.C. (Tommy) Douglas in 1944, began an incremental march towards universal health insurance. Saskatchewan had suffered the double challenge of a small and dispersed population combined with the devastation of the economic depression and years of drought in the 1930s. In response, the provincial government had experimented with a patchwork of municipal doctor programs and rural health units.[49] Consolidating and expanding these community-based programs was high on the agenda of Douglas's new government. In collaboration with the provincial College of Physicians and Surgeons, the CCF government created a special health plan for indigent persons and those on social assistance.[50] Having taken care of the poor and most marginalized parts of the population, Douglas and his cabinet undertook the task of broadening the range of services to the entire population.

From the beginning, Douglas and his ministers consulted widely, seeking national and international advisors, and drawing explicitly on British and American models of care and planning. Henry Sigerist, chair in medical history at Johns Hopkins and one of the leading American-trained proponents of state-run medical services, famously visited Saskatchewan in the 1940s, offering insight into and moral support of the Saskatchewan experiment.[51] In addition, as Jim Connor has demonstrated, the brains behind the rolling out of health insurance in Saskatchewan was another American, Frederick Mott, who had written the "bible" on rural health care in the United States in the 1930s. *Rural Health and Medical Care* became an ideological flashpoint in the United States but acted as a blueprint for the early experiments in Saskatchewan.[52] The British connection was equally important, as hundreds of decommissioned Commonwealth medical doctors returned from World War II with knowledge of the Beveridge Report and its proposals for universal health care that had circulated in medical circles during the war.[53] As Esyllt Jones has recently demonstrated, community health clinics occupied a cardinal position within the transnational circulation of ideas of the political left in the 1930s and 1940s.[54]

In 1945, the CCF government implemented the Saskatchewan Social Assistance Plan, which offered a comprehensive health services program for recipients of social assistance.[55] Without restrictions on choice of hospital or duration of stay, the plan paid for both medical and hospital services as well as treatment for cancer and for mental illness.[56] In January 1947, compulsory hospital care insurance was extended to all citizens under the same terms and included public ward care, X-ray and laboratory services, and common drugs.[57] There was even coverage to offset the cost of out-of-province hospitalization.[58] Additionally, physician services for diagnosis and treatment for cancer, tuberculosis, and venereal disease were covered under a distinct part of the act; in 1946 this included psychiatric services including, by 1947, all outpatient care. The Saskatchewan government also experimented with covering physician services through pilot community care clinics. The largest and most ambitious of these was located at Swift Current, a town at the centre of Health Region No. 1, in the southwest corner of the province. At the time, the town of Swift Current had a population of only 7,200 people, but including the outlying six small towns, thirty-two villages, and thirty-eight rural municipalities, the total population of the region was close to 55,000. Nevertheless, the health region had fewer than five persons per square mile, most of whom were part of households engaged in farming and ranching. At Swift Current, the regional board that was struck to oversee the program made arrangements to expand the original remit of preventive care and offer a wider array of medical, hospital, dental, nursing, and other health services.

At the time, it was already recognizable that Saskatchewan was breaking new ground. In an address to the American Public Health Association in 1948, the American born and McGill-trained Frederick Mott, who chaired the Saskatchewan Health Services Planning Commission for the provincial government, laid out the details of the plan to his American colleagues, highlighting early successes as well as challenges.[59] The scheme at Swift Current, an outgrowth of Henry Sigerist's health survey of 1944,[60] provided a municipal doctor contract arrangement for the service providers for about one-third of the population of the area. The rest of the physicians were organized into a group practice but through a centralized clinic, with community members on the board; they were recruited and organized to provide a wide range of general and specialist services.[61] Mott explained that a health region was "built on the concept of a natural trading area surrounding a trading centre."[62] He hypothesized that the trauma of the 1930s left the farming population sympathetic, or at least open, to "socialized medicine" as a means of survival. Unsurprisingly, given his position and political sympathies, Mott hailed it as a "courageous pioneering effort with spreading influence."[63]

Reporting two years later, CMA secretary A.D. Kelly surveyed the services at Swift Current and offered a grudging, and less enthusiastic, review. He recognized this plan as compulsory health insurance, operating "on a more extensive scale than exists for a total population elsewhere in Canada" – the only exclusion being pharmaceutical services.[64] He also forecast that "the patterns being established [at Swift Current] may well serve as a guide for future developments."[65] His concern, as representative of the CMA, was how the members of the medical profession fared financially and professionally under the terms of the new service. All thirty-four resident physicians of the region participated in the provision of medical care, and, save for the fact that the bills were sent to the secretary of the health region instead of the patient, Kelly observed, with satisfaction and relief, that "the pattern of private practice is preserved."[66] Apart from the fact that physicians did not play a leadership role in the administration of the health region board, his assessment was generally positive, except for one caveat: medical manpower.[67] He observed that the demand for services had increased dramatically and that the workload of the physicians was punitive. "[D]octors," he reported, "are carrying the maximum load which is desirable in the interests of their health and efficiency."[68]

Staffing in the Saskatchewan system posed significant problems from the outset. The public health office, for instance, had "an active program in full swing" for several months and these were offered on a full-time basis despite what they admitted were "personnel shortages." According to Mott, the board was very interested, even one year into the new service, in improving and expanding hospital and diagnostic facilities at regional and district centres. "They are fully aware of the personnel problems," Mott concluded, "ranging from the chronic shortage of nurses to gaps in their physician resources, and their latest action was to guarantee a doctor $6,000 to move into a remote area of the region."[69] Still, all was not bleak: Swift Current had managed to augment its physicians in the region as the number of practitioners jumped from nineteen to thirty-three within the first year. In A.D. Kelly's more critical review of health services from July 1946 to December 1947 he also concluded that the medical population of the region increased from twenty-one to thirty-four, with a

physician–population ratio in the order of 1:1530.[70] Kelly, however, did
revisit the area in 1960, on the eve of the implementation of a province-
wide system of prepaid universal health care, and reported to the CMA
that the number of resident physicians had risen further to forty-one
even though the population of the region was largely unchanged. Yet,
Kelly indicated that, despite the gains in absolute numbers, there was a
high rate of turnover: "one gathers the impression that the representatives
of the profession have been very mobile and that the tenure of individual
doctors has been brief."[71]

The impact on the structure and availability of health services changed
the way that medicine was practiced, centralizing in the hospital setting
care that was normally provided by a general practitioner in the community. Mott himself had observed most people in the region received medical attention in hospital now, although he claimed this was characteristic
of sparsely settled territories where the number of doctors remained low
and the supply of hospital beds was reasonably adequate. In the Swift
Current health region, five new hospitals had opened over the previous
three years, giving a region-wide ratio of 5.2 beds per 1,000 by bed capacity in the fourteen hospitals. The rates of hospital usage were very high,
"[e]ven in the prairies," Mott observed, "where the nature of medical
practice has been to go to the physician or the district hospital, rather
than call the doctor to the home."[72] Ten years after implementation, several medical practitioners criticized this hospital-centric system. Free
hospitalization, according to one disgruntled Saskatchewan specialist, put
unnecessary pressures on practicing physicians. "Patients have been
known to 'shop around,'" he complained, "until rewarded by a physician
who will hospitalize them irrespective of the merit of legitimate need."[73]
For the most part, however, physicians of Saskatchewan accommodated
themselves to the hospital insurance scheme.

The Douglas government recognized that the Prairie province would
face significant challenges finding sufficient doctors and nurses to fulfil
this first step toward state-run health insurance. The problem was in part
self-made, as the province lacked a medical school providing a comprehensive undergraduate medical program. Cognizant of this constraint,
Douglas expanded the two-year medical program at the University of Saskatchewan's medical school to a full four-year program, the first full cohort of which was scheduled to graduate in 1958. Until that time, the

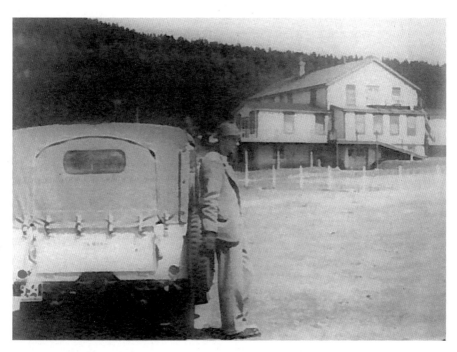

Figure 1.4 Dr Olds of Twillingate, Newfoundland, 1952
The Cottage Hospital System was created in Newfoundland during the 1930s as an attempt to service outport communities that could otherwise not support an independent private medical practitioner. The system of salaried doctors and provincial hospitals was modelled on a similar initiative in place in the Scottish Hebrides. Here Dr Olds, an American-trained doctor, stands in front of the local cottage hospital.

province relied on foreign-trained doctors and nurses to staff the emerging health insurance system. During this time, it issued 826 new licensees to practice medicine; of these, almost one half went to foreign-trained doctors. A small number came to teach in the newly expanded medical school in Saskatoon, but most were recruited to the municipal doctor schemes and, as we will show in chapters to come, initially came to practice in rural regions of the province.

Although we tend to associate the early initiatives in universal health care with the province of Saskatchewan, there were, in fact, other provinces that were experimenting with similar proposals in the 1930s and 1940s. Newfoundland shared the challenges of providing medical services to small and dispersed communities. Although the capital city of St John's did support some centralization of government administration, the provision of services for the rest of the island remained extremely difficult. For nurses, the outport communities were often isolating, and chronic shortages and turnovers characterised their precarious existence.[74] For doctors, private medical practice in small communities proved to be unprofitable. As a consequence, many communities operated without medical practitioners for considerable periods of time, providing challenges, as well as opportunities, to allied health care practitioners, such as midwives.[75]

In response to the chronic lack of medical practitioners and nonviability of private practice, the British government responded, in the interwar period, by implementing a novel system of community hospitals that had been pioneered in the north of Scotland. Over the course of the 1930s and 1940s, nineteen hospitals were created.[76] They were municipal hospitals, funded directly by the government, where doctors and nurses (usually one each per hospital) were paid a salary to provide primary care to the local population. The model was to pay by salary solo medical practitioners accompanied by community nurses and equip them with modest surgical facilities for the small communities. Since Newfoundland had no medical school, the doctors and nurses would, by necessity, either come from (mainland) Canada, from the northeast of the United States, or from Britain and Ireland.[77] Not unlike the rural hospitals under Saskatchewan's system, the Newfoundland cottage hospitals functioned as a geographical "hub" in which to concentrate scarce medical resources. Serving approximately 115,000 people, thirty physicians based in fourteen small hospitals spread out across the island – twelve newly built by the government – provided medical care both before and after Newfoundland joined the rest of Canada in 1949. Indeed, by 1957 almost half of all Newfoundland medical services were provided through fourteen cottage hospitals.[78] Jim Connor concludes that, in large part due to the cottage hospital system, rural and remote medicine constituted a "colonial success story."[79]

The health policy initiatives in Saskatchewan and Newfoundland were a response to the crisis in rural and remote medical care that existed throughout the country. Speaking on behalf of rural practitioners in Ontario, William Victor Johnson, a practitioner who would played a key role in making general practice a specialty in Canada, declared that some sort of state-administered health insurance was "inevitable" if rural areas of

Canada would be successful in recruiting physicians to serve sparsely populated areas.[80] Various voices within the medical profession began to accept the notion of state involvement in the provision of all health services, not just public health initiatives or the care of certain segments of the population like injured workers or the urban poor. An initial plan for postwar expansion, developed during the war by the Heagerty Committee in 1942, benefitted from the full participation and support of the Canadian Medical Association. At a 1943 meeting the CMA had cautiously adopted a stance in favour of health insurance, as long as "such plan be fair both to the insured and to all those rendering the service."[81]

CONCLUSIONS

The 1950s witnessed rising tensions between a system of provincially administered medical education, a federal immigration act that continued to emphasize immigrants from traditional countries, and the growing pressures of a postwar economic and demographic boom. For the first postwar decade Canada made do by supplementing its domestic supply of medical practitioners with doctors and nurses from the British Isles. Some, following the tradition of Leatherbarrow, would easily transition into small town and rural practice. However, others would find life as a doctor in rural Manitoba or the outports of Newfoundland too hard, relocating after short periods of time to more hospitable and financially viable climes. As contemporary commentators lamented, foreign doctors were often transient, temporary solutions to systemic problems of medical provision and access. This set the stage for a half-century-long debate over the retention of medical practitioners in many parts of the country. During these early years of provincial experiments in universal health insurance, Canada would face two principal challenges. On the one hand, provincial governments urgently required more doctors and nurses to make the system operational, a need fulfilled, at least for the first decades, by a steady flow of British- and Irish-trained practitioners. On the other hand, the increasing tendency of provincial and national medical societies to actively engage in determining the direction of health policy would create political tensions and conflict. As the next chapter will demonstrate, there was no little irony in the scores of British doctors "escaping" the National Health Service who would find themselves, in the case of Saskatchewan, in the middle of emergent debates over socialized medicine. Such tensions would arise in various forms long before the famous doctors' strike captured the nation's attention in 1962.

Changes in medical education and training would also elevate the demand for health care personnel and concentrate resources increasingly in urban areas. Although graduate training before the Second World War tended to be informal, with travel to Britain and domestic diplomas supplementing the traditional MD degree, changes were afoot. By the late 1940s and early 1950s, medical specializations became formalized into residency programs and increasingly prized by the profession. Canada witnessed the establishment of stand-alone specialty associations, such as the founding of the Canadian Psychiatric Association in 1951, that also advocated for the formalization of "specialist" training through university-affiliated programs. Such specialization required more and more training in medical institutions, which were, in Canada at least, all located in the principal urban centres of the country. Medical students thus gravitated to the city for medical education and increasingly stayed there for training purposes and employment opportunities, exacerbating the urban–rural distribution of medical practitioners.

The federal government also contributed to the centralization of medical training and technology in the growing urban cities of postwar Canada. Flush with cash, but constrained by constitutional responsibilities, the federal government in Ottawa created federal health grants (1948) that assisted in the rapid expansion of general and specialist hospitals in the country. With federal assistance, hospital capacity exploded in the 1950s, while domestic medical education, controlled by the provinces, plateaued. Hospitals faced a chronic human resource crisis calling out for exceptions to the immigration regulations. With some degree of ambivalence, immigration officials began to admit select numbers of health care practitioners from countries not traditionally granted admission to Canada. As a consequence, by the end of the 1950s, a new generation of Afro-Caribbean nurses, Indian doctors, and Filipina caregivers would appear on the health care landscape.

Chapter Two

Commonwealth Connections

Stanislaw Kryszek grew up in a prosperous middle-class Polish household during the interwar years. After graduating from secondary school in 1934, he entered medicine at the University of Warsaw at the tender age of sixteen. However, his medical studies were interrupted shortly before he was due to graduate. After the so-called Non-Aggression Treaty between Soviet Russia and Germany in 1939, Poland scrambled to mobilize. The Nazi–Soviet Pact was in effect a partition of his native Poland, and the country was soon squeezed between the invading Nazi forces from the west and Soviet forces advancing from the east. As the Germans began bombing Warsaw in September of 1939, Stanislaw began an improbable journey. He and another medical student escaped southward, walking by foot for dozens of miles, hitching a ride with an ambulance, jumping on a flatbed truck, before finally making it to Lublin about 50 miles to the southeast of where they began. Shortly after arriving, he was sent further south, travelling by horse and buggy and then train to assist at a military hospital. Knowing that Russian troops were closing in, he crossed the border into Slovakia and then Romania, with a plan to continue to Turkey. After a brief detainment at the Romanian border, he and a handful of other fellow nationals arrived in Bucharest. The Polish embassy there was still operational, and he received a temporary passport and a visa for France. The young medical trainee then boarded a train to Zagreb and then on to France via the Italian and French Rivera. The palm trees, he marvelled, "were beautiful."[1]

Eventually he reached Paris and was ordered to join other displaced troops with French regulars at an infantry officer's school in Brittany during the winter of 1939–40. Unfortunately, his dim view of the quality of the French troops with whom he was cohabiting was soon justified. France was quickly overrun by German troops in May of 1940, forcing him to flee once again, this time due south through Bordeaux. In Bayonne, he and some other displaced Polish officers bribed the captain of a French trawler to take them around the Iberian Peninsula to Gibraltar. After two tense days, the Polish troops (and some displaced Czech troops) were ordered to Britain. They arrived in Liverpool where they were greeted with sandwiches and tea and where ultimately relocated to Scotland. It was during this time that Stanley formally completed the last year of his medical degree at the so-called Polish Medical School, which had been established by expats in conjunction with the University of Edinburgh (see figure 2.1).

By the time of his graduation in 1942, continental Europe was under Axis control. Stanislaw was assigned as a medical liaison officer to a British base in the Middle East town of Habbaniyah (in what is now Iraq), where he subsequently contracted malaria. He convalesced for two months in a British hospital in Egypt and, upon recovery, worked in a hospital in Ismailia. In early May 1944, after what he considered a peaceful year in Egypt, he was assigned to the Italian campaign in May of 1944, as Polish and British units fought vicious battles alongside Canadians and Americans as they worked their way up the peninsula. Stanley was a mobile medic, moving with aid stations about 200 yards from the ever-changing front line. After the invasion of Normandy and the liberation of Paris, he travelled northward into France and across the channel back to England. There he reunited with extended members of his family in London. The family reunion, however, was bittersweet. It was there that he learned that his mother, sister, and fiancé had all been murdered in the Warsaw uprising.[2]

By the close of the war he had married a fellow medical student, but Kryzsek decided that he needed to relocate once again. Poland was now under the Soviet sphere, and his experience in the British hospital system had not been positive. He obtained a visa for South Africa and filed for his decommission. Nearly penniless, the young doctor arrived in Cape Town and then Durban, and desperately searched for work, eventually opted for an obscure job as a medical officer for Choke Timber Concessions in Bechuanaland (now Botswana). There, on the edge of the fading British Empire, he practiced medicine for five years. Upon receiving news that Polish graduates of Edinburgh would be recognized as practicing physicians – but only if they were resident on 1 January 1949 – he rushed back

Figure 2.1 Graduation photo
of Stanislaw Kryszek, 1942
Britain would prove to be a central
hub in the international migration
of physicians in the English-speaking
world. In this personal photograph,
Stanislaw Kryszek poses with a fellow
student upon graduating from the
Polish Medical School in Edinburgh.
Dr Kryszek, a Polish refugee who escaped the Nazi–Soviet occupation of
his country, ultimately found himself
in Scotland during the war where he
completed his medical school training
in exile at the University of Edinburgh. Some medical refugees stayed
in Britain and still others – like Dr
Kryszek – continued their migration
to settle and practice in Canada.

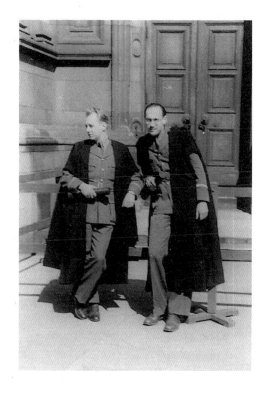

to Britain in late 1948 to be fully register with the GMC and complete internship requirements. After two more years in Africa, he received his British naturalization certificate in 1951. He continued his relocations through the British Commonwealth, working with his obstetrician wife in Nyasaland (Malawi) until she suddenly and tragically died of a brain hae-morrhage. Stanislaw sent his four-year-old daughter to relatives in Kenya while working on yellow fever in Zomba (Malawi), returning several months later to pick up his daughter and then to rejoin relatives in Eng-land. By this time, the peripatetic Polish expat had options. It was the early 1950s and many GMC qualified doctors – both British and non-British-born – were crossing the Atlantic to North America. Stanislaw joined the exodus, taking a ship to Newfoundland without any letter of offer. When no desirable positions presented themselves on the island he ultimately purchased what he later described as a "terrible practice" in a small town near Wolfville, Nova Scotia. It didn't have the elephants, wildebeest, and eland of Bechuanaland, but it was a stable and pleasant environment to raise his young daughter.[3]

NATIONAL HEALTH SERVICE

The British National Health Service had come into being in July, 1948, the result of wartime debates over the role of government in providing social services. It built on earlier precedents, including the 1911 Health Insurance Act, which provided limited sickness and disability insurance to working men and their families.[4] Following the war, a sweeping array of administration changes was launched by Aneurin Bevan, the minister of health in the Labour government of Clement Attlee, including the nationalisation of hospitals under the responsibility of local health boards and the regulation of general medical and dental practices. The guiding principle was that medical services would be provided based on need rather than the ability to pay. A small market of private care, however, was still permitted to continue alongside state-run health insurance, and a minority of hospitals maintained a certain degree of autonomy if they were predominantly research establishments. By any measure, however, the advent of the National Health Service in 1948 was revolutionary in scope and impact, reorienting medical practice and health care for Britain and evolving into a symbol of postwar social justice and national identity.[5]

The very creation of the NHS unleashed a demand for medical services in Britain that the pre-existing supply of doctors and nurses simply could not meet. Personnel had been severely depleted by the war, causing unskilled, semiskilled, and professional labour shortages. Tens of thousands of workers arrived in Britain in the 1950s to fulfil jobs such as bus drivers in London and textile workers in the Midlands, many arriving from the British Caribbean and Indian subcontinent.[6] Irish and Caribbean nurses were also recruited en masse to the expanding health care system.[7] Concurrent to this influx of working-class immigrants was also a steady arrival of hundreds of foreign doctors. The regional medical boards that were responsible for administering the new public system were only too eager to tap into the large pool of English-speaking Commonwealth doctors in order to fill holes in underserviced areas and to staff the junior ranks (house officers and house surgeons) of their local hospitals.[8] As a consequence, by the second half of the 1950s, England's physician supply was becoming heavily dependent on non-British and non-Irish medical practitioners, many of whom were arriving with the intention of staying only for a few years of training. Overseas doctors arrived predominantly from India and Pakistan, practitioners whose status as medical "outsiders" was compounded by racial, linguistic, and religious differences from the host communities.[9]

Of course, Britain's role as a central node in a complicated network of international medical education and transnational migration was hardly novel to the immediate post-WWII world. Historians of medicine have documented the fluid circulation of medical practitioners that was occasioned by the expansion and consolidation of the French and British empires. During the eighteenth and nineteenth centuries, military and naval surgeons accompanied military and merchant vessels across the vast expanse of the oceans to the far reaches of the globe. In an uncertain medical marketplace at home, being a naval surgeon at least provided some degree of job security, even if the pay was poor, the conditions appalling, and the physical environments dangerous. Indeed, the first cohort of European medical practitioners in Canada were French naval surgeons who decided to settle in New France.[10] With the expansion of British North America in the eighteenth and nineteenth centuries, a similar phenomenon was witnessed in the British colonies of Nova Scotia, Newfoundland, and Upper Canada.[11]

Within the British Empire more broadly, the pattern of medical migration, and remigration, took various forms. Some British and Irish doctors would ultimately settle in Cape Town, Auckland, Bombay, Halifax, Nairobi, or Kingston. But their connection with British medical education would scarcely end with resettlement across the globe. These doctors continued to engage in a dialogue with British medical practice and ideas, reading periodicals such as the *British Medical Journal* and travelling, when possible, to national or international conferences to reconnect with the wider British-trained medical diaspora. Some would help establish British Medical Association branches in their adopted countries that would attempt to interweave the medical practices of the West with local traditions, remedies, and clinical customs.[12] The sons of many transplanted doctors would themselves often aspire to be medical practitioners, returning to Britain for undergraduate or postgraduate medical training. In this manner, a circulation of generations of medical practitioners from colony to Britain and back to colony began to take shape, as is well documented by the demographic analyses of the graduating classes of the Glasgow and Edinburgh medical schools in the nineteenth century.[13]

As countries like Canada, New Zealand, Australia, South Africa, and India developed their own undergraduate medical programs by the dawn of the twentieth century, there emerged a tradition of "completing" medical training in Britain, whereby aspiring young graduates would travel to England and Scotland (and to a lesser extent Ireland) for what was still considered by many to be the most prestigious training programs on offer. In smaller countries like New Zealand, this became almost a rite of passage for new specialists.[14] For other larger and diverse countries, like India, it was an opportunity to distinguish and differentiate oneself from the medical practice of thousands of competitors who did not have the opportunity to travel and train abroad. For other British colonies too small for their own medical schools, the lucky few who had, or could secure, the funds continued to return to Britain for undergraduate medical training until World War II, even if, somewhat ironically, they would still face discrimination when they returned home by (white) British colonial authorities.[15]

The presence and comingling of Commonwealth doctors – doctors of a variety of races, religions, and ethnicities – training in British teaching hospitals was far from unusual before World War II. However, the immediate post-WWII era witnessed a fundamentally new phenomenon superimposed on this older circulation of practitioners. Postwar reconstruction and the rupture of the National Health Service opened up a new, accelerated period of medical out-migration as thousands of British-born and British-trained doctors began to quietly emigrate in significant numbers. The Royal Society (of Britain) sounded the alarm about the out-migration of British scientists to the United States and Canada. In no short order, the concern over research scientists was widened to included doctors. The issue soon became politicized, as exemplified in the establishment of the Willink Committee, a British Parliamentary committee struck in 1955 in response to claims that Britain was haemorrhaging doctors to North America.[16]

The Willink Committee became embroiled in two interrelated medical phenomena. First, the members were charged with investigating the apparent out-migration of British-trained doctors; however, their investigations also became preoccupied with the related phenomenon of the growing presence of foreign-doctors in the NHS. The committee observed that approximately one in eight NHS doctors were "overseas trained," by which they meant that these young doctors had completed their undergraduate training outside of Britain and Ireland. It is unclear what proportion of these were originally refugee doctors who arrived in the late 1930s and 1940s.[17] However, with the undeniable inflow of Indian- and Pakistani-born doctors, the Willink Committee concluded that there were sufficient medical practitioners in the "system" and that, in fact, British medical schools were probably producing too many doctors. Much to the shock of medical leaders, the committee report recommended a reduction of medical school places by 10 per cent.[18] The number of medical school student placements consequently declined in Britain, from 2,220 in 1955–56 to 2,030 in 1958–59.[19] A subsequent Royal Commission on Doctors' and Dentists' Pay (1960) endorsed the Willink Committee's conclusion that there was no apparent crisis in medical personnel and added, for good measure, that the levels of remuneration were appropriate.[20]

The concern over the migration of British-trained doctors to Canada and the United States, however, did not fade away. Rather, it became the subject of retrospective studies in the early 1960s. A research project, for example, focusing on Birmingham medical graduates from 1955 to 1959 concluded that the outmigration of British-trained doctors was real and had serious implications for the NHS; if extrapolated to Britain as a whole, the Birmingham study suggested that Britain had lost more than 1,000 doctors to Canada alone during this five-year period (a figure which exceeded the Willink estimate of doctor emigration to all countries combined).[21] Studies such as this also identified an interrelated phenomenon – there was a dramatic substitution underway. The aggregate number of doctors was indeed stable but that was only because of the backfilling of medical posts by foreign-trained doctors. As British doctors left for Canada, the NHS was becoming more and more dependent on "Asian" doctors (a British term referring to what North Americans would have called "East Indians" at the time). Needless to say, the volatile combination of race and the stresses of the NHS particularly vexed politicians and senior ranks of the British medical establishment. By 1961 a heated dialogue erupted in medical journals over the clinical training of these new doctors as well as their "language skills," coded language for anxieties over, and prejudices about, race and religion. Medical journals teemed with articles commenting on the large number of "Asian" doctors working in junior posts in the National Health Service.[22]

Canadian sources support these British studies that concluded that hundreds of British-born and British-trained doctors were leaving the NHS for Canada on an annual basis. Canadian Medical Association figures, submitted to the Royal Commission on Health Services (1961–64) estimated that Canadian provinces had admitted about 400 foreign-trained doctors *per year* in the period 1954–60, of which about 40 per cent were British and 20 per cent (continental) European. In other words, approximately 160 British-born doctors were entering the country on an annual basis during most of the 1950s. If one also factors in that some of the European and Commonwealth doctors may have worked in the National Health Service prior to coming to Canada, an approximate figure of at least 200 NHS doctors leaving annually for Canada in the 1950s emerges. Put in context, this was one quarter of the equivalent output of Canadian medical schools. Data, published in Canada in 1964, concluded that of nearly 15,000 newly registered physicians in the 1950s approximately 5,000 were international medical graduates (IMGs), and of these 2,000 were GMC-qualified.[23] Although exact numbers remain elusive, the wave of "NHS refugees" was undeniable. As one British medical commentator concluded, doctors were clearly "voting with their feet." Drawing on Canada's own decennial census returns, John Seale, a searing critic of the NHS, estimated that the number of British-born doctors resident in Canada had trebled from 557 (in 1951) to 1,638 (in 1961).[24]

"VOTING WITH THEIR FEET"

The migration of professionals across national borders has been a widespread and longstanding phenomenon, one informed by a variety of personal motivations. But there were also deep, structural issues that transformed a general circulation of medical practitioners into a surge of postwar transnational migration. Much had to do with the organizational structure of the National Health Service itself. As laid out in the Spens Report of 1948, the NHS was designed as a "ladder" that medical graduates

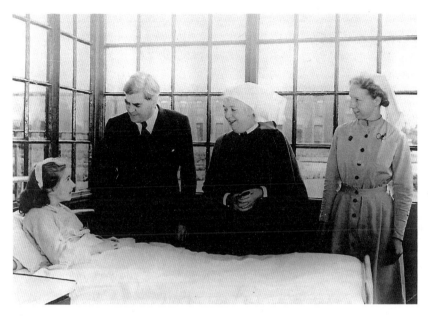

Figure 2.2 Aneurin Bevan, British minister of health, 1948
Emergency control of medical services during the Second World War led to renewed
calls for state-run health insurance and hospital administration, once hostilities ended.
The inauguration of the British National Health Service (NHS) in 1948 proved to be an
inspiration for many leftwing activists, who wanted to see a similar system in Canada.
However, dischentment with, and the lack of professional advancement within, the NHS
led to an exodus of hundreds of young doctors who made their way to Canada and the
United States in the 1950s. Here Aneurin Bevan poses with nurses and patient on the
first day of the NHS.

would progressively climb over a period of approximately seven years.
The first postgraduate year would be spent as a preregistration house
officer after which the doctor's name was admitted to the national medical register. The next year a candidate would work as a senior house
officer, followed by two years as a junior registrar and three as a senior
registrar or chief assistant. Finally, British doctors would be (in theory)
appointed to a prestigious (and highly remunerated) consultant post, at
which point their specialist status would be fully recognized. Rising to the
post of consultant was thus the goal, and indeed expectation, of all graduating specialists.[25]

Some historians believe the hierarchical configuration of the NHS doomed it from the start, while others argue that the imperfect structure of professional progression was exacerbated by chronic underfunding by the consecutive Conservative governments that returned to power in 1951.[26] According to Rosemary Stevens, the pyramidal structure of the NHS was derived from traditional teaching patterns rather than a contemporary analysis of actual service needs. Technological advances and the migration of almost all specialist services to urban-based hospitals produced unique staffing needs that were different from those of pre-NHS times. Additionally, because the system was established as a series of defined posts, labour mobility was constrained; individuals could only move forward when there was a vacancy to be filled, thereby creating an unsustainable inflexibility in the physician labour market. By 1950 the staffing of consultant positions appeared to be severely unbalanced: with 2,800 registrars and senior registrars in place it would be necessary to have a turnover of 2,800 consultants *every five years*, yet the number of consultant posts was only 5,600 and the average consultant tenure was in fact *thirty* years (these numbers did not even include the 2,000 senior hospital medical officers [SHMOS] who could also aspire to consultant positions).[27] The only way to become recognized as a specialist by the NHS was to attain consultant status, and there was little market for private practices (outside of the NHS) in the community; therefore, senior registrars were being faced with turning to general practice or entering a different, less competitive, specialty. Or waiting and waiting and waiting. Due to significant lobbying by the medical profession, some concessions were granted. The registrar grade was redesignated as a staffing grade in 1951, the senior registrar post was lengthened from three to four years in 1952, and in 1954 concessions were made for "time-expired" senior registrars on a year-to-year basis while they searched for a new position.

Still, the structural problem remained; there was simply a huge excess of junior doctors "stuck" in registrar and senior registrar positions in 1950s Britain. The time required to achieve consultant status was becoming much longer than the originally intended seven years, and every year as a "time-expired" senior registrar made it more difficult to either achieve a consultant post or move to a different specialty. Indeed, by 1958 more than 75 per cent of senior registrars were thirty-three years or older, thirty-three years being the age when the Spens Report had predicted that they *should* have become consultants.[28] That same year, the situation was so acute that a joint Parliamentary working party (the Platt Committee) was established to reappraise hospital staffing issues. In addition to the excess of registrars and senior registrars, the committee observed that the number of junior staff was insufficient to meet the new demands placed on them by technological advances. Furthermore, there was significant discontent with the SHMO position; as its role was undefined, many SHMOs felt they were simply performing the same job as a consultant but for a much smaller salary. While the most immediate concern was clearly the excess of registrars and senior registrars, it was also apparent that staffing as a whole would need to be considered.[29] While emigration necessarily involves complicated professional and personal decisions, as the interviews below suggest, the perceived lack of timely professional advancement with the NHS, combined with the attractiveness of Canada as a comfortable alternative, figured large in the thinking of those who left, regardless of whether they were British born or non-British medical practitioners who were working in the NHS.

The challenges of professional advancement within the National Health Service were further exacerbated by what some researchers have suggested was an unrealistic expectation of the cost of the new National Health Service. The NHS had been implemented by a postwar Labour government based on expenditure goals articulated during wartime but then overseen by more than a decade of Conservative governments in the 1950s that viewed the new system with some degree of suspicion. As Tony Cutler has argued, there emerged a mismatch between perceptions of a service whose expenditure was out of control and the actual reality of very modest public investment that translated as a diminishing share of national income. For Cutler, the British government had been constrained by the "flawed" wartime estimates of the cost of the National Health Service.[30] One of the many consequences of the decade of austerity was the low level of remuneration. According to one report, British general practitioners were being paid approximately one third the salary of their comparable German and Scandinavian counterparts.[31] As many would quickly realize, the difference between Canadian and British medical incomes, at least for the junior staff, was equally stark.

GOODBYE TO ALL THAT

As mentioned above, Canada was the top destination for hundreds of doctors leaving the British National Health Service. As revealed in oral interviews, some of the cultural reasons behind this choice were unsurprising. British-trained doctors found Canada to be a "happy medium" between the open and freewheeling life of the United States and what many saw as the class-ridden and hierarchical nature of British society. "It was easier ... to come to Canada," admitted one medical practitioner: "Canada seemed sort of half way between some of the extremes of the States and some of what was then ... the stagnation of Britain. Canada seemed to be about half way ... sort of reasonable, progressive, yet not quite as crazy as the States."[32] Geography also played an important role. When asked about the possibility of having chosen Australia or New Zealand, many concluded that they were simply too far to have been a viable option. Some had families that they wanted to keep in touch with; transportation being what it was, Australia or New Zealand would mean effectively isolating themselves from kith and kin. Thus geography, language, and culture all coalesced to make Canada a comfortable choice.

Many foreign-trained doctors who had worked in the NHS were in their thirties and had young families. The perception that Canada was a much safer destination to raise a family figured large in their deliberations, particularly in the context of the Vietnam War, as discussed later in this book. Professional reasons also loomed large. The structure of the British National Health Service was perceived as overly bureaucratic, hierarchical, and outdated – a "decrepit organization" to use the words of an Oxford-trained physician. Although he had returned to England after one year in Nova Scotia, he could not get used to the NHS. Working as a locum back in western England, he found conditions unsatisfactory.

Figure 2.3 *Opposite* Advertisements for overseas positions, *British Medical Journal*, 1955 In the era before professional recruiters, doctors in Britain and elsewhere scanned the pages of English-language medical journals to see what foreign positions were on offer. The market was very much open within the Commwealth, as the advertisements in the *British Medical Journal* below demonstrate. A longstanding policy of reciprocity between the General Medical Council of Britain and former colonies meant that accreditation within the Commonwealth was a relatively smooth process.

"You were very much the slaves of your patients," he explained, "there were huge clinics and a lot of house calls and lots of bureaucracy. It wasn't like practice in Nova Scotia, which was very free. You could do it the way you wanted to do it. And in terms of pay there was no comparison, I was much better paid here [Nova Scotia] … [and] you were nobody else's servant, it was more, you were more able to control your destiny."[33] "What got to me," lamented another European-born, but British-trained doctor, "really in a way you see was the British system and how it was organized is that once you have a practice under National Health Service well basically at that time, maybe it is still like that I don't know, but anyway certainly at that time for a long time it was worse than being married. If your marriage didn't work you could always get a divorce, but if you had a practice, that was it."[34]

One doctor, who considered himself to be of a lower middle-class background, spoke at length about his uneasiness about the status-preoccupied culture of British medical life:

I think medicine probably, at the time, was more of a snobbish sort of profession than my friend in physics experienced. We … actually went through university together until obviously he graduated before I did, we shared the same lodging rooms and apartments and things like that. We had the physicians' sons who had gone to public schools [private schools] the whole atmosphere [of medical education] was you know was kind of a bit snobbish and you know the consultant would ask who's father is a doctor, you know, and all that chummy old boys stuff. So I just felt that was one factor that kind of class structure in Britain, and then the pyramidal career structure which you surely know about.[35]

Others were put off by the demoralized attitude of other physicians working in the system: "The [junior] doctors lived in residences. So you pick up a lot about what it is like to be a doctor and there was a lot of grumbling, they were not a happy group … You know over coffee or so, here I was interacting with these doctors a few years ahead of me and they were not a happy lot, grumbling about you know, the Ministry of Health and other things."[36]

Seen in this context, the more egalitarian structure of the Canadian medical profession became appealing to many disgruntled NHS doctors. With the advent of different provincial hospitalization insurance systems, all doctors in Canada who had completed their residency were granted fellowship (FRCP/FRCS) status and were paid at the same billing rate as more senior physicians. Faced with an indeterminate number of years as a junior or senior registrar in the NHS, waiting for a consultant's position to free up, the option to go to Canada, set up practice almost anywhere and be a self-standing "consultant" was extremely attractive. As one doctor, who first emigrated to the United States before settling in Toronto, characterised the training programs on both sides of the Atlantic, "When I finished my training in England … people drifted around for years in junior registrar positions and you just hoped for some fifteen beds in this hospital or that hospital to open up because he or she had died and that you could be appointed and given these beds."[37] One Scottish physician agreed that Canada offered many more professional options:

> In those days, [under the NHS] you couldn't really choose where you were, where you set up a medical practice, if you were specializing as I was an intending at that stage. In general practice, you just had to go where the opportunities were, and I had done a couple of locums in family practice in Glasgow and I really didn't like it too much, I wasn't really impressed with the National Health Service … if one specialized fully, again, you couldn't choose where you were going to work. You had to more or less apply for jobs and the chance of getting them were fairly remote unless you were well connected. And for that reason I decided I didn't really want to stay in Britain.[38]

Despite their criticisms of the NHS, many foreign-trained doctors had no clear intention of staying permanently in Canada. Many thought, like the physician quoted above, that they had many options in the English-speaking world. Canada was a country they could "try out" for a year, do some travelling, and, if they did not enjoy it, return to Britain or select another destination. This applied to both male and female doctors interviewed, who embraced travel for career goals bot0.h as part of a couple or a family, as well as unmarried single professionals looking for a fresh

start and new experiences.[39] The geographic vastness of Canada offered
many different regions to try out as well. Another Scottish-born doctor
interviewed was glad to leave behind a culture of discontent that plagued
the National Health Service, but at the same time he hadn't quite given
up the idea of making a career in Scotland. But he embarked upon what
would be a veritable Canada-wide career in general medicine, joining a
group practice in a hardscrabble mining town situated in the northern
borders of Manitoba and the Northwest Territories, tending fishers and
their families in a cottage hospital established on a remote island off the
coast of already-remote Newfoundland, and serving farm families in
bucolic Prince Edward Island. Finally, toward the end of his working life,
he secured a plum government position with the province of Nova Scotia.
The idea of returning to practice family medicine in Scotland presented
itself as an option to consider with every move he and his family made,
but he got caught up in a busy life as a rural general practitioner, and the
variety of work and seemingly endless opportunities in many Canadian
provinces meant he never would return.[40]

Although the foreign-trained doctors interviewed talked at great
length about the ease (or difficulty) of registration, they talked surprisingly little about remuneration – either in terms of what attracted them
to practice in Canada or what made them stay or what made them leave
the National Health Service. Much more time was devoted to geographical mobility, the impermeability of hierarchies, and cultural factors.
Only one openly disclosed his starting salary as a "company" doctor in
an industrial Nova Scotia town.[41] Most referred often to the high "quality
of life" – a proxy that may well relate to income but might just as well
refer to the quality of schooling, social inclusiveness, low cost of living,
and the natural environment. One doctor stated earnestly that it was his
ability to sail almost on a daily basis that was the clincher; another, an
avid fisherman, was drawn to the size of the fish in the advertisements
placed by a hospital in the *British Medical Journal* looking to recruit an
overseas physician for medical positions. Whatever drew them initially,
staying in Canada was often a matter of finding both professional opportunities and community connection.

What emerges from the oral interviews of British-trained practitioners
is how little formal "recruitment" took place for the period under study.
Rather there was a lingering sense of medical mobility among newly

minted postwar NHS physicians. And so most of the physicians who would ultimately migrate to Canada from Britain commented that there were absolutely no recruiting agents and all that existed were simple advertisements placed by individual hospitals and health authorities in relevant British medical publications. Some interviewees alluded to the social and professional culture of identifying possible colleagues "back home" who might be interested in coming to Canada, indicating the presence of chain migration patterns. Other push and pull factors played roles in determining the final location. For instance, the married women physicians who were interviewed tended to follow their husband's career path, perhaps because their most mobile years as young professionals coincided with childbearing and child rearing.[42] The greater openness and potential for career advancement in Canada often meant that both partners would find rewarding work in the same city or even the same hospital. It seems that the expansion of the health system in Canada through the fee-for-service system permitted a certain flexibility for the management of both career and family life when two doctors were looking for work together. Many physicians interviewed remarked with surprise how many of their British classmates had ultimately made careers abroad, when they eventually reconnected at class reunions a few decades later.[43]

BRITAIN'S COMMONWEALTH CITIZENSHIP

The flow of NHS doctors to Canada may well have been motivated by a complicated mix of professional and personal factors. However, the actual process of migrating from Britain to Canada was structured by changing immigration regulations in the two countries. The British Nationality Act of 1948, passed the same year that the National Health Services took effect, established the right of Commonwealth citizens to live and work in the United Kingdom under the category of Citizen of the United Kingdom and Colonies (CUKC).[44] This category of "imperial citizenship" had long-lasting effects that disrupted subsequent legislative efforts to exclude the in-migration of certain "undesirable" Commonwealth citizens.[45] As mentioned above, the postwar labour shortage combined with the right of Commonwealth citizens to work in Britain facilitated the arrival of tens of thousands of South Asian and Afro-Caribbean workers in the 1950s.

Their arrival is noteworthy considering that countries like Canada made it extraordinarily difficult for nonwhite Commonwealth citizens to immigrate before 1962, unless exceptions were made for them or they were part of sanctioned scientific exchange programs.

In response to this "return to the metropole," anti-immigrant sentiment was ascendant in Britain by the dawn of the 1960s. The British government responded, in part, by passing the Commonwealth Immigrants Act of 1962, which aimed to impose immigration controls on all Commonwealth citizens (except for those from the UK) or bearing a passport issued by London (as opposed to a UK passport issued by colonial governments).[46] Hereafter, the British government distinguished between those who were "born British" and those who were bearers of London-issued passports.[47] A three-tiered, quota-restricted "employment voucher scheme" was introduced as an attempt to reduce the settlement of "Black" and "Asian" immigrants, broad nonwhite groups that might include individuals from as diverse locations as Trinidad, Uganda, Malaysia, or Sri Lanka.[48] The following year quotas were further reduced and "additional qualifications" added to each category to deliberately cut down on potential applicants, particularly applicants of colour.[49]

While the 1962 Act restricted working-class Afro-Caribbean migration to Britain, there continued a flow of skilled male professionals – predominantly engineers and doctors – from the Indian subcontinent.[50] Doctors were notably excluded from the new voucher system.[51] Although the then Conservative minister of health, Enoch Powell, did his best to downplay the arrival of "Asian" doctors, their presence in local hospitals was evident across the country and indeed back in India. Using General Medical Council data, researchers for the *Journal of the Indian Medical Association* estimated that there were approximately 1,600 Indian doctors in training courses in Britain in 1962.[52] Some medical editorials in Britain focused on the dramatic rise in the number of foreign doctors as house officers (some quoting a figure as high as 40 per cent of all house officers by 1960); others decried the flight of British doctors to North America that, they alleged, had caused the growing dependence on foreign doctors in the first place.[53] Given their presence, the growing backlash against nonwhite immigrants in Britain placed Indian and Pakistani doctors in a rather unenviable situation. During the rest of the decade, the British government developed

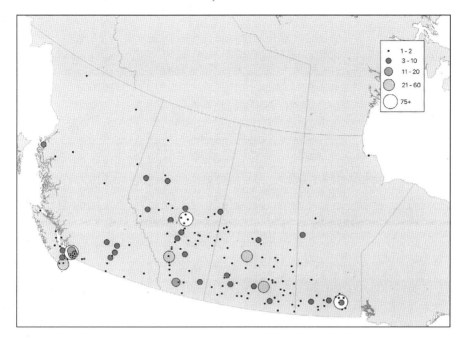

Figure 2.4 UK-trained doctors in western Canada, 1961
Two thousand doctors who completed their undergraduate training in the United
Kingdom would emigrate to Canada in the 1950s, the top destination for self-styled
"NHS refugees." This map, generated from the 1961 *Canadian Medical Directory*,
illustrates the geographical dispersement of 800 of these practitioners throughout
the Western provinces.

ever more restrictive immigration regulations according to the model of
"limitation-integration."[54] Meanwhile, at exactly the same time, Canada
and the United States were moving slowly to a system of immigration
that was, in theory at least, not based on religion or race.

Concern over racial discrimination in government agencies and policies in Canada was heightened under the Progressive Conservative government of John Diefenbaker. Diefenbaker had long championed human
rights and considered one of his crowning achievements the passing of
Canada's first Bill of Rights in 1960. As discussed further in the next
chapter, the Progressive Conservative government, in 1962, stated that no
immigration officer was permitted to discriminate against applicants
based on religion or race. The new immigration regulations called for a
person to be admitted to Canada "who by reason of his education, training, skills or other special qualifications is likely to be able to establish

himself successfully in Canada."[55] The changes in Canada and similar changes in the United States (in 1965) signalled to nonwhite English-speaking practitioners in Britain that North America was now a realistic option for medical migrants from South and East Asia, the Caribbean and Africa. Many young Commonwealth doctors practicing in Britain took the opportunity occasioned by their "medical passport" to resettle their young families.

CONCLUSIONS

By the end of the 1950s, Canada and Britain were entangled in a complicated web of medical migration and state health insurance. On a policy level, progressive politicians in Canada looked to the National Health Service for inspiration, suggesting that Britain had pioneered a new postwar system of universal health care provision that was just, equitable, and effective. Although stymied at home by the constitutional challenge of health care being a provincial prerogative, many progressive politicians dreamed of a pan-Canadian system similar to the principles, if not the precise delivery mechanisms, of the British NHS. The connections were not just ideological but also demographic. Concurrent to the political debates over state-run medical services, British-born and Irish-born doctors were entering Canada following the 1952 Immigration Act. Literally hundreds of NHS doctors scattered across the vast expanse of Canada and disproportionately in parts of the country where they could quickly establish practices. There were 800 alone in the western provinces at the end of the 1950s (see figure 2.4). By 1964, the *Financial Post* reported that half of Saskatchewan's licensed physicians were trained outside of Canada and most of these were from Britain.[56]

Back in Britain, the question as to the extent of the exodus of British doctors had been more or less settled. In 1964, Brian Abel-Smith of the London School of Economics and his research associate Kathleen Gales would publish the results of a comprehensive qualitative study of the out-migration of British-trained doctors. Their investigation, drawn from a random 5 per cent sample of names appearing in the Medical Register for the years 1925–59, aimed to both document the extent of and uncover the reasons behind physician emigration from Britain. Published as *British*

Doctors at Home and Abroad,[57] the book cemented Abel-Smith's reputation as a leading scholar in what was then commonly called social administration. The book also added fuel to a political firestorm in Britain, prompting the then Conservative minister of health, Enoch Powell, to denounce what he characterised as exaggerated claims circulated by "opponents" of the NHS.[58] But Powell himself must have been only too aware that a serious problem of physician out-migration threated the very existence of the National Health Service itself. In retrospect, it is hard to argue with Abel-Smith's conclusion that "The hospital service [in Britain] would have collapsed had it not been for the enormous influx of junior doctors from such countries as India and Pakistan."[59] Some of these "Asian" doctors would, of course, settle permanently in Britain; others, however, would continue their migration to Canada and the United States.

The arrival of so many foreign doctors in Canada was greeted with ambivalence and muted enthusiasm by the Canadian Medical Association (CMA). By the late 1950s, however, the "medical nativism" of the CMA that had lingered in certain quarters would be overwhelmed by the popular demand for health care practitioners unleased by hospitalization insurance. Not only were rural and remote areas of the country acutely short of doctors and nurses, the rapid construction of shiny new downtown medical facilities were also short of staff, despite the continued influx of British and Irish doctors, nurses, and midwives. This demand within Canada, as Karen Flynn has demonstrated, forced the hands of the federal government, which gave immigration officers greater latitude to admit individuals from nontraditional backgrounds or countries if they demonstrated "exceptional merit" – meaning, in practice, that they were skilled in occupations in high demand that could not otherwise be filled by Canadians.[60] Black nurses thus began to be admitted into the country from the late 1950s, although professional practice and advancement remained very difficult for them.[61]

British-trained doctors found themselves in an unusual situation upon arriving in Canada in the 1950s. Having left the NHS, many were ambivalent about the proposals for universal hospitalization and medical insurance circulating in Canada. Writing in from Winnipeg, British physician John Etherington had come to Canada because he disagreed with the principles and practice of the NHS. He offered a cautionary word to the CMA and on the issue of state-sponsored health care, warning, "The profession in Canada should take careful note of what has happened in Britain, and should see that the same mistakes are never repeated here." For him, these included ensuring that patients should be free to choose and change physicians. He emphasized that payment along fee-for-service lines was "an essential part of any medical service which is to offer the best in medical care to the patient."[62] Nonetheless, he was of the opinion that such health care schemes were not inherently flawed, pointing out how patients were rather well-served under the NHS, the service removing the financial stress and worry from illness, despite the waits for nonemergency service that resulted.[63] Other British expat physicians were not so conciliatory. J.A. Armstrong, newly arrived in Edmonton, weighed in one year later with an even more strongly worded view. Coming to Canada offered "a new way of life and one which gives the great majority a standard of living, a chance to better themselves and a chance to enjoy satisfying work conditions, such as this generation of Britons has never known in its own country." This spirit of free enterprise and the rewards for hard work and initiative in Canada was refreshing. This, in his opinion, made Canada "a less frustrating and happier place to live."[64]

Chapter Three

Medical Manpower

Dr Iain MacDonald[1] was born in a shipbuilding town of Scotland, the son of a Gaelic-speaking shopkeeper and teacher. Like many young Scottish students, he profited from the excellent comprehensive education and ultimately enrolled in medical school at the University of Glasgow. However, he became deeply discontented with the National Health Service at the end of the 1950s. He bristled at the lack of opportunities and professional mobility. After two or three years spent completing his diploma in obstetrics and performing his mandatory internship, he looked for other possibilities. New Zealand was "too far," the United States "too American"; he ultimately chanced upon an advertisement in a British medical journal for a vacancy in a new clinic in Manitoba. There, he joined another Scottish-trained doctor in a small-town practice. But, even for a Scotsman, the weather was cruel. "You spend the winter longing for summer and the summer longing for winter," he recalled laughing.[2] After two years, he relocated to be the resident doctor at a cottage hospital in Newfoundland, where the weather, it must be said, was scarcely better. "There was a snow storm that lasted three and a half days," he recalled, startled by discovering that one could "lean on the wind – I mean, you could just lean forward, and, uh … The wind would prop you up."[3] No doubt, however, the community he served was happy to see him and the modest hospital facilities. "[T]he locals appreciated it [the cottage hospital system]," he emphasized, "because [before it was established] they were used to not having a hospital at all."[4] Nevertheless, medical practice and community life had their challenges. It was "a quiet remote place" even for a Scottish expat from a smaller community. The isolation, in particular, required adjustment: "It was shut off at times for, uh, a day or two, with the ice, the wind in the valley, and the little hospital, and you had to cope as best you could."[5]

The Scottish doctor's practice on the island was all encompassing. At the cottage hospital there were two doctors and a small number of nurses. Due to vacation, sickness, or the departure of the other doctor, he was often working for weeks at a time as the sole medical practitioner. Still, the flip side was that he had almost complete freedom, the work was not (at least to him) physically gruelling – indeed he recalled that the afternoons were quiet and relaxing. It was a life of local respect and comfort amidst very modest surroundings. Poverty was ubiquitous, and local economies waxed and waned on the vagaries of seasonal work. Most houses had no running water, and many had no electricity. Since his own doctor's house was physically attached to the cottage hospital, he had both, and thus considered himself to be rather "spoiled." Unsurprisingly, the local general practitioner in such a setting was a respected figure in the community, someone who, even if they were "from away," was quickly integrated into community rituals, such as weddings, to which everyone was invited. Moreover, unusual for most of the rest of Canada, and perhaps maybe a good number of his medical colleagues, Dr MacDonald enjoyed the stability of being on a salary.[6] After three years in Newfoundland, the itinerant doctor, now with two young children, relocated to Prince Edward Island, which he found (to his pleasure) to be less windy and more "Scottish." He worked in a small (ten- to fourteen-bed) local hospital as Prince Edward Island transitioned into the era of Medicare in the early 1970s.

HOSPITAL INSURANCE

The multiple journeys and small-town hospital experience of Dr MacDonald highlights the fluid movements of foreign-trained doctors as they entered Canada during an important time in hospital construction, expansion, and insurance. For the experiments with hospitalization insurance and provincially administered cottage hospitals did not go unnoticed in Ottawa. Successive governments in a bipartisan consensus introduced a range of postwar health and welfare programs that involved extending social assistance to the general public. Family allowances were first, whereby the federal government sent households monthly cheques for all children under the age of sixteen. Veterans' benefits (mostly targeted for vocational training) followed, as did more modest support for public housing. More dramatic was the introduction of pensions in 1951 for all those over seventy, and the Unemployment Insurance Act of 1956, a compulsory scheme with contributions from employees, employers, and the government. Needless to say, some provinces, Quebec and Ontario included, chafed at the federal intrusion into spheres generally considered to be the prerogative of the individual provinces, but many of the measures proved to be deeply popular, ensuring the continued electoral success of the federal Liberal party.[7]

As the government of Louis St Laurent neared the end of its third mandate, it looked to build on the evident popularity of these federal initiatives. Inspired by the repeated success of the CCF in Saskatchewan, many leaders in the federal Liberal Party believed that hospitalization insurance would ensure yet another majority victory in the looming election of 1957. Health care had long been discussed as part of the federal Liberal Party platform at the national level, but federal–provincial wrangling had made its implementation problematic. The postwar federal Liberals, under federal Health Minister Paul Martin (Senior), began gingerly by introducing health grants (from 1948) for targeted public health initiatives (such as trials for the Salk vaccine for polio) as well as government support for basic medical research and the construction of new hospitals.[8] Payments for medical services, however, would be riskier. Maurice Duplessis, the Union Nationale premier in Quebec, for one, made it clear that he would not tolerate any intrusion in the management of hospitals, which were almost all run by Catholic orders in his province.

Addressing a joint session of the British and Canadian Medical Associations in 1955, Paul Martin Sr remarked on the wide array of prepayment plans then in operation, pointing out that in four provinces governments were already involved in a variety of schemes intended to subsidize hospital care.[9] Focussing on doctors in particular, Martin observed how Canada boasted "one of the highest ratios of physicians to population of any country in the world," a workforce which then numbered approximately 16,000. Perhaps as a gentle jab at the British Medical Association representatives in attendance, he highlighted the more than 700 physicians and surgeons trained in the United Kingdom who had arrived since the passage of the Immigration Act of 1952. Without such foreign-trained doctors, Martin mused, Canadian health care would have been hard pressed to meet the growing demand for physician services that was emerging from these provincial plans.[10] As the Liberals geared up for another federal election in which they wished to continue their decades long run as the "natural" governing party, the federal minister of health and welfare was persuaded that hospitalization insurance should occupy a central plank of the federal election. However, due to allegations of corruption and a downturn in the economy, the St Laurent Liberals fell to the Progressive Conservatives in 1957, before a new hospitalization insurance bill was passed into law.

It is noteworthy that the new minority Progressive Conservative government under John Diefenbaker would reintroduce the hospitalization insurance bill and see its passage as one of its first major accomplishments. The Hospital Insurance and Diagnostic Services Act provided matching federal government funding for acute hospital care and diagnostic services.[11] The legislation went much further than the tepid federal health grants of the Liberals, which had provided funding assistance in the less contentious fields of research and hospital infrastructure. HIDS, as the legislation became to be known in policy circles, directly intruded into the contested field of the delivery of health care services. This joint undertaking came with strings attached, of course, conditions that signalled the federal government's desire to ensure universality for state-sponsored plans. Provinces that elected to participate were required to develop plans that were available to all residents "upon uniform terms and conditions" and include a comprehensive slate of services for standard inpatient services and amenities, including meals, accommodation, and nursing services but also encompassing drugs, therapeutic procedures, and follow-up services such as physiotherapy. Physician services would be a part of the coverage insofar as hospital services engaged physicians in a diagnostic capacity or otherwise as a health provider who received remuneration from the hospital for services provided, such as radiology and surgery. Although the contribution of Ottawa has been characterised as reimbursing provinces 50 per cent for the annual costs of hospitalization, the actual funding formula, unsurprisingly, was more complicated.[12] One notable clause, presaging constitutional debates later in the century, was that no contributions were supposed to be paid out until at least six provinces, containing at least one half of the population of Canada, entered into the agreement. However, in the face of Duplessis's continued resistance, this stipulation was quietly withdrawn the following year.

The 1950s had a remarkable diversity of medical institutions that could potentially qualify under the appellation of "hospitals." In the end, the federal government chose a limited definition, excluding the reimbursement of several types of medical institutions that were deemed to be designed for long-term care, including tuberculosis sanatoria, provincial mental hospitals, nursing homes, and homes for the aged. The "insured services" associated with hospitalization referred to the inpatient and outpatient services to which residents of a province were entitled to under provincial law without charge.[13] Inpatient services included free accommodation and meals at the "standard" or "public ward" level, as well as "necessary" nursing and medical care. In addition, all laboratory, radiological, and other diagnostic procedures necessary for the purpose of maintaining health, preventing disease, and assisting in the diagnosis and treatment of any injury, illness, or disability; drugs, biologicals, and related preparations as provided in an agreement; use of operating room, case room, and anaesthetic facilities, including necessary equipment and supplies; routine surgical supplies; use of radiotherapy and physiotherapy facilities where available; and services rendered by persons who received remuneration from the hospital were covered. The outpatient hospital services included all of the aforementioned inpatient services, with the exception of the accommodation and meals at the standard or public ward level.[14]

The advent of federally subsidized hospitalization insurance prompted a mixed reaction from medical organizations, labour unions, and politicians of various stripes. By passing this legislation, the federal government had indirectly guaranteed the payment of hospitalization for poor patients, a principal demand of the Canadian Medical Association dating from the 1930s. And they had done so without "nationalizing" hospitals or restricting private practice in the communities, two critical issues that had been a factor in the disaffection with the NHS in Britain and fears that similar measures would find their way into Canada. Given these concessions, a certain number of physicians in rural and remote parts of the country saw the change as welcome. Writing from his medical practice in Lamont, Alberta, Morley Young observed that hospital insurance in places like Saskatchewan proved popular among both clinicians and patients. He forecast several ways the new federal legislation would influence physicians' work, but he expressed more concern about the structure of his own work and billing practices as part of an extended hospital-based team.[15] Newfoundland, with its cottage hospital system was also quick to sign on, eager to reap some of the federal assistance benefits that were supposed to have been the principal incentive for joining Confederation in the first place. Ontario, Alberta, and British Columbia, which had all been experimenting with subsidies for poor patients, grudgingly accepted.

The medical societies, however, did not see HIDS as either inevitable or necessary. Rather, they considered it a dangerous first step towards the control of *all* aspects of health care delivery by the state and the end to professional independence and clinical autonomy. Certain aspects of the bill itself were particular cause for concern – such as how the "politicization of admitting privileges" might threaten professional cohesion unless it were carefully managed by provincial medical colleges and not by bureaucrats. Writing from Nova Scotia, J.A. MacMillan, vice president and director of the Maritime Hospital Service Association, foresaw financial problems for physicians who were used to offering and billing for diagnostic services like x-rays and various lab work. He also predicted a crisis of administrative personnel: "Actuaries, accountants, statisticians, I.B.M. [computer] operators, tabulating clerks – all these people [who] have been trained in the operation of prepayment plans," he observed ruefully, "will become fair bait for hospital insurance commissions."[16]

Hospitalization insurance, however, proved immensely popular throughout the country amongst the general public, owing in no part due to the reality that, despite the postwar boom times, a sizeable minority of Canadians lacked proper insurance for hospitalization. The Royal Commission on Health Services (1961–64) estimated that 40 per cent of Canadians had no or inadequate health care for medical services (in general) at the time of their inquiry.[17] A reasonable inference is that a considerable proportion of Canadians on the eve of the 1957 act relied on a patchwork of free municipal hospital care, partial coverage from prepaid services, and paying out of pocket when they or a member of their family required hospital care. As a consequence, the new public hospitalization and diagnostic services led to an explosion in demand for these new clinical services that were now "free" at the point of delivery. Surveying urban and rural health care clinics and hospitals on behalf of the provincial College of Physicians and Surgeons of Alberta in 1958, the year in which HIDS took effect, H.V. Morgan reported that the waiting lists for diagnostic services had lengthened considerably and "pressure from the public for admission to hospital for investigation services has greatly increased."[18] Just as in the National Health Services, the extension of hospitalization insurance unleashed a surge of demand that required a dramatic expansion of trained medical personnel.

By 1959, the principle of federally cofounded, but provincially run, medical services had been established, if not embraced enthusiastically. Meanwhile, as explained in the previous chapter, Saskatchewan had been the crucible of experimentation, piloting projects to extend hospitalization insurance to health insurance for all medically necessary services. As the CCF government geared up for another provincial election, they expressed their goal of establishing "Medicare" in the province. With the increasing cost of medical care and the positive examples provided by provincial experiments, there was a strong sense that an expansion of the cofunding structure and principles embodied in HIDS to cover all medical services was not only possible but also desirable. The CCF, fresh off yet another provincial victory in June of 1960, began to finalize plans for universal health insurance in the province in the fall and winter of 1960–61. So great was the expectation that such a proposal might reach the federal level that the Canadian Medical Association, perhaps tired of playing defence, requested Prime Minister Diefenbaker strike an independent commission to evaluate the "future of health services." At the very least, it would buy a few years' time for the medical profession to find ways to avoid the perceived catastrophe of state-run medicine. Caught between the popularity of hospitalization insurance and his own conservative constituencies, Diefenbaker obliged.[19]

ROYAL COMMISSION ON HEALTH SERVICES

The Royal Commission on Health Services began its work in June of 1961, charged with inquiring into and reporting on "the existing facilities and the future need for health services for the people of Canada." Cognizant of provincial sensitivities, the mandate required the commission to "recommend such measures, consistent with the constitutional division of legislative power in Canada."[20] The group tasked with this challenging undertaking involved seven members, chaired by Saskatchewan Justice Emmett M. Hall. Hall was not only a justice of the Court of Appeal from Saskatchewan but was a former fellow law student with Diefenbaker. The other six commissioners included a francophone nurse administrator from Montreal, an economist, an industrialist, a dentist, and two physicians.[21] Between the summer of 1961 and the late spring of 1962, the commission toured the country, holding hearings in all ten Canadian provinces and the Yukon, and receiving submissions from more than 400 organizations. They also commissioned their researchers to report on medical programs and practices in countries around the world. In total, a further twenty-six research studies were commissioned from Canadian scholars on a variety of topics from "Medical Education," to "Trends in Psychiatric Care," to the "Economics of Health."[22] One of these studies specifically investigated "Medical Manpower" in Canada.[23] The commission thus represents a remarkably timely investigation into the immigration of foreign-trained doctors, at the very moment of the Fairclough Directive, the hardening of the immigration regulations in Britain, as well the eve of the Saskatchewan doctors' strike of the summer of 1962.

The growing preoccupation with the interface of medical manpower and universal health insurance reflected deep structural problems in medical education and staffing that had emerged over the previous decade and reflected one of the many anomalies of the division of powers under Confederation. Put simply, there was a disconnect between the domestic production of medical practitioners (which occurred in provincially regulated medical schools) and the growing population of Canada (indirectly affected by the federal immigration regulations of the country). The postwar population of Canada was booming, resulting from net immigration and the reversal of the generations-long decline in the birth rate. Immigration, the baby boom, and rural depopulation all led to the accelerated growth of cities and that new postwar phenomenon – suburbia. And many of the new suburbs were not yet well supported by the same kind of hospital structure that had been centred in the older parts of Canada's major cities, neither were they well served by a medical school system that had barely changed in several decades.

Despite the growing population, medical school enrolment had remained stable for the decade between the censuses of 1951 and 1961, at

Table 3.1

Medical student enrolment in Canada, 1947–48 to 1960–61

Year	Medical school enrolment	Canadian population '000	Enrolment per 100,000 general population
1947–48	3,100	12,551	24.7
1948–49	3,233	12,823	25.2
1949–50	3,278	13,447	24.4
1950–51	3,489	13,712	25.4
1951–52	3,458	14,009	24.7
1952–53	3,444	14,459	23.8
1953–54	3,643	14,845	24.5
1954–55	3,589	15,287	23.5
1955–56	3,651	15,698	23.3
1956–57	3,655	16,081	22.7
1957–58	3,686	16,610	22.2
1958–59	3,668	17,080	21.5
1959–60	3,549	17,483	20.3
1960–61	3,508	17,870	19.6

Source: Adapted from Stanislaw Judek, *Medical Manpower in Canada*
(Ottawa: Queen's Printer, 1964), 64.

about 800 per year (or 3,100–3,500 "steady state" – that is, all medical students under training at any particular moment in time). The failure of medical education to expand in tandem with the increase in the general population meant that the ratio of medical school enrolment *per population* was actually decreasing during the 1950s, the decade during which all of these provincial subsidies were taking place (see table 3.1). Compounding the real decline in medical school enrolment was the by then well-documented phenomenon of Canadian doctors relocating south of the border. As table 3.2 demonstrates, and contemporary medical observers knew well, Canada was a net exporter of physicians to the United States, about 200 (on average) per year. Thus, during the 1950s Canada lost approximately 2,000 Canadian-trained medical practitioners to the United States, well over 10 per cent of its medical workforce. In the face of these two factors Canada only managed to maintain, and indeed needed to improve, its physician-to-population ratios through the immigration of 4,000 foreign-trained doctors.

One might assume that the situation was stable, with the net loss (and underproduction) of medical practitioners being more than offset by the influx of foreign-trained doctors, but this was not entirely the case. For two other factors had become pronounced in the 1950s – namely the rapid increase in the *demand* for medical services unleashed by provincial (and later) federal hospitalization subsidies and secondly the *maldistribution* of doctors within the country. Put simply, more and more doctors (both Canadian-trained and foreign-trained) were settling in the cities, leaving rural and remote areas relatively underserviced. For those rural communities in Atlantic Canada and the Prairies the situation was dire, and newspapers across the country began to report on a national doctor and nurse "shortage," despite the absolute increase in licensed physicians reported by medical associations and decennial censuses. For example, in 1960 the town of St Albans (population 3,000 persons) made national headlines as they petitioned the Newfoundland government to station either a doctor or nurse in their community, as they had no one to look after them. The nearest medical practitioner to the town was some twenty miles away; the nearest hospital was fifty. Since there were no reliable roads in the area, patients had to be ferried out by boat when they were sick.[24] Similarly the *Financial Post* reported that Manitoba College of Physicians and Surgeons complained that only one-third of their graduating medical class remained in Manitoba (one third left for the United States and another third for another part of Canada).[25]

So why were more and more medical graduates settling in urban and suburban areas? There were multiple, interrelated reasons for this trend. One factor that fed into the increasing urbanization of physicians was the growing importance of medical technology to clinical practice. Physicians practicing in rural areas lacked hospital access, laboratory, and clinical facilities, whereas larger urban centres often possessed more advanced medical facilities as well as the medical schools themselves. Indeed, the situation of medical schools in the principal cities of Canada had a direct sociodemographic impact. It was a well-known phenomenon that physicians tended to begin their practice in communities of similar *or greater* size than those in which they resided prior to entry into medical school.

Table 3.2
Migration of physicians into and out of Canada

Year	Immigration From USA	Immigration Other countries	Total	Emigration To USA	Immigration -emigration	Net loss to USA
1950	–	68	68	260	-192	**-260**
1951	–	166	166	173	-7	**-173**
1952	–	293	293	186	107	**-186**
1953	55	347	402	105	297	**-50**
1954	39	272	311	135	176	**-96**
1955	33	300	333	127	206	**-94**
1956	29	386	415	96	319	**-67**
1957	46	589	635	265	370	**-219**
1958	52	342	394	179	215	**-127**
1959	66	373	439	229	210	**-163**
1960	84	357	441	262	179	**-178**
1961	67	378	445	296	149	**-229**
Total	**471**	**4181**	**4652**	**2313**	**2339**	**-1842**

Source: Adapted from Stanislaw Judek, *Medical Manpower in Canada* (Ottawa: Queen's Printer, 1964), 38.

Medical schools disproportionately drew their students from the urban middle class.[26] Social and cultural expectations to live in suburban or urban environments were reinforced by financial considerations. Rural regions tended to be characterized by an overall lower income than urban centres, and after investing a great deal of not only time but also money into a medical education, there were certainly incentives for new graduates to settle in areas where patients were better able to afford their fees or where higher volumes of patients were achievable.[27]

The uneven distribution of physicians between urban and rural areas mirrored a disparity of physicians *between* provinces.[28] While physician–population ratios are an imperfect measure of health care utilization and access, they do provide for some interprovincial comparison.[29] The Atlantic provinces had physician–population ratios much lower than the national average, with none breaking the barrier of one physician per 1,000 residents by the time of the Hall Commission. Newfoundland's ratio, in fact, still hovered around one per 2,000 residents. British Columbia, Quebec, Ontario, and Manitoba's ratios were below the national average, trending towards one physician per 800 residents (see table 3.3), a figure then consistent with World Health Organization's estimate of the recommended physician-to-resident ratios in industrialized countries.

In summary, several trends had emerged in the 1950s. First, Canadian provinces were losing hundreds of doctors to the United States and back-filling with doctors either born in Britain or Ireland or who were Commonwealth doctors previously working in the National Health Service. The overall number of doctors in the Canadian health care system thus looked like it was increasing comfortably, but this augmentation was largely due to foreign doctors and characterised by stark disparities between urban and rural areas and between have and have-not provinces. Furthermore, a large proportion of Canadian-trained physicians were migrating to the United States; this offset the number of foreign-trained physicians setting up practice in Canada and increased Canada's reliance on doctors trained elsewhere. Of course, if all of the foreign-trained doctors were migrating uniformly to rural and remote areas of the country this may well have "solved" the problem of the maldistribution of doctors. However, as chapter 6 will explore, it appears that the settlement of foreign-trained physicians in Canada did not occur uniformly and was far from stable.[30]

Table 3.3
Provincial physician–population ratios, 1911–61 (residents per doctor)

Province	Year					
	1911	1921	1931	1941	1951	1961
Newfoundland	-	-	-	-	2,524	1,991
Prince Edward Island	1,306	1,309	1,397	1,418	1,342	1,149
Nova Scotia	1,206	1,147	1,153	1,350	1,094	1,044
New Brunswick	1,253	1,448	1,517	1,693	1,445	1,314
Quebec	1,003	1,065	1,046	1,054	990	853
Ontario	828	848	872	903	857	776
Manitoba	1,065	1,095	1,051	1,108	926	823
Saskatchewan	1,298	1,445	1,579	1,700	1,278	973
Alberta	1,014	1,073	1,256	1,320	1,118	982
British Columbia	945	862	952	1,010	847	758
Canada	*970*	*1,008*	*1,034*	*1,072*	*976*	*857*

Source: Adapted from Stanislaw Judek, *Medical Manpower in Canada*
(Ottawa: Queen's Printer, 1964), 27.

Despite the fact that the absolute number of licensed doctors grew steadily from 1941 to 1961 a growing discourse of a "doctor shortage" in the country came to dominate, one that added fuel to the passionate debates during the Saskatchewan doctors' strike and informed discussions of immigration reform.

THE SASKATCHEWAN DOCTORS' STRIKE

Within this volatile context of competing provincial and national visions for health insurance one of most controversial events of postwar Canadian history occurred – the 1962 Saskatchewan doctors' strike. The conflict arose from a culmination of clashes between the Saskatchewan College of Physicians and Surgeons (scps)[31] and the Cooperative Commonwealth Federation (ccf) government of the province. As discussed earlier, Sas-

Table 3.4
Proportion of physicians and surgeons living in communities of >10,000 as
compared to proportion of the Canadian population living in communities
of >10,000

Year	% Physicians and surgeons in communities >10,000	% Canadian population in communities >10,000
1947	70.8	-
1951	73.2	48.2
1962	85.8	58.7

Source: Stanislaw Judek, *Medical Manpower in Canada*
(Ottawa: Queen's Printer, 1964), 131–3.

katchewan had been one of the flashpoints of experimentation with health
insurance schemes in the immediate postwar period. The scps, however,
maintained its longstanding opposition to a government-controlled universal medical care program from its announcement in December 1959
(during the lead-up to the 1960 provincial election).[32] With the successful
re-election of the ccf in 1960, a campaign that some have described as
being a "referendum" on provincially run universal health insurance, the
provincial ccf government was ready to go it alone instead of waiting for
the results of the Royal Commission on Health Services.

The provincial government in Saskatchewan moved quickly to pass the
new Medicare bill. The bill was hastily introduced in October 1961, without granting the scps opportunity to review the details before it was
tabled, an act interpreted as a breach of faith by the doctors of the province.[33] Its implementation was also swift. Several weeks later the Saskatchewan Medical Care Insurance Act received royal assent on 17 November
1961 and a Medical Care Insurance Commission (mcic) was created in
January 1962 to administer the new health system.[34] Unsurprisingly, the
first half of 1962 witnessed a pitched battle between the provincial government and the scps, during which time the government offered an
array of concessions.[35] For example, the government proposed to allow
physician-based private plans to continue (under certain conditions) and

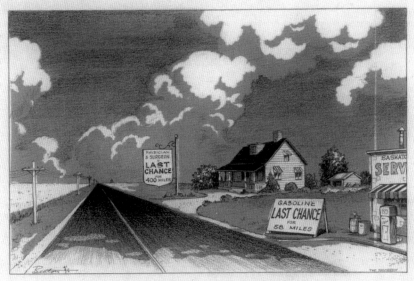

Figure 3.1 "Physician and Surgeon: Last Chance for 400 Miles"
The problem of staffing small scattered communities on the prairies was a perennial problem for provincial governments. During the 1962 doctors' strike, national newspapers overflowed with cartoons about the imminent exodus of doctors from Saskatchewan, including this one that appeared in the now-defunct *Toronto Telegram*.

to permit doctors to opt out entirely of the provincial plan. The scps, for its part, continued to lobby for government subsidization of private insurance plans, consistently rejecting a public, single-payer option.[36] The college's unwillingness to play ball delayed implementation of health care reforms from April to July 1962.[37]

According to some scholars, the government expected some doctors "to ignore the medical care plan and to continue to bill patients directly" rather than actually engage in a comprehensive withholding of services.[38] However, when in April of 1962 amendments to the act were interpreted by the profession as a ban on opting out, the scps prepared for strike action.[39] Nearly 600 of the province's 900 doctors attended a two-day meeting in Regina in May 1962 "to demonstrate membership support." The premier spoke for an hour in defence of the new system, but to no avail: all but five doctors present agreed to go on strike.[40] The government and the profession then did not meet for seven weeks, while the provincial hospital association attempted to mediate between the two sides. Three

days of meetings were held beginning 22 June, at which time the government unsuccessfully attempted to reassure doctors by guaranteeing the
professional independence of physicians, their right to practice outside
the new system, and local administration by individual health regions.[41]
This failed to placate the doctors' federation, which finally agreed to go
out on strike, effective 1 July.

Within this dramatic standoff, foreign-trained doctors were active on
both sides of the dispute. In the decade leading up the crisis, more than half
of new registrants in Saskatchewan were foreign graduates.[42] Indeed, by
1960 an estimated 250 of the province's 750 physicians were so-called "refugees" from the NHS, bolstering opposition among the province's doctors
to "state medicine." A *New York Times* journalist observed that the "hard
core of the striking doctors" were British expats.[43] Meanwhile, the MCIC
proactively recruited British and American doctors to help undermine the
imminent labour action. The arrival of 110 British and North American
(American and out-of-province Canadian) doctor recruits doubled the
number of physicians in a new "emergency service force."[44] Although precise numbers are difficult to determine, the Saskatchewan Federation of
Labour estimated that, in total, ninety recruits from Britain arrived to staff
emergency services.[45] The near daily landings of strikebreaking foreign doctors became a regular news item, an unusual medical parallel to supply
flights arriving in Berlin after the Soviet blockade a decade earlier.[46]

The use of sympathetic, strikebreaking doctors had been discussed in
advance by the provincial government. The province had already dis-
patched one administrator to London "to recruit British doctors willing
to take full-time posts in rural areas to help temporarily during the strike."[47]
Initially this was framed as recruitment only for "existing rural practice
vacancies"; as of 18 June, however, it was expanded explicitly to recruit as
many strike replacements as possible. Reports put the number at approximately 200.[48] But, for this reason, recruits had actually landed before the
strike even began.[49] Temporary (one to three month) posts in locations
bereft of physician services were advertised to General Medical Council
qualified doctors with one of more year of experience.[50] Remuneration
was purportedly three times that offered for comparable work in Britain.[51]
One newspaper reported that a doctor with more than seven years of experience might earn C$1,400 a month and would be provided with "an
automobile, a cash allowance for gasoline, an office, and a daily living

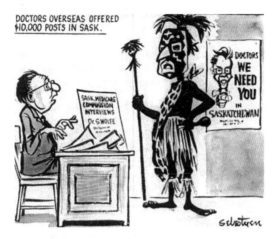

Figure 3.2 "Doctors Overseas Offered $10,000 Posts in Saskatchewan"
As the doctors strike captured headlines across the country, anger and frustration
were directed against the Saskatchewan government's initiave to license dozens of
strike-breaking doctors from outside of the country. This racist cartoon, depicting
the recruitment of foreign doctors as akin to hiring "African witch doctors," was one
of many tropes used to denigrate nonwhite foreign doctors in the 1960s. The practice
of cartooning had parallels in Britain as well, where the depiction of nonwhite foreign-
trained doctors reflected a public backlash over the growing presence of South Asian
doctors in the NHS hospital system.

allowance until he starts work."[52] American-based doctors were also on
standby. As Sam Wolfe recalled, "by July 10 [ten days into the strike] plans
had also been completed to mobilize doctors who could have replaced the
entire emergency service within forty-eight hours. Specialist teams were
on stand-by arrangements in Pittsburgh, Chicago, New York, Los Angeles,
and Detroit."[53]

The arrival of British-based doctors had fostered tensions between the
profession and the government as well as between the Canadian and British
medical communities. The British Medical Association, dismayed by the
efforts of the Saskatchewan government to bring in strikebreaking doctors, cautioned medical practitioners to contact the CMA's Saskatchewan
office before going to the province.[54] The CMA, for its part, attempted to
discourage the recruitment efforts by placing circulars in British medical
journals.[55] The British Medical Practitioners Union denounced any strikes
by doctors and gave the green light for British practitioners to serve in

Saskatchewan,[56] so long as they "[did] not involve themselves in any way in the dispute and restrict[ed] their activities to medical relief work."[57] With a divided medical profession at home, the British Medical Association attempted to remain neutral and voted down a motion to debate and take a formal position on "the role of the British doctors in the Canadian dispute."[58] As if there was not enough British involvement, Lord Stephen Taylor (a medical practitioner by training and former Labour MP involved in the creation of the NHS) arrived at the behest of the Saskatchewan premier on 17 July to mediate.[59] The British peer apparently came on the agreement that he would receive no pay, simply a reimbursement for expenses and a weeklong fishing trip at the conclusion of negotiations.[60] After eight days of "intensive negotiations," the two sides compromised in the Saskatoon Agreement.[61]

The doctors' strike has become a deeply symbolic event in Canadian history. Many argue there was never a total strike, even during the short duration of three weeks. In July, it was customary for as many as one third of the doctors to go on annual holidays anyway,[62] so it wasn't at all clear who was actually striking and who was choosing to take holidays as a sign of neither supporting a formal strike nor endorsing the government's plans. Emergency services continued, and the SCPS determined which hospitals would remain open.[63] It would appear that, throughout the strike, approximately 200 doctors continued to work in thirty different hospitals.[64] From 10 July to 23 July – the last formal day of the strike – the number of open hospitals had actually increased, from fifty-nine to 121 (of 148 total). Similarly, the number of practicing physicians increased from 243 to 316 during the same period (although emergency services physicians dropped from 204 to 190, "due to exhaustion"). Of these, between eighty and one hundred were "MCIC-recruited" doctors.[65] Community clinics emerged through the intervention of citizens, staffed by those doctors willing to practise and supported by government "seed money."[66] By the end of the strike, there were five such clinics, with ten on the verge of opening.[67] Throughout, the government maintained 110 physicians "employed in full time health services" as well as the Air Ambulance Service. The government purportedly "never seriously considered" back-to-work legislation.[68]

During the strike, the media coverage grew heated, engendering much mudslinging and ill will towards foreign doctors. The Keep Our Doctors

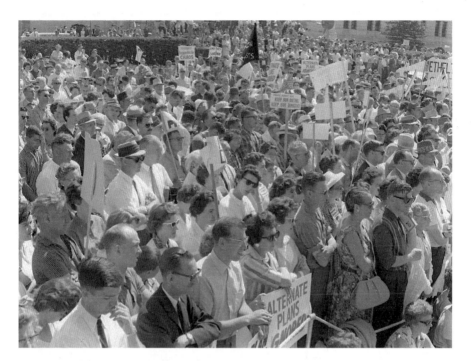

Figure 3.3 Anti-Medicare protest
There was strong opposition, amongst Saskwatchewan doctors and the lay public, to the
new Saskatchewan Medical Care Insurance Act of that province, which would extend
universal health insurance to all citizens of the province. As the Saskathewan government flew in strike-breaking doctors from Britain, several incidents of professional
harassment resulted in an official inquiry. Eventually a compromise was reached
maintaining the fee-for-service billing system and the professional independence
of doctors as private professional contractors.

campaign opposed the foreign-trained recruits and rallies fostered antipa-
thy towards foreign physicians who seemed to be assisting the "other side."
These could turn ugly. At one rally, a protester dressed in "large semitic
nose, Chinese pig-tail, and middle-east style of clothing" while carrying
a sign reading "Sask Gov't Medicare Import." [69] In a similar manner, the
Regina's *Leader Post* and Saskatoon's *Star Phoenix* featured a cartoon
showing "a painted African tribal witch doctor applying for a job" (see
image 3.2) and were, in turn, "castigated [by the premier] for impugning
the motives and competencies of doctors from the United Kingdom." [70]
Badgley and Wolfe, sympathetic to the province's side, reported that
"Many doctors expressed their antagonism openly when they learned that
the government was preparing to import doctors to break their boycott.

One doctor in Rosetown snapped: 'the only reason these jokers are here is that they can't make a living on the other side.'"[71]

One doctor quoted in the *Toronto Telegram* claimed that "They'll have to fill up the profession with the garbage of Europe … Some of the European doctors who come out here are so bad we wonder if they ever practised medicine."[72] One early recruit, Dr Ida Fisher, a "forty-five-year-old Irish-born physician from a group practice in London and the mother of five children," came for ethical reasons and was placed in charge of a hospital in Biggar. Her competencies were harshly criticized, and she was removed from her post and left for Saskatoon, returning to London at the end of July. Two other British doctors then joined a "new co-operative medical clinic" in Biggar, posing competition to physicians after the strike.[73] After several doctors were harassed by local groups and Drs Ida Fisher and Joseph Montgomery were dismissed under disputed circumstances, the provincial government pledged that British recruits would be protected and created a state commission to follow up on allegations of harassment and interference in practice.[74] Given the tension, it is noteworthy that as part of the Saskatoon Agreement the provincial government agreed to stop recruiting foreign-trained doctors, "except for those needed in under-doctored areas."[75] Those serving temporary contracts could choose to go home or remain for the duration of their contract. Reportedly, "several doctors [had] indicated that they wish[ed] to settle in Saskatchewan."[76] Meanwhile, the threat of Saskatchewan doctors leaving the province en masse proved to be exaggerated and somewhat short lived. In total, sixty-eight doctors left the province in the first half of 1962; however, by June 1964 the physician complement in the province had rebounded to 955, providing Saskatchewan with the highest physician-to-resident ratio it had ever enjoyed.[77]

MEDICAL MANPOWER

The commissioners enlisted by the Royal Commission on Health Services were touring the country in the winter of 1961–62, taking testimony from community leaders, doctors, and other stakeholders in the months leading up to the Saskatchewan strike. Any expectations, however, that they would be hesitant in their recommendations in light of the mounting frustration of provincial medical elites were soon dashed. They tabled their report in 1964 and recommended, in effect, extending the Saskatchewan model to the entire country. The Royal Commission report, however, recognized that, if access to physicians was tight in the pre-Medicare area, it would become much more problematic with the establishment of universal health insurance, as more and more pent-up demand was unleashed. The authors drew upon the experience of HIDS. When hospital care became essentially "free" to the general population, the number of people seeking hospital care rose rapidly.[78] Clearly the commissioners felt that, upon introduction of a broader "Health Services Programme," a similar accelerator effect would be likely for physician services in the community. They predicted as much as a doubling of the number of persons seeking health services if universal health insurance were to be introduced free at the point of delivery. As a result, commissioners feared for the "the capacity of medical schools in Canada to graduate a sufficient supply of well-qualified physicians."[79] Any new system of universal health insurance would require dramatically ramping up the physician workforce in the country, in case any new system collapse under the weight of the pent-up demand.

The commissioners were well aware of the reliance on foreign-trained doctors. Indeed, not only did they feel that Canada was too dependent upon immigrant physicians but they expressed concern that the steady stream of foreign doctors might dry up in the future.[80] They expected that immigration from Europe would decline by the early 1970s and that emigration to the United States would increase, leaving Canada in the very serious situation of being acutely understaffed. To meet future needs, the Royal Commission suggested that several new medical schools be built over the next decade. Specifically, it advised that funds be provided to cover one-half the cost of constructing a new medical school practically every year, starting with University of Sherbrooke (Sherbrooke, Quebec) in 1966, McMaster University (Hamilton, Ontario) in 1968, an unnamed university in the Toronto area in 1969 (widely believed to be at the new York University), the University of Calgary in 1971, the University of Victoria in 1973, Moncton University in the mid-1970s, and potentially at Memorial University if such a project could be demonstrated to be feasible. Political wrangling and the intervention of the University of Toronto scuttled the second medical school in the Toronto area.[81] In addition,

Moncton lost out to St John's as the second medical school in the Atlantic provinces, a decision that no doubt went down poorly with New Brunswick's Acadian population. McMaster and Calgary went ahead as planned (with unusual, avant-garde three-year undergraduate medical programs), but the University of Victoria medical school failed to materialize. In addition to the infrastructure support, federal funding was also recommended for the expansion and renovation of existing medical schools to support a greater number of students and the provision of financial incentives – both bursaries and higher salaries for interns and residents – were suggested. As part of the seven-year crash program, for example, training grants of $5,000 per year were recommended for students undertaking postgraduate studies in high-demand specialties.[82] In addition to the four new medical schools across the country, individual universities left out of the spoils jockeyed for new programs in nursing and dentistry, particularly as nursing began to move away from hospital-based to college- and university-based instruction.

It should be underlined that while nursing historians have identified an acute nursing shortage during this time[83] the Hall Commission devoted comparably less time to the national "nurse shortage." Attention focused on the shortage of qualified instructors at nursing training facilities and the need for a vast overhaul of the nursing education system in general. It was recommended that two categories of nursing education be created: (1) a four- to five-year university-based program and (2) a two-year college diploma program to train clinical or bedside nurses. Furthermore, it was suggested that nursing assistants be used to promote the more efficient use of fully trained nurses. The specific recommendations of the commission included not only these changes to nursing education but also the provision of financial incentives and bursaries to nursing students and the establishment of at least ten more university schools of nursing as the old hospital-based nursing schools would be phased out. While future physician supply and demand was predicted up until 1991, nursing projections were made only until 1971 and indicated that if the recommendations regarding nursing education were put into place there would be an excess of nurses by that time. No mention was made of how to improve distribution of nurses across the country, although it was recognized that some communities seemed to be experiencing a nursing shortage.[84]

Table 3.5

New medical and dental schools opened in the wake of the 1964 Royal
Commission on Health Services

Medical schools	Year of admission of first students	Dental schools	Year of admission of first students
Sherbrooke	1966	UBC	1964
McMaster	1969	Western Ontario	1966
Memorial	1969	Saskatchewan	1968
Calgary	1970	Laval	1971

Sources: P. Ralph Crawford, *The Canadian Dental Association: A Century Of Service,
1902–2002* (Ottawa: Canadian Dental Association, 2002); D.W. Gullet, *A History of
Dentistry in Canada* (published for the Canadian Dental Association by UTP 1971),
appendix J, Canadian Dental Schools; N. Tait McPhedran, *Canadian Medical Schools:
Two Centuries Of Medical History, 1822 to 1992* (Montreal: Harvest House, 1993);
Geoffrey Tesson, Geoffrey Hudson, Roger Strasser, and Dan Hunt, eds., *The Making
of the Northern Ontario School of Medicine* (Montreal and Kingston: McGill-Queen's
University Press, 2009). Laval: Section de chirurgie dentaire; Full Faculty in 1993.

A principal recommendation of the Royal Commission on Health Services, then, was to dramatically ramp up the domestic production of medical and allied health practitioners, acknowledging that "a significant
characteristic of the composition of Canadian medical manpower is the
large proportion of immigrant physicians in the postwar years."[85] Such
discourse framed Canada's reliance on foreign-trained doctors as inherently
risky and counterproductive. Indeed, as mentioned above, the Royal Commission report, assuming that immigrants would always come predominantly from Britain, Ireland, and the United States, predicted gloomily
that immigration from these counties would begin to decline over the decade to come.[86] Instead, their solutions to the anticipated physician shortage
lay in the aforementioned construction of new medical schools, expansion
of existing ones, and financial incentives to attract potential medical students.[25] While the report discussed the rural/urban divide in great detail,
few recommendations addressed the maldistribution of doctors. The suggestion that "with respect to the urban/rural situation, the establishment

of group practices and a strong system of communication may ameliorate the situation" seems, in retrospect, half-hearted.[87]

The final report of the Royal Commission on Health Services was submitted in July 1964. As historians have well documented, the Canadian Medical Association felt sideswiped by the very Royal Commission that it had requested in the first place. The report recommended federally co-funded, provincially administered universal health insurance throughout the country. Provinces that passed enabling legislation pursuant to four principles of Medicare would receive 50 per cent of insured services in a health transfer at the end of the year. Emphasising the "Canadian" nature of the program, the government insisted on "portability" between provinces and that all residents be covered. Despite the resistance of some provinces to the intrusion of the federal government into provincial constitutional domains, the deal was too good – even for Quebec – to turn down. As a final reframing of health care as a part of a larger project of nation building, Pearson vowed to launch the program on the centenary of the country (1 July 1967), though this was delayed for one year for administrative reasons. Despite the anger of medical associations across the country, organized medicine's wings had been clipped by the lack of support for the doctors' strike in Saskatchewan in 1962 and by the popularity of public health insurance across the country. Between 1967 and 1972, all provinces fell into line and passed enabling legislation. This process was only temporarily disrupted by a weak and long-forgotten specialists' strike in Quebec in 1970, the timing of which could have been better: It occurred only days before the October Crisis of that year which completely diverted all political attention to the terrorist kidnappings in Montreal.

CONCLUSIONS

Medicare constituted a watershed moment in Canadian history, an audacious policy gamble that would affect all Canadians in intimate ways, as well as providing an important component of our identity as a nation over the next two generations. As Antonia Maioni has argued, although Canadian and American policy makers had been discussing similar opportunities for state-run or state-subsidized health care, Canada ultimately adopted a "socialist" system while the Americans opted for more targeted assistance to the elderly and indigent. The majority of middle-class Americans would be offered the choice between private or occupational plans, which might be administered by for-profit or not-for-profit organizations. Maioni attributes this "parting of the ways" of the two countries to multiple factors, the most important of which were the flexibility of the Canadian parliamentary system as well as the lack of a third national party in the United States. It seems undeniable that the organization of a national social-democratic party in Canada, from 1960, proved important in pushing the Pearson Liberals into introducing universal health insurance as part of a broader mandate of the postwar welfare state.[88]

It is also worth reflecting, however, how Canada also parted ways with the health insurance systems in Europe and, most notably, Britain. For while the National Health Service permitted a parallel private system, the Canadian legislation marginalized private delivery of medically necessary services in this country. The Medical Care Act of 1966 did not make private medical care illegal. However, by preventing doctors from working in both the private system *and* the public system, it rendered the conditions of opting out so financially unattractive that only a marginal number of doctors ever chose to work outside of the new provincial plans. To be sure, extra billing would be tolerated for the short term (except in Quebec where contemporary provincial legislation prohibited the practice) but even that concession to doctors' independence would wither away over the next two decades. Thus, from the end of the 1960s Canada would gradually embrace a health care system based upon independent medical practitioners billing to a single payer – the provincial government. What's more, unlike the British system, with differential salaries based upon rank, the Canadian fee-for-service system was in some ways strikingly egalitarian. Qualified specialists all billed the same amount (within provinces), regardless of seniority.[89] This would prove deeply attractive to many young foreign-trained doctors coming from countries where differential salaries and remuneration were the professional norm.

The Royal Commission on Health Services was under no illusion about the challenges posed by implementing Medicare, a huge undertaking requiring an enormous financial investment by the federal government. But it was an investment that, in the heady days of the 1960s, seemed affordable. Under the Medical Care Act, the federal government agreed to provide annual health transfers to provinces that had passed enabling legislation that abided by the guiding principles. Concurrently, the Health Research Infrastructure Grant program (started in 1965) pumped out a staggering $500 million dollars to assist provinces in the construction of new medical, dental, and nursing schools. In partial accordance with the Royal Commission's recommendations, new medical schools were established at Memorial University, McMaster University, the University of Sherbrooke, and the University of Calgary. However, the time taken to identify teaching faculty, to construct programs, to build new infrastructure, to recruit students, and to teach the students both at the undergraduate and postgraduate level resulted in a ten-year delay before the complete flow of doctors would reach communities. As a consequence, between 1966 and 1976 there would be a decade-long gap, at the very moment of the inception of Medicare, one that, as following chapters will demonstrate, would be filled by foreign-trained medical practitioners.

The key to the success of Medicare was thus inextricably linked to immigration. When the federal Liberals returned to power in 1963, far from reversing the Progressive Conservative focus on "highly skilled" manpower, they quietly embraced and extended the system, formulating a new White Paper on Immigration in 1966, which would usher in a new act the following year. Although entitled the Immigration (Appeals Board) Act of 1967, more profound than an appeals mechanism for the history of immigration to Canada was the introduction of a new, purportedly objective and transparent system of ranking candidates, known to this day as the "points" system. Within a few short years, immigration from "traditional" countries – Britain, the United States, France, Italy – would be overtaken by immigration from India, Pakistan, China, and the Philippines. Leading this remarkable surge of immigrants would be highly skilled, English-speaking "medical manpower" – doctors and medical scientists from the nonwhite British Commonwealth who would have a transformative effect on the rolling out of Medicare in this country. For a remarkable six years following the passing of the Medicare Care Act, Canada would admit more than 7,000 foreign-trained doctors, even more doctors than it graduated domestically. It would be an era without precedent in Canadian history. In the words of one medical school dean of the time, foreign doctors rescued Medicare from dying at birth.

Chapter Four

The Points System

On 12 June 1972, the new minister of manpower and immigration, Bryce Mackasey, officially welcomed the ten millionth immigrant to Canada. Richard Swinson, a British psychiatrist trained in Liverpool, had recently accepted an offer to work at St Michael's Hospital, one of the University of Toronto teaching affiliates in the downtown core of the city. Although early reports implied that he had been selected randomly, the process, in fact, was one very much loaded in certain demographic ways. The bureaucrats in the Department of Manpower and Immigration created a short list of newly accepted immigrants based on age, occupation, and intended place of residence. The perfect candidate, they agreed, should be a married man with children, under the age of thirty-five, looking to settle in the Toronto area. Ultimately, Swinson was chosen amongst seven finalists. As one (unnamed) official readily disclosed, the choice of a foreign-trained doctor was an easy one: "We didn't want to [select] a guy who will be unemployed in two months or take a job from a Canadian."[1] Although the government was evidently pleased with their selection of a British doctor, one bureaucrat mused that "it might have been more appropriate if number 10 million had been a heart surgeon from Houston"[2] due to the large number of Americans who had emigrated to Canada in the previous year.

Choosing a foreign doctor for this ceremony was deeply symbolic. Swinson emigrated from Britain to Canada at the apex of a remarkable influx of foreign-trained professionals. Doctors, engineers, university professors, and nurses entered the country by the thousands to support national infrastructure projects, staff the expanding university system,[3] and underpin the new era of universal health insurance. Indeed, the absolute number of new Canadians who self-identified as "physicians or surgeons" exceeded the number of graduating doctors from Canadian medical schools for five straight years leading up to the year in which Swinson arrived. However, by 1972 the mood of the general public towards immigration had begun to sour. Critics felt that immigration had spiralled out of control. Reports on the record number of "illegal immigrants" filled the pages of newspapers and magazines the very year in which the ten millionth arrival was being feted.[4]

THE FAIRCLOUGH DIRECTIVE

The origins of the dramatic influx of "highly skilled manpower" date back more than a decade earlier. John Diefenbaker had made several hyperbolic pronouncements during the 1958 election, stating, for example, that Canada had to "populate or perish."[5] However, according to some scholars, the new prime minister in fact had no real interest in engaging in controversial new proposals governing those entering the country.[6] Immigration was always a hot-button issue, and some members of the Canadian press observed ruefully that southern European immigration to Canada had exceeded British by the end of the 1950s; more racially explicit complaints included repeated allegations of fake identities for Chinese immigrants coming from Hong Kong.[7] As the economy sank under a mild recession, Diefenbaker handed the portfolio to Ellen Fairclough, whom he was confident could steer discussion away from growing resentment around sponsored relatives as well as the embarrassing backlog of more than 100,000 applicants for landed immigrant status.[8]

Ellen Fairclough, however, proved to be far more than a caretaker minister or someone who was gently suppressing immigration with a reassuring smile. Largely ignoring the ambivalence about the acceptance of refugees from Europe, she took the bold step of admitting "tubercular refugees" during World Refugee Year of 1959–60, bold because Canada had not yet signed the United Nations Convention on Refugees and had a long-standing policy of rejecting immigrants based on pre-existing medical conditions.[9] What is more, Fairclough enacted a change to immigration regulations that forbade discrimination against landed immigrant candidates on the basis of "race, colour, or nation of origin." Now known as the Fairclough Directive, this 1962 Order in Council[10] followed naturally from Diefenbaker's much-cherished Bill of Rights, which had been passed by

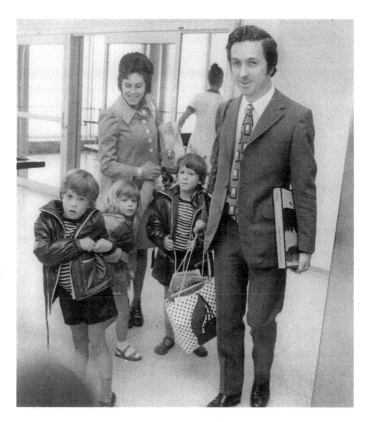

Figure 4.1 Canada's ten millionth immigrant
In 1972, the Department of Immigration and Manpower selected the ten millionth immigrant to the country, in part as a public relations initiative to ease growing disquiet about nonwhite immigration in the years following the introduction of the 1967 points system. Here, Dr Richard Swinson, a British-trained psychiatrist from Liverpool, arrives at Pearson Airport with his wife Carolyn and three children to be welcomed by the minister of immigration and other dignatories as the nation's ten millionth immigrant.

Parliament in 1960. With this statement of principles, Canada, at least on paper, became the first major industrialized, immigrant-receiving country to eliminate "race" as a basis for immigration assessment. Of course, individual immigration officers continued to be influenced by their own judgment as to the "suitability" and "adaptability" of particular candidates.[11] And race continued to figure prominently in the asymmetrical application of immigration regulations, whereby only sponsored relatives living in preferred European, Middle Eastern, and Latin American countries were permitted.[12] However, in terms of professionals applying as "independent class" candidates, Fairclough's new guidelines would foreshadow further changes during the next decade that would profoundly affect health care provision across the country.

During her brief tenure as the first woman federal cabinet minister in Canadian history, Fairclough became accustomed to two complaints about immigration: (1) that the arrival of "sponsored" or "nominated" relatives – the family members of Canadian citizens or permanent residents – represented a drain on social services and (2) that foreign workers were arriving in a haphazard manner, taking jobs from ordinary Canadians. In response, the minister of immigration, who was an MP for Hamilton (incorporating large Italian and working-class constituencies), attempted to reframe federal immigration to Canada as the scientific pursuit of *highly skilled* immigrants filling positions desperately needed by the country and that no native-born Canadian could fill. Her gambit was largely successful. The resulting Parliamentary debates of the early 1960s reflected a flip-flopping of immigration positions in the country. The Liberal Party, formerly the party more sympathetic to immigration, increasingly criticized the Progressive Conservative government for the arrival of professionals from "Third World" countries. Taking a suspiciously convenient stand of the moral high ground, the Liberal immigration critic decried Canada for welcoming "talent" from poor countries. The *Globe and Mail* weighed in, quoting a trade union leader who complained that Canada was engaged in "poaching" skilled labour from Asia, Africa, and the Middle East. The editors opined that Canada should only accept foreign trainees if the intention was to provide them with enhanced skills which they could then take back with them to their home countries.[13]

Nevertheless, when the federal Liberal Party returned to power in 1963 under Lester Pearson, the two parties switched sides. Buffeted by the renewal of economic expansion that began just before they took office, the federal Liberals embraced a novel "meritocratic" approach to the selection of new immigrants, while the Progressive Conservatives, now in opposition, argued that federal regulations were increasingly marginalizing basic humanitarian considerations for the sake of filling occupational gaps in the economy. For example, the Progressive Conservative MP Michael Starr attempted to shame the Liberals for contemplating policies where "immigrants were allowed in [solely] according to the demand for labour."[14] The

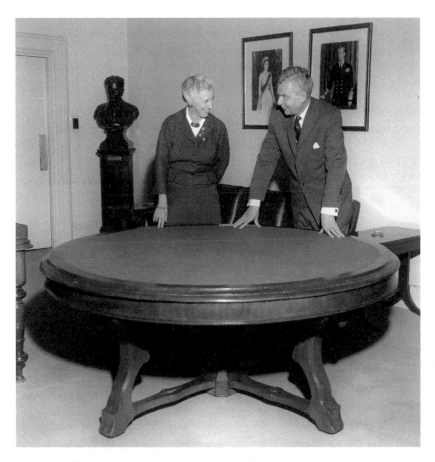

Figure 4.2 Ellen Fairclough with Prime Minister John Diefenbaker
In her role as the federal minister of immigration, Ellen Fairclough was responsible for introducing a 1962 directive forbidding Canadian immigrant agents from using race or religion as a factor in the selection of candidates. It was the first step towards opening the country up to immigrants from a wider range of nations. Amongst the first immigrants to arrive from diverse nations as the Philippines, Egypt, Jamaica, and Pakistain were health care workers.

Liberal minister of manpower and immigration, Jean Marchand, reassured parliament that while "immigration must surely ... be related in some way to the requirements of the labour market," to "restrict immigration *exclusively* to the labour market in Canada would make for an inhumane and unacceptable policy."[15] Building on Fairclough's earlier initiatives, Marchand and the federal Liberals sought to make immigration selection less subjective and more "scientific," creating a new framework in the Immigration White Paper of 1966. Gone were the days where the judgment of the suitability of candidates lay largely at the discretion of individual immigration officers. In its place, bureaucrats hatched a new, seemingly objective, plan that would score potential immigrants in a more systematic manner. Immigration agents would henceforth score "independent" (that is, nonsponsored) class candidates on a standardized *pro forma* sheet of qualifications.[16] Prospective immigrants could earn the following points (formally called "units"), with the maximum number listed in parentheses: for education and training (twenty units), for occupational demand (fifteen units), for occupational skill (ten units), for age (ten units), for arranged employment (ten units), for language skills (ten units), relatives in the country willing to assist (five units), and employment opportunities in the area or region of settlement (five units). The final fifteen units depended upon an individual assessment of the candidate's "adaptability, motivation, initiative and resourcefulness" during an interview. The new points system assigned aspiring immigrants to Canada a mark, accepting those who "passed" with a score of fifty or higher.[17]

The points system, which became operational in 1967, had not been intended as a mechanism to prioritize the acceptance of immigrants from nontraditional countries or as an early impetus towards official multiculturalism. It was very much put in place as a response to "manpower" challenges in the country. There was no coincidence that the Liberals had renamed the Department of Citizenship and Immigration, the Department of *Manpower* and Immigration. As deputy minister of the new renamed ministry Tom Kent later acknowledged that the points system was a social scientific attempt to "identify and define the various factors affecting a person's ability to settle successfully in Canada, and attach relative weights to them [so that] immigration officers would have a consistent basis on which to assess potential immigrants."[18]

One immigration officer, who had been seconded to the task force in 1967 to finalize and implement the new point system, recalls that some members were sensitive that, if implemented too comprehensively, "we would empty countries such as Hong Kong, Jamaica, etc."[19] The challenge, this immigration officer acknowledged, was to devise a system that was "universal" in application but allowed a mechanism for selection, of "getting newcomers who could rapidly enhance our labour force but at the same time control numbers."[20] After discussions with visa officers in Canadian consulates around the world, they agreed to retain the discretion of refusing certain applicants who passed with fifty units or more if their occupational demand was nonetheless considered marginal.[21]

The new points system thus provided a framework for assessing immigrants that was more transparent but also flexible. For example, the determination of occupational demand could be adjusted on an annual basis in response to changing labour demands. One immigrant officer recalls that the adjustment of points thus worked as a "thermostat," controlling overall numbers from year to year. With respect to the medical practitioners, with the launch date of Medicare moved from 1 July 1967 to 1 July 1968, there was little debate that doctors be assigned the maximum fifteen points for occupational demand.[22] Indeed, the maximum amount was directly tied to the Hall Commission's concern about the dearth of doctors and nurses. This maximum point assignment would continue until 1972, then diminish until 1976, at which point the occupational demand of doctors fell to zero. However, in the context of the late 1960s, it is little surprise that English- or French-speaking medical practitioners, with their high level of education, their training, and their occupational demand in the wake of the Hall Report, were virtually guaranteed to rank high enough for admission.

The demographic impact of these cumulative immigration changes was dramatic. Total immigration under Diefenbaker's government had dropped to a postwar low of only 72,000 and continued to be relatively restrained during the economic malaise of 1957–60.[23] A decade later the absolute number of immigrants entering the country had trebled, reaching 218,000 in 1974.[24] Noticeable amongst the tens of thousands of arrivals were families from such countries that had either been barred or subject to formal and informal quotas: from Pakistan to the Philippines, from Hong Kong to Haiti. During this time, a contemporary report observed that the percentage of "visible minorities" – a rather vague and problematic term generally referring to nonwhite, non-European immigrants – more than doubled to more than 30 per cent.[25] Figure 4.3 summarizes the annual arrival of immigrants from four regions of the world that had previously been largely excluded from providing immigrants in significant numbers in the preceding decades. The dramatic uptick from 1962

onwards is readily noticeable. The importance of these new source countries was not only a function of the new points system, however; by 1967,
Canada had opened new immigration offices in Egypt, Japan, Lebanon,
the Philippines, the West Indies, and Pakistan, tripling the number of
immigration offices outside of Europe from before the 1962 Fairclough
Directive.[26] The practical aspects of actually attending an immigration
office, securing an interview, and completing the necessary paperwork
should not be underestimated in the processing of potential foreign-
trained doctors accessing the Canadian immigration system.

The 1967 Immigration Act, sometimes referred to as the Appeals Board
Act, incorporated the points system. This legislation has been rightly
identified by historians as an important turning point towards a multi-
ethnic society that would be formalized in official multiculturalism in
1971. For the purposes of this book, however, the immigration changes
that occurred in the 1960s paved the way for an extraordinary surge of
foreign-trained health care practitioners, many of whom hailed from outside the British Isles. Indeed, the changes to immigration regulations intersected inevitably with the introduction of universal health insurance.
The Fairclough Directive, for example, occurred at the same time as the
conclusion of the Royal Commission of Health Services hearings (1962);
the White Paper on Immigration was also being drafted in the same year
(1966) as the passage of the Medical Care Act. The latter wound its way
through Parliament in the autumn of 1966, receiving royal assent just days
before Christmas. Figure 4.4 reflects citizenship and immigration data on
the number of landed immigrants stating "physician or surgeon" as their
intended occupation. The annual number of doctors as landed immigrants more than tripled, from 400 in 1960 to more than 1,300 in 1969.
Hundreds of doctors, like Swinson, continued to arrive from Britain and
Ireland, as per the previous decades, but in addition, hundreds also came
from the aforementioned source countries where they had previously
been denied entry to the country and where new immigration offices had
been opened.

The particularities of the arrival, settlement, and practice of select "national" groups will be discussed in greater detail in chapters 5 and 6. But
it is worth pointing out here the aggregate impact of this remarkable
period on health care. As the Royal Commission on Health Care Services
(1961–64) had predicted, the greatest challenge for Medicare would be

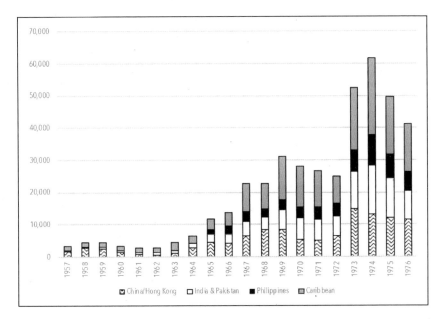

Figure 4.3 Annual immigration to Canada: select nontraditional source regions, 1957–76
Source: Statistics Canada: Immigration Statistics, 1957–76.

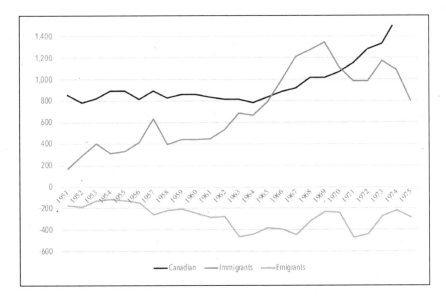

Figure 4.4 The production, inflow, and outflow of medical practitioners to and from Canada, 1957–76
Source: Statistics Canada: Immigration Statistics, 1957–76.

staffing the new system of universal health insurance. Four new medical schools had been established at the dawn of Medicare, but training the undergraduate medical students, including specialist training, would take close to a decade to turn out a new flow of Canadian-trained physicians. In the interim, hospitals and local health authorities took advantage of the supply of doctors and nurses on the move. The practical result was an unprecedented wave of immigrant medics. From the outports of Newfoundland to rural Manitoba, foreign-trained doctors arrived to settle, often temporarily, in communities that were desperately short of health care practitioners, thus maximizing the points for doctors going to areas in which their occupation was most in demand. Foreign doctors also secured key positions in university-affiliated hospitals, as these institutions expanded their research remit and evolved into transdisciplinary health sciences centres. Physician immigration during this period was augmented by an equally dramatic influx of foreign-trained nurses. From a steady state in the 1950s of a loss of 1,500 nurses to the United States, balanced by a gain of 1,500 nurses from elsewhere, Canada began to accept more nurses than it was losing. Indeed, by the middle of the 1960s, Canada was granting landed immigrant status to more than 3,000 foreign-trained immigrants who indicated their intended occupation was "nursing," peaking at 4,200 in the centennial year of 1967. For the decade leading up to 1970, Canada ranked third (behind Britain and the United States) in terms of the absolute number of nurse immigrants and was the largest in terms of *per capita* reception of immigration of nurses amongst major industrialized countries.[27]

FOUR PRINCIPLES OF MEDICARE

The Medical Care Act of 1966 was a preeminent piece of legislation in the history of public policy in the country, creating the legislative, regulatory, and financial framework for universal public health insurance, or what is now known in Canada as "Medicare." At its heart was a funding mechanism that committed the federal government in Ottawa to contribute annual payments to the provinces to reimburse them approximately half of the costs for insurable medical services. Due to the fact that health care was a provincial jurisdiction, the most important aspect of the federal health insurance legislation was the fact that it was a *voluntary* program. Of course, whether receiving taxes from Canadians across the country and then remitting to their provincial government annual health grants only under certain conditions was truly voluntary was a matter of political opinion. Nevertheless, the federal plan was framed in such a way as to defuse some (though not all) of the inevitable constitutional complaints. For federal cofunding to take place, the Medical Care Act required subsequent provincial legislation that would be consistent with the four principles of Medicare: universality (that all, or nearly all, of the permanent residents of a province be covered), portability (whereby those with health insurance in one province would be covered while visiting another), comprehensiveness (that insurable services cover all medically necessary interventions), and public administration (that the system be run by the provincial government itself). Unlike its predecessor legislation of cofunded hospitalization insurance in 1957, there were no provisions requiring a minimum number of provinces sign on to the agreement; as a consequence, each individual province debated and passed their own legislation, sometimes enthusiastically, often begrudgingly, between 1967 and 1972.[28]

The federal government thus constructed a program that goaded the provinces into providing a similar level of medical services across the country, despite the differences of wealth, geography, and medical traditions. This was accomplished by *universality* (where the uniformity of service provisions was to be provided to all citizens and permanent residents[29] regardless of age or geographical location). Minimum thresholds of coverage (90 per cent, later 95 per cent, of individuals insured) were also put in place to ensure broad compliance. It was also indirectly guaranteed by the requirements of *portability*, which took two forms: (1) provisions for emergency care for individuals who were covered in one province to be treated in another (which would then be subsequently reimbursed by the province of residence), and (2) whereby individuals who moved to another province (say for new employment) would be covered by their previous province during the waiting time to qualify as a new "resident" in the new province. The coercive nature was embedded in the voluntarism itself. As provinces began to sign onto Medicare, the ones who delayed were faced with the prospect of subsidizing health care transfers to other (participating) provinces. Nevertheless, in a matter of a few years, virtually the entire country was insured for *comprehensive* medical care, defined as including all clinical interventions that were considered to be medically necessary. The federal government wisely avoided defining these necessary interventions and, rather, trusted the provincial governments to make decision of what was "in" and "out" based on their own respective provincial health care plans. Doctors maintained a significant degree of professional autonomy under the new system by continuing as independent professionals billing the provincial government (the so-called single payer) and by determining their own scope of practice as defined by their own professional regulatory bodies.

Because the new principles were open to some degree of interpretation, and some provinces already had subsidized health insurance in place, the transition to Medicare took several years. By the 1960s, many provincial governments had devised alternate systems of extending health insurance to citizens while preserving the then delivery of other services by for-profit and not-for-profit health insurance companies. Dubbed Manningcare or Bennetcare (after the respective premiers of Alberta and British Columbia), these alternate systems subsidized the purchase of private health insurance by those too poor to afford health insurance themselves. In the Alberta model, these health care deliverers could be for-profit; in the British Columbian system, the insurers had to operate on a not-for-profit basis. The Medical Care Act of 1966 rejected the Alberta option as falling outside the four principles of Medicare but permitted the British Columbian one to continue in the short term under strict government oversight.[30]

Over time, the ten provincial health care systems would merge into a networked "Canadian" Medicare system and would evolve into the most comprehensive – some might say, the most "socialist" – of all of the health care systems in the industrialized world. While Britain, France, and many European countries permitted parallel public and private systems (allowing individuals and doctors to, in effect, work in both systems concurrently), the Canadian system that emerged from the 1966 act would marginalize, to the point of nonexistence, private medical care for core medical services. Doctors in Canada were not permitted to work in *both* the new public system and in independent private practice. Doctors could legally opt out of provincial health insurance plans entirely but they would, in effect, be forced to support medical practices in which they were charging hundreds or thousands of dollars for clinical services that the public could secure elsewhere, at no direct cost to themselves. Although there remained a tiny clientele willing to pay for expedited private care, the market was so small that only a handful of practitioners in the entire country ever opted out. In reality the demand for private care could easily be secured in the United States, thus further undermining any potential for a residual, independent private market in Canada. As a consequence, close to 100 per cent of all licensed medical practitioners in Canada were soon working in the new public system of Medicare from the early 1970s onwards.

Within this new single-payer system, fee-for-service remuneration would dominate the payment of medical practitioners. The implementation of Medicare was largely (though not uniformly) based on the model of private practice with public payment, to borrow the title of David Naylor's book.[31] Doctors retained their status as independent professional practitioners that decided (within professional scope of expertise) their clinical decisions and billing hours. Although some bureaucrats across the country would have preferred placing doctors on salaries, politicians bowed to the obvious: in a new universal health care system, governments realized that a fee-for-service system would incentivize doctors to see a maximum number of patients in their practice, thus assisting the provinces with the potential explosion of waiting lists that universal health insurance might create. The downside was the expectation of relentless negotiation, and renegotiation, of the provincial fee schedules. Salaried doctors were found only in niche sectors, such as those working in government-appointed positions (medical officers of health, for example), those working in long-stay psychiatric hospitals, and, in some places, those working on contract providing medical services to Indigenous communities.[32]

Many contentious items, however, were left unresolved, not the least of which was whether individual practitioners were free to charge top-up fees from their patients for insured services in addition to the government fee payment, a practice known as "extra-billing." The federal government did not explicitly eliminate this practice in the 1966 Medical Care Act (though the Quebec legislation pursuant to the act would abolish extra billing in that province from the outset).[33] Similarly, the grey area of additional charges by hospitals for private rooms, parking, and in-room amenities lingered in the background. Workers' compensation evaluations and other medical interventions related to occupational injuries also remained outside of the structure of Medicare. Furthermore, other health care services not provided by medical doctors – such as those rendered by dentists, optometrists, psychologists, and physiotherapists – posed further problems. The Canadian Medical Association opposed nonphysician services being reimbursed under Medicare as opposed to being funded and regulated in a separate system entirely; as a consequence, Parliament moved forward with a compromise. Dental and optometry services would be reimbursable only if they were covered under the respective provincial plan[34] and the governor-in-council would be "empowered to authorize federal contributions toward such coverage if deemed advisable."[35] In practice, however, many provinces opted to provide these nonphysician services to targeted groups (children, the aged, and those on welfare, for example) via the Canada Assistance Plan.[36]

Although one would have expected that reimbursing provinces for 50 per cent of the cost of insured health services would be administratively straightforward, that too became highly politicized. Some argued at the time that higher cost health services, provided in wealthy provinces, would be met by equally high federal transfers, while the converse would result in smaller per-capita copayments to have-not provinces. This could have been construed as simply a system of making the richer provinces, richer. Could a national program of Medicare be truly "national" if the quality and availability of care differed dramatically between provinces? As a consequence, federal bureaucrats devised a mischievous plan that interjected a degree of equalization into the annual health transfers. Put simply, the annual federal reimbursement involved a formula based on the average health care costs *for the entire country*, thereby topping up poorer provinces that tended to spend less at the expense of richer ones that could afford to pay more.[37]

Finally, the checks and balances of the new system lay in the provision that they had to be publicly administered. Unlike the giant health care organizations that had emerged in postwar United States, some of which were for-profit, others not-for-profit, Medicare stipulated that provincial plans needed to be publicly administered and run by the provincial governments. This ensured that if decisions over the provision of medical care fell out of line with the expectations of the electorate (for example, by being too restrictive), the government in power would be subsequently held accountable.[38] The stipulation of public administration led to the delay in more than one province, as nongovernmental agencies responsible for the administration of health insurance had to be rechristened as formal government departments and units. Ultimately, the insistence on a publicly administered system itself introduced a fundamental tension within the delivery of medical services under Medicare. The public perceived doctors to be acting in a *public* system – providing public services like civil servants or the provision of primary education – and yet medical practitioners remained independent, private contractors.

The years immediately following the Medical Care Act were dizzying ones. A flurry of national infrastructure projects and municipal initiatives celebrated the country's centenary anniversary. The world exposition, of course, was only the most outrageous, and lauded, of the year's events. Montreal had literally built an island in the St Lawrence for Expo 1967, as well as greatly expanded its own metro system to assist with the twenty million expected visitors (in the end, close to fifty million crossed the turnstiles). Centennials halls, centennial parks, centennial high schools, centennial bridges were being constructed across the country. Amidst this orgy of self-congratulation and nation building, soil was also being broken for four new medical schools across the country and dozens of new health science centres to inaugurate that other centennial project – Medicare – which after all had been considered so important to the country that its launch date had been symbolically scheduled for 1 July 1967 itself.

"AN IRREGULAR FOREIGN LEGION"

The Hall Commission report had predicted that Canada would need to rely on immigrant physicians until the country ramped up the domestic production of doctors to a point of national self-sufficiency. Depositions and witnesses to the cross-country hearings spoke of a doctor and nurse shortage that was only partly being met by foreign-trained health care practitioners. But expanding domestic capacity was an enormous national undertaking, riddled with the politics of where these new medical training facilities would be located and how they would be financed. Hundreds of millions of dollars were at stake. What is more, the university sector in Canada was already in overdrive: during the 1960s, thirteen new universities across the country were being created, as well as five new campuses of the Université du Québec network that arose out of the Parent Commission.[39] The money was there, but could the doctors and nurses be produced to supply the new system of Medicare?

The scramble for federal funding was officially unleashed by a much-anticipated federal Health Resources Fund (HRF) in 1965, created to assist provincial funding for new medical, nursing, and dental schools and the expansion and modernization of existing ones. The federal government committed a whopping $500 million to cover up to 50 per cent of the capital costs for a projected fifteen-year period scheduled to start in 1966.[40] Provincial governments selected eligible projects to support, on the condition that "some other agency, such as the provincial government or the university," would provide the remaining 50 per cent of the capital.[41] The fund was augmented by "special additional capital programs" for hospitals and higher education in the provinces.[42] The draft plan was first presented to premiers in July 1965 and Pearson's announcement of the fund splashed across the front page of the *Globe and Mail* in September of that same year.[43] A technical committee was formed to organize distribution of the fund and submitted its report in December.[44] Apportionment was agreed at the federal–provincial conference in late January 1966, where the federal government committed to extend the federal Hospital Construction Grant until 1970.[45] Official parliamentary approval and royal assent to the Health Resources Fund were given in the summer of 1966.[46] By late 1967, all provincial projects had been approved in principle by the Health Resources Advisory Committee, the federal committee overseeing the new fund.[47] The fund was itself relatively uncontroversial and greeted with near unanimous support. The loudest critiques were that the proposed sum was too modest; Tommy Douglas, for example, called it "pitifully inadequate."[48]

The Health Resources Fund led to the establishment of four new medical schools, six new dental schools, the expansion of existing medical and dental schools (which were sometimes combined), and the creation of a vast network of health sciences centres to underpin these programs and embody the new commitment to medical research. New nursing schools were also established, made urgent (and more complicated) by the fact that nursing education in many parts of the country was being transferred from hospital- to university-based training.[49] In terms of new medical schools, the Hall Commission had recommended cities and regions for new schools and external advisory committees evaluated their feasibility.[50] Ultimately, four new medical schools had been approved, two of which had already had significant planning in the years leading up to the approval of the fund. They included, in order of establishment: (1) Université de Sherbrooke, a much needed new francophone medical school in Quebec's Eastern Townships; (2) McMaster University, which won out over York University as the second medical school within driving distance of Toronto; (3) Calgary, the second medical school for the province of Alberta; and (4) Memorial University (in St John's Newfoundland), the second medical school located in the Atlantic Provinces. Of these McMaster and Calgary were particularly noteworthy, inasmuch as they embraced radical medical pedagogies like the "Case Western Reserve" system of medical education and offered a three-year rather than four-year undergraduate MD program.[51] McMaster University soon garnered the reputation as the most innovative of all Canadian medical schools and prided itself on not being called a medical school at all but rather a program within a Health Sciences Faculty that offered an undergraduate MD degree as well as nursing and occupational therapy training. Calgary, by contrast, was initially created with a mandate to focus primarily on the training of family practitioners.[52]

One of the controversial (though unsurprising) aspects of the new federal funding was that it was solely for bricks and mortar and not operating costs.[53] Despite complaints, ongoing federal funding for provincially run medical schools was probably never in the cards. However, another criticism that did gain greater traction involved a complaint that the federal government was fast-tracking funding for medical education at the expense of federal research funds. Medical school deans asked for the federal government to boost medical research, a key factor, to their minds, in the hundreds of Canadian-trained physicians who had drifted to larger, research-intensive universities south of the border.[54] An article in *Canadian Doctor* suggested that enhanced research support would help "bring home doctors who have fled to US facilities and funds."[55] Some medical administrators contended that the government's neglect of medical research funding would doom recruitment efforts to the new medical schools.[56]

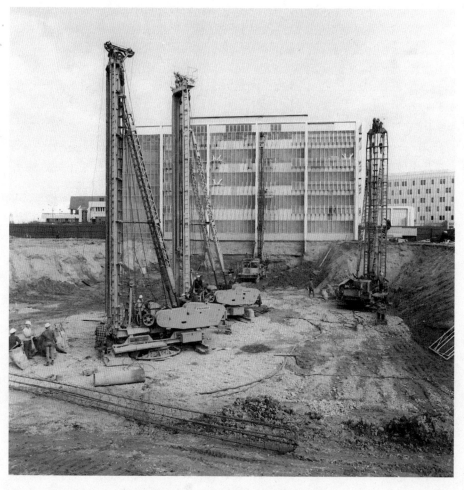

Figure 4.5 Construction of the new Health Sciences Centre in Calgary
The Royal Commission on Health Services (Hall Commission) report warned, in 1964, that universal health insurance would unleash a pent-up demand for medical services that could not be met with the existing cohort of doctors. As a consequence, it recommended a large federal fund to assist with the construction of four new medical schools. The new medical schools would take almost a decade to complete. Here, construction is underway in Calgary for Alberta's second medical school.

Their calls soon reached the corridors of power: "You can build as many buildings as you want in this country, and you can call them medical schools, but they will not work unless you have the personnel to staff them. That is the thing that is completely ignored by the Government – completely ignored!" thundered one indignant Senator reviewing the HRF bill in the upper chamber.[57]

The challenges of attracting faculty turned out to be no mere political grandstanding. It was clear that Canada did not have the critical mass of medical educators needed to staff the new and expanded medical schools. In retrospect, many of the founding deans and department chairs reflected on the irony that they needed to look abroad for foreign-trained clinician scientists to teach the next generation of Canadian doctors and become self-sufficient in the production of Canadian-born doctors. At Sherbrooke's new medical school, for example, one-third of the 160 medical faculty had obtained their qualifications outside of Canada, including thirty-four in Europe, seven in South America, four in the US, two in Egypt, and one each in South Africa, Jerusalem, India, Vietnam, and the Philippines.[58] At McMaster, John Evans, the first dean of the Faculty of Health Sciences wryly observed, "To date, in true colonial fashion, Canada has imported a large proportion of its skilled manpower from the United Kingdom, the United States and Europe, and has never been pressed to rely exclusively on its own resources for any length of time."[59] The recruitment of clinical teachers had turned out to be fierce, not least because the United States was also engaged in a massive expansion of medical education, where thirty new medical schools opened between 1968 and 1978.[60]

In contrast to those based in the United States, Commonwealth doctors, particularly those disenchanted with the National Health Service, found the conditions in Canada to be relatively agreeable. And the new medical schools scored some initial successes. The recruitment of Moran Campbell in 1968, for example, was seen as a coup for McMaster and a blow to British medicine and renewed fears of another medical exodus from that country to North America:

News that Moran Campbell was leaving the Hammersmith Hospital to come to McMaster caused shock waves in academic circles in Britain. The press got wind of the move, heightening the concern of the British that the country was losing too many able people. Eager to tell its readers why an entrenched member of the academic medical establishment should take off for an unknown, fledgling medical school in Canada, the London *Times* published an extensive interview with Dr Campbell. Many, many doctors had emigrated from Britain to escape what they saw as the restrictions of the National Health Service. Now there was danger that strengths in academic medicine might be seriously eroded by another migratory wave.[61]

Campbell reportedly accepted a department chairmanship at McMaster because he failed four times to gain a senior appointment in Britain. A half dozen research associates followed him, "thereby depleting Britain of a top medical team."[62] Campbell, attracted by the challenge of creating a new school, later reportedly described it as the "educational equivalent of invading Normandy."[63] Campbell's activities to recruit others highlighted these challenges and were detailed in his own autobiography. The first candidate he interviewed was "a brilliant young Canadian neurologist now working in the States who, in principle, wanted to return to Canada but only to a job that guaranteed his ability to pursue his research."[64] Visiting Melbourne in 1969, Campbell managed to "interest a number of very able Australian doctors in visiting or moving to Hamilton."[65] Edinburgh-trained Peter Cockshott, chair of radiology at Ibadan, Nigeria, was in 1967 "one of the earliest faculty members to be appointed." At the time, he had never heard of McMaster; he was recruited with the encouragement of his Burlington-based former medical resident. In a rare instance of persuading an American clinician scientist, psychiatrist Alex Adsett was enthusiastically recruited from the United States. Despite the mixed success, Campbell recalled that "it was difficult to recruit residents, to establish the traditions that we found in places like McGill or Toronto. Our first years were a sort of irregular foreign legion."[66]

A similar situation was witnessed across the country. At the Regina campus of the University of Saskatchewan in 1969–70, only one half of faculty had obtained their first degree in Canada; at the older Saskatoon campus, the figure had barely reached 60 per cent.[67] In London (Ontario), in response to the creation of a new health sciences centre (in part to underpin the new dental school), only one half of the 180 medical faculty at the University of Western Ontario were solely Canadian-trained, according to their 1970–71 calendar. At least thirty presented both Canadian and foreign

THERE IS OPPORTUNITY FOR YOU IN YOUNG DYNAMIC CANADA

If you have a skill, trade or profession, the time is right, the mood is right for you and Canada to get together. Industrial production in Canada has more than doubled in the last 15 years and is still forging ahead. For years to come Canada will be a country of growth.

You will enjoy life in this young land of opportunity. Wages and salaries are high. Canadians enjoy one of the highest standards of living in the world.

Your children will have the best possible start in life—free secondary and primary education and every chance of going on to University or to a modern Technical Institute. You and your family will be protected too, by a social welfare programme: family allowances, hospital insurance, unemployment insurance and retirement pension.

Canadians are friendly, down-to-earth people—and remember—emigrating to Canada is not like going to the far corners of the globe, you are only six hours away by air, six days by sea.

Go and grow with **CANADA** *the land of opportunity*

CANADA Needs Doctors

Expansion in Canada creates many opportunities for medical personnel—Physicians, Surgeons, Pathologists, also Laboratory Technicians and Radiographers.

Write today for further information about Canada to:

CANADIAN GOVERNMENT Immigration Service, Dept. 6 B.M.J.17/2, 38 Grosvenor Street, London W.1.

(16503)

Figure 4.6 "Canada Needs Doctors" By 1968, countries like Canada became more aggressive in their recruitment of highly skilled professionals, as depicted in this advertisement, paid for by the Canadian government during the inaugural year of Medicare. Note the unsubtle jab at New Zealand and Australia – competitor countries for migrant doctors – as being located in the "far corners of the globe."

(mainly British and US) credentials, of which ten were British and nine American, while a dozen were from countries as diverse as Japan, Egypt, and India.[68] If securing medical faculty at McMaster and Western proved challenging, they were comparatively better positioned than the new medical school in St John's. Memorial's founding dean of medicine, Ian

Rusted, appreciative of the longstanding challenge of attracting and more importantly retaining, medical practitioners on the island, approached the problem of faculty recruitment aggressively, forming international advisory committees "consist[ing] of three individuals from Canada, two from the United States, and two from Great Britain. This meant that within a few weeks fifty to seventy well-known leaders in medicine had details of [Memorial's] plans and were providing valuable advice and assistance."[69] As a result, "a credible faculty was attracted as planned, and on schedule[.]"[70] According to Rusted, the initial goal was to develop a faculty that was "one-third Canadian, one-third from the United States, and the remainder from Britain or elsewhere." His strategy turned out to be largely prophetic, with clusters of Canadians, of Americans, and a third heterogeneous group of faculty initially educated in Egypt, Germany, India, and Czechoslovakia. He was delighted that, by 1974, the medical school could boast that almost half of their faculty were Canadian.[71]

Not all regions were winners under the new HRF scheme. For example, there were calls in some quarters for a medical school in New Brunswick, namely by the mayor of Saint John in the face of a hospital bed shortage in the city. There were also fears that New Brunswick students "would find it increasingly difficult to enter medical schools" as other provinces changed admission requirements.[72] However, a Provincial Medical School Survey Committee ruled that there was inadequate financial support and too few potential applicants.[73] The university sponsored an international conference on the topic of new medical schools in September 1966 and, despite an appeal from the Acadian community for a medical school in Moncton, recommended support for the new medical school at Memorial.[74] York University, having missed its first attempt to secure a medical school, tried again, making ambitious plans for a new medical school, a bachelor of health sciences program, and nurse practitioner training. However, in 1971 an Ontario provincial report recommended against the creation of yet another health science complex in the GTA.[75] The failure of York to convince Queen's Park as to the need of another medical school in Toronto would be longstanding; when the province of Ontario looked around for a new medical school at the dawn of the twenty-first century, York was once again denied, as the government chose to establish the Northern Ontario School of Medicine in the northwest of the province, shared between Sudbury and Thunder Bay.[76]

The HRF was not only about creating *new* medical schools but also about dramatically expanding and modernizing existing ones. Since funding could only be used for bricks and mortar, there was a surge of construction of new, research-intensive, and transdisciplinary "health sciences centres" that combined patient care, teaching, and research. At the University of Alberta, for example, the fund enabled the construction of a new clinical sciences building and basic medical sciences building.[77] Class sizes subsequently jumped to 118 in 1967 from fifty a decade earlier.[78] In addition to a new medical sciences building and dental sciences building in Saskatoon, the Health Resources Fund was also used to construct a second teaching hospital in Regina, called the Plains Hospital.[79] In Toronto, HRF funds supported the conversion of Sunnybrook from a veterans' hospital into a University of Toronto-affiliated teaching hospital.[80] At Laval medical school in Quebec City, the fund supported facility expansion and the hiring of full-time faculty cross appointed to affiliated hospitals.[81]

Providing adequate research facilities was, in the minds of leading medical educators, key to recruiting foreign-trained medical educators and enticing back leading Canadian-trained clinician scientists. In order to drive home the point, the profession coalesced around an initiative whereby Toronto's Hospital for Sick Children chairman C.L. Gundy coordinated a national report on the shortage of funds for medical research. Gundy commissioned a management consultant team – Woods, Gordon & Co. – to prepare a study on the relationship between research and clinical training. Known then as the Gundy Report, its findings and recommendations were personally endorsed by more than 600 medical scientists, by the deans of the medical schools, and by the country's medical and biological societies. It contended that the federal government's approach to medical research compromised recruitment efforts to the new and expanded medical schools.[82] Professional groups argued vehemently that expansion of medical graduate classes could not occur without stronger research support.[83] Fraser Mustard did not mince his words in 1966; the choice for the future of health care in Canada was clear, he declared to the Empire Club of Canada. Either we strive for "excellence" or resign ourselves to "mediocrity."[84]

As foreign medical educators streamed into the medical schools, they were under increasing pressures to squeeze out non-Canadian students. The percentage of foreign students in Canadian medical schools (as undergraduates) dropped precipitously, from 15 per cent in 1959–60[85] to less than 2 per cent in 1974–75. Of these remaining foreign medical students, the majority were Americans enrolled at McGill.[86] Medical school deans recognized the pressure to restrict undergraduate medical school enrolment to Canadians and landed immigrants, with occasional exceptions to student refugees, such as those displaced by the events in Czechoslovakia and Uganda.[87] A second, indirect effect was the dramatic increase in the absolute and proportionate female medical school enrolment in Canada. During this time period, the percentage of female students increased substantially, doubling from 7 per cent in 1957–58 to 13 per cent in 1965–66, and then almost tripling to 33 per cent ten years after the Medical Care Act. Given the *absolute* increase in student numbers mentioned above, this represented a near fivefold increase in absolute female undergraduate medical enrolment in the first ten years of the HRF.[88]

CONCLUSIONS

The Medical Care Act of 1966 and the Immigration (Appeals Board) Act of 1967 were turning points in the history of contemporary Canada. Both have taken on cultural meaning in the broad history of nation building, bolstering two symbolic centrepieces of twentieth century Canadian identity: Medicare and multiculturalism. Although they were not drafted as complementary or twinned legislation, their entanglement and interaction cannot be overlooked. The points system opened the door to health practitioners from nontraditional countries who proved only too willing to emigrate to Canada either to set up practice in underserviced areas or to help staff the new medical facilities facilitated by the HRF. From 1960 to 1973–74 (the midway point of the HRF and the time at which the new medical school graduates were appearing), Canadian first-year medical school enrolment had jumped from 970 to 1,774, an 83 per cent increase. This even outpaced the United States (69 per cent increase over the same period).[89] Total (steady state) enrolment doubled in the period 1960–75, from 3,508 to 7,012 medical students.[90] It represented the largest increase in human resource capacity in twentieth-century Canadian medical history.

Although the Fairclough Directive and the subsequent points system have often been framed in racial terms – ushering in a new era of multi-ethnic immigration – in other respects, Canada's shift to "merit" can also be seen as entirely opportunistic: just as the government had encouraged hardworking European farmers to immigrate and populate the prairies in the early twentieth century, the 1960s system reoriented immigration toward the new needs of the postwar economy. Occupational demand fluctuated in direct response to the needs of the Canadian economy, with only a passing thought as to the impact on the countries from whence these doctors came. And when there were enough doctors, nurses, and technicians in the country, the federal government, with the encouragement of provincial ministers of health, simply "turned off the tap." As Frank Miller, the Ontario minister of health and future premier, concluded in 1975 as the grand era of medical migration was drawing to an end, "We've drained the poorer nations of very valuable assets for a long time because we needed them and we did it openly and we were happy to steal them."[91] In the chapters that follow, we will see that although foreign politicians would from time to time complain about the impact of the West's shift to "highly skilled manpower," those complaints were often drowned out by other international and national concerns.

Chapter Five

Medical Diasporas

THE PRAGUE SPRING

Mirko Havlas was born in Pisek, a middle-sized town in Bohemia, just months after the outbreak of the First World War. Fatherless from the age of two, he lived with his grandmother until his mother remarried eight years later. He would have only been starting primary school when the Allies carved out the state of Czechoslovakia from the remains of the Austro-Hungarian and German empires in 1919. During the 1920s, a young Mirko attended elementary school and high school in the eastern Czech town of Hradec Kralove before moving to Prague to enrol in medical school at Charles University. Charles University, although largely unknown in Canada, was one of the oldest and most famous universities in Europe, founded in 1348 by the Holy Roman Emperor Charles IV. By the dawn of the twentieth century it had become a flashpoint for the respective German- and Czech-speaking populations of Bohemia, to such an extent that the university was actually split into two with a "German" as well as a "Czech" half functioning concurrently and semi-independently.[1]

Mirko began medical school sometime in the turbulent mid-1930s after Hitler had consolidated power in Germany and began to make ominous claims over ethnic German areas of Bohemia in the west of Czechoslovakia. Early in his medical program, the young doctor-in-training met Vlasta Bozena, a fellow medical student, whom he would later marry during their studies. Although the record is unclear, the young couple's degrees would have undoubtedly been interrupted by the Nazi occupation of the Sudentenland in 1939 and suspension of the Czech universities during the war.[2] Some of their fellow medical students escaped to England where they completed their medical degrees (under the name of

Charles University) at the University of Oxford.[3] The now married couple remained in occupied Prague and officially graduated in 1945 and 1946 respectively, completing their internships in the war-ravaged hospitals of the postwar Czech capital. The time must have been unsettling: most of the Germans (and remaining Jews) migrated north and westward as this part of Bohemia became repatriated as ethnically Czech territory at the end of the war.[4] According to their obituaries, the Drs Havlas set up separate medical practices in the small town of Doksy, known as a summer vacation resort on Lake Macha; Vlasta as a paediatrician and Mirko as a family practitioner.[5]

In the wake of the Second World War and the division of Europe (and Germany) into competing blocs, Czechoslovakia occupied an uneasy position straddling East and West in the heart of the European continent. Ultimately, Czechoslovakia would turn toward communism and the Soviet alliance. Appealing strategically to nationalist sentiments and riding a wave of leftist enthusiasm, the Communist Party won the 1946 elections with 38 per cent of the vote.[6] A Communist-majority government then subsequently emerged through a "bloodless coup" in 1948. What ensued was a widespread social experiment of re-establishing Czech ethnicity within the structure of a Soviet-bloc state. In its first decade in power, the Czech Communist Party pursued the nationalization of industries, agricultural collectivization, and the installation of a command economy.[7] The government also engaged in suppression of the Catholic Church and a widespread purging of students and professors, expelling 21.7 per cent of enrolled university students in 1948–49 alone. A disdain for traditional bourgeois pursuits was reflected in the relatively low status and remuneration of professionals, including doctors, whose private practices were abolished by the state. "By the mid-1960s," John Connelly observes, "a locksmith earned more than a lawyer, and a turner more than a physician."[8] Indeed, young men who aspired to practice medicine but were perceived too bourgeois were obliged to work as manual labourers and prove they were dedicated citizens of the new socialist republic. One interviewee recalls digging ditches at a chemical plant for a year before, with letter in hand validating his proletarian experience, he was permitted to apply for medical school.[9]

The consolidation of the Communist Party led to the widespread emigration of Czechs in two distinct waves, the first of which was mostly ten

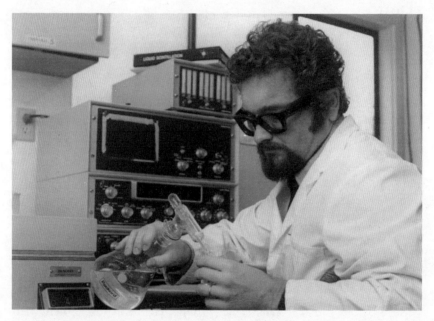

Figure 5.1 Dr Josef Skála
Dr Josef Skála was born and raised in Prague, Czechoslovakia. After being imprisoned
in 1948, he worked in the steel works Poldovka near Kladno before completing his
studies in medicine. Like many thousands of his conationals, he fled the country in
August of 1968, first to Sweden and in 1969 to Vancouver. Apart from the significant
career in medicine, he helped establish the Czech Theatre Around the Corner.

thousand professionals in the early years of the consolidation of Communist power.[10] After that time, the Czech state obstructed general travel
abroad, permitting only "supporters and protégés" to cross its borders.[11]
By the 1960s, however, the state began allowing Czechs to obtain passports
to travel beyond the bloc in a more liberal fashion.[12] At the same time, Czechoslovakia was home to the emergence of youth activism and something
resembling a counterculture, which criticized their perceived shortcomings of socialist society.[13] The press, too, became more daring and critical
of the regime in the 1960s. The era of liberalization crystalized in early
1968 when reformist elements of the Communist Party, headed by Alexander Dubček, came to lead the party. Party reformists aimed at opening
up the country through the decentralization of political planning and
greater freedom of speech. Their actions had a snowballing effect: "The

more reforms they instituted, the more they mobilized an excited population, which in turn pressed for further liberalization."[14] Spooked by the uncoordinated uprising, the Warsaw Pact allowed for the USSR's invasion of Prague in August of 1968. In brief, Moscow regarded the reformist measures as "a destabilizing example to citizens in neighbouring communist countries, a virus that might spread and undermine [Soviet] control."[15]

The suppression of the political uprising triggered a second wave of emigration, one that paradoxically was abetted by the government itself. As Jan Raska summarizes, "In hopes of getting rid of the proponents of Communist reform, Czechoslovakia's borders remained open in the early hours, weeks, and months after the invasion."[16] According to the obituaries of the Drs Havlas, they were part of this exodus, leaving during the August invasion with their two teenage children. Two months later they were accepted as political refugees by Canada and arrived in Peterborough, Ontario. This is where the doctors studied English and wrote medical equivalency exams to be able to practice medicine in Canada.[17] They would ultimately take up employment in a psychiatric facility in southwestern Ontario. They were one family of an estimated 11,000 Czechs who would arrive in Canada in 1968, with an equal number in the United States, and approximately 6,000 in Australia.[18] Armed with the experience of receiving political refugees fleeing the failed Hungarian uprising in 1956, the Canadian government colluded in enticing Czech émigrés by "manipulat[ing] the conventional definition of a refugee and consciously adopt[ing] policies" in order to facilitate the admission of Czechoslovakian migrants.[19]

Czech doctors fleeing the country during the Prague Spring formed an important cohort in the émigré doctor community. In total there were 285 Czechoslovakian-trained doctors who appeared at least once in the select four editions of the *Canadian Medical Directory*. In addition to an unusual cluster in provincially run psychiatric institutions, they were listed as practicing in a diverse array of specialties. They graduated from the principal universities across the Czech and Slovak divisions of the country, including the aforementioned Charles University, Brno University, and Palacky University; a further dozen graduated from Bratislava University (Comenius University) in Slovakia. Czech and Slovak graduates could be found across Canada, with strong rural representations in the Prairie provinces and in the Maritimes (see table 5.1). As for the

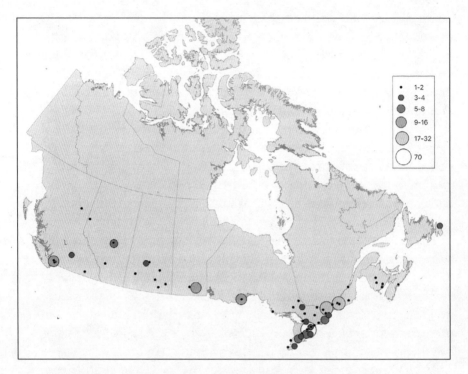

Figure 5.2 Czechoslovakian-trained doctors in Canada, 1961–76

Haslavs, an obituary states that Mirko vowed never to return to his native Czechoslovakia while it remained Communist.[20] There was also a practical concern as well as an ideological one: in the wake of the Prague Spring, refugees who left in 1968 were tried in absentia and thus could be arrested if they returned as visitors.

The Havlas arrived in 1968, the year Medicare was launched, and in the midst of an unprecedented surge in medical immigration. By 1976 there were 34,669 practicing licensed practitioners in the country, according to the *Canadian Medical Directory* of that year, 10,732 (31 per cent) of whom were listed as having received their undergraduate medical training outside of Canada.[21] By contrast, only 3,756 foreign-trained doctors appeared in the 1961 CMD, constituting only 16 per cent of the medical workforce. Of the 10,000 foreign-trained doctors scattered across the country in the mid-1970s, as many as 6,000 had arrived in the critical first decade after

Table 5.1
Thirteen continental European countries, including Czechoslovakia, that had graduated fifty or more CMD-listed doctors, by place of undergraduate medical training, as listed in the 1976 *Canadian Medical Directory*

(West) Germany	327	Italy	123
Czechoslovakia	**253**	Austria	127
France	230	Switzerland	107
Hungary	227	Belgium	72
Spain	143	Romania	76
Poland	126	Yugoslavia	75
Netherlands	122		

Source: *Canadian Medical Directory, 1976.*

the passage of the Medicare Act (1966) and the introduction of the points system. As older, Canadian-born doctors retired, by the late-1970s, the proportion of foreign-trained doctors practicing as physicians or surgeons in the country would rise to one-third of the total workforce.[22] Taken as a whole, the Canadian physician workforce expanded dramatically during this period, far outpacing the growth of the general population, which was itself augmenting rapidly as a result of the twin effects of the final years of the baby boom and general immigration.

Aggregate numbers mask some fundamental transformations in the composition, country of origin, and geographical distribution of the medical workforce. Certainly, the medical schools of the British Isles continued to produce the greatest number of foreign-trained doctors, though one must keep in mind that a minority would have been non-Canadian and non-British nationals who graduated from British or Irish medical schools. About 5,000 doctors practicing in the early 1970s had graduated from medical schools in the United Kingdom and almost 1,000 more from medical schools in the Irish republic. Many residents of the settler communities in smaller commonwealth nations also got caught up in the trend towards North American practice: for example, almost one hundred graduates of Otago Medical School in New Zealand were practicing in Canada in 1976, accompanied by 200 graduates of Australian medical schools. The majority of these Antipodean doctors would likely have remigrated from Britain after postgraduate training.

By 1976, however, the source countries of doctors had diversified in a substantial manner beyond the "white" Commonwealth. Indeed, more than 200 medical schools in eighty separate countries were listed as places of undergraduate education in the *Canadian Medical Directory* of that year. A staggering three dozen separate countries contributed at least fifty practitioners to the Canadian medical workforce. Here and the following chapter will examine physicians from select countries to dig deeper into the growing diversity of medical practitioners and their impact on the rolling out of Medicare. These countries are united by their shared experience of the period as one of great social and political upheaval in their home countries. As bureaucrats were putting the final touches on the Medical Care Act and negotiating the entry of provinces under Medicare, tumultuous events in other parts of the world would provide the social and political backdrop to the creation of medical diasporas that would reach the shores, and the clinics, of Canada.

SIX DAYS THAT SHOOK THE WORLD

Just months before Dubček came to power in Czechoslovakia, a brief war broke out between Egypt and Israel over the Suez Canal, the vital waterway linking Europe through the Mediterranean to the Red Sea and ultimately the Indian Ocean. The strategic importance of the Suez Canal cannot be underestimated. For Western colonial powers, the canal had long remained central to military and economic power in the Middle East and South Asia. After direct British colonial rule ended in the Paris Peace Conference of 1919, the Kingdom of Egypt operated during the interwar years under King Fuad and later his son the young King Farouk. Both kings assured Western access to the canal in return for military support from Britain. However, in 1952 a coup changed the political dynamic of the region. A year later, Gamal Abd al-Nasir (Abdel Nasser) assumed executive power, which he would maintain until his death in 1970. His nationalization of the Suez Canal in 1956 proved to be the justification of the invasion of Egypt by Israel, Britain, and France. Israel overran the Sinai with ground troops, while British and French paratroopers attempted to secure the Suez shipping routes.[23] The subsequent standoff was finally resolved by pressure from the United States and the United Nations and the timely intervention of Canadian minister of external affairs Lester Pearson. Pearson, of course, would receive the Nobel Peace Prize for his role in defusing an international crisis in 1956 and in "inventing" a new unit – the blue-helmeted UN peacekeepers – to intervene as neutral and stabilizing agents in such international conflicts.[24]

Pearson's peace, however, would be short-lived. Tensions remained high between Egypt and Israel over the territory of the Sinai Peninsula and Gaza. Nasser repeatedly threatened to close down the Suez to international shipping during the 1960s, prompting a so-called pre-emptive strike by the Israeli air force in 1967 and a ground invasion that saw Israeli troops quickly take over the Sinai Peninsula. The brief conflict – referred to by some as the Six-Day War – proved to be a disaster for Egyptian morale, the military, and the economy.[25] The nationalization of the Suez Canal, however, was far from a capricious move; it had been part of a strategy of Egyptian nationalism, as the new government of Nasser attempted to rid itself of foreign influences and control. The state initiated wide-ranging nationalization among all major businesses, industrial regulation, income redistribution, and more impactful land reform as part of an experiment in "Arab socialism."[26] There was a political cost however: throughout and beyond this period, freedom of speech, the press, and assembly were suppressed.[27]

The expansion of a highly educated middle class was a central pillar of self-sufficiency and independence from external interference in the 1960s. The Egyptian government expanded public education and ensured that all university graduates were guaranteed a position in governmental departments and state-owned firms.[28] As well, the government offered scholarships for study abroad.[29] The number of university graduates quadrupled between 1952 and 1969, and while the government sought to provide opportunities, scholars have concluded that the number of graduates far exceeded the number the country's economy could absorb.[30] The growing Egyptian middle class of the 1960s was deeply attached to the security of guaranteed government employment, though this dependence declined in the early 1970s when government salaries did not keep pace with inflation.[31] This only worsened the situation of the surplus university graduates who were "faced with long-term military service upon graduating."[32]

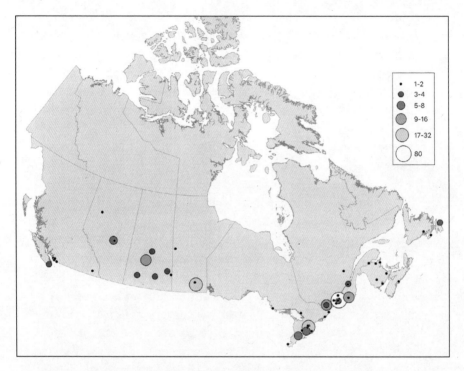

Figure 5.3 Egyptian-trained doctors in Canada, 1961–76

Under Nasser, anticolonialism and political Islamism were major aspects of a political climate that facilitated and forced the emigration of minority groups, many of whom had been successful members of the Egyptian commercial and professional classes.[33] For the decade leading up to 1967 a series of laws relating to work, employment, and businesses targeted non-Egyptians including Jews, Greeks, British, French, Armenians, Lebanese, and Syrians.[34] Thomas Philipp concludes that "by the mid-1960s the non-Coptic minorities in Egypt had for all practical purposes vanished from the Egyptian scene."[35] Amidst this exodus of commercial interests and ethnic minorities, doctors and medical researchers occupied an important and sensitive position. Through the 1960s, the Egyptian government maintained a restrictive policy that made emigration challenging for certain professionals in demand. Like many countries of the time, the government also maintained laws conscripting various professionals, including doctors, for periods of national or military service.[36] While the migration policy grew more ambivalent during the late 1960s,[37] and some procedures relaxed, the government continued to require exit visas. Following Nasser's death in 1970, however, the uncertainty and restrictions over immigration were lifted.[38] The Sadat government, promoting its new *infitah*, or open-door policy, enshrined Egyptians' right to migrate in the new 1971 constitution.[39]

In total, 262 Egyptian-trained doctors appeared at least once in the four editions of the *Canadian Medical Directory*, 90 per cent of whom arrived *after* the changes to Canadian immigration in 1967 and coinciding with the Egyptian open-door era. About one-half of the doctors graduated from the University of Cairo, one-quarter from the University of Alexandria,[40] and the final quarter from the new medical school of Ain Shams University, a nonsectarian public university founded in 1950 in Cairo.[41] The strong tradition of learning French amongst the educated sons of the Egyptian middle class made them ideal candidates for emigration to Canada under the new points system and particularly for practice in Quebec. Indeed, more Egyptian-trained doctors settled in Quebec than in any other province, with notable clusters in Sherbrooke where some took part as teaching and research faculty in the new medical school. Their specialties stand out as configuring around the operating table: no fewer than 10 per cent who arrived in Canada were anaesthesiologists, a further 10 per cent were urologists, complementing a surprising cluster of neurosurgeons and handfuls of ear, nose and throat surgeons, orthopods, and ophthalmologists.

Despite the large number of Egyptian doctors who would settle in Ontario in the 1970s, their arrival in the most populous province was anything but smooth. As in other provinces, it was the provincial College of Physicians and Surgeons that had the authority to grant enabling certificates to write the Medical College of Canada exams for foreign-trained physicians.[42] As doctors began to arrive from a wider range of countries following the Fairclough Directive, the CPSO announced in 1964 that it could *not* guarantee that graduates of medical schools in Germany, Greece, Hungary, India, Italy, or Pakistan would be eligible for full registration "until such time as the College has reviewed the standard of training provided

Table 5.2
Countries of the Eastern Mediterranean and West Asia that had graduated
fifty or more CMD-listed doctors, by place of undergraduate medical training,
as listed in the 1976 *Canadian Medical Directory*

Egypt	229	Turkey	66
Lebanon	94	Iran	56

Source: *Canadian Medical Directory, 1976.*

by schools in these countries and is satisfied that it is equivalent to that
provided by Canadian medical schools."[43] Following a multiyear assessment of foreign medical schools, the college introduced new regulations
that recognized degrees from seventeen European countries and the US[44]
but excluded graduates of Indian and Pakistani medical colleges from acceptance for full registration.[45] Graduates of schools in Turkey, Egypt,
Japan, and the Philippines were likewise barred.[46] As a consequence, doctors who were eligible to write the Medical Council of Canada exam
(LMCC) in the mid-1960s in some other provinces were barred from doing
so in Ontario.[47] It is unclear how many doctors were prohibited from gaining licensure in Ontario. Some reports said that the ban affected between
sixty and one hundred doctors;[48] *Maclean's* estimated as many as 300 practitioners were affected.[49]

Needless to say, in the aftermath of the Royal Commission Report of
1964 – which predicted significant shortfalls in doctors – the unilateral approach of Ontario took many by surprise. In 1965, four Indian, one Japanese, and one Turkish doctor accused the CPSO of discrimination for
"refusing to license for general practice graduates from non-white Commonwealth medical schools."[50] These doctors "accused the college of attempting to maintain a supply of cheap, foreign-born labor for hospitals"[51]
in order to "kee[p] the fees of local doctors high and the salaries of doctors
in residence at hospitals low."[52] Reportedly, there were almost 200 immigrant doctors – "mostly Asians" – who would be relegated to supervised
hospital work.[53] An editorial in the *Toronto Star* described them rather
vividly as "the medical equivalent to the Chinese coolies who were imported to build the Canadian Pacific Railway."[54] The CPSO, unconvincingly,

MACLEAN'S REPORTS

SEPTEMBER 18, 1965   VOLUME 78 NUMBER 18

FOREIGN DOCTORS WHO "AREN'T GOOD ENOUGH"

Dr. Krishna Baichwal, a specialist in cardiovascular surgery, is eligible to hang out his shingle in Britain, British Columbia and Nova Scotia. However, since he happens to prefer to live in Ontario, he holds a salaried job as a resident surgeon and research fellow at Toronto Western Hospital. There he teaches interns and regularly performs operations. Much of this surgery is minor, but if Dr. Baichwal were not competent, he might easily maim or kill his patients.

By such practical standards as this, Krishna Baichwal is a skilled and experienced physician and surgeon. Yet as long as he chooses to live in Ontario, he can never establish a practice of his own. The most he can hope for is the kind of job he has now, as a hospital resident — for which salaries average four thousand dollars a year.

How bad can Bombay be?

Dr. Baichwal's problem is that he got his medical training in Bombay. And, under the blanket ruling laid down by the Ontario College of Physicians and Surgeons, he therefore has such a poor academic background that he is not fit to practise privately in the province where he has chosen to live. This is not a ruling requiring Dr. Baichwal to gain additional experience in Canada or to pass certain Ontario tests. It is a rule that says, in effect, that no matter where he works, what operations he performs, or how many examinations he might be able to pass, he will never overcome the deficiencies of the undergraduate training he got in Bombay.

If Dr. Baichwal wants to establish himself in private practice in Ontario, he must forget he is already a cardiovascular specialist and sign up for medical school. Since he is already thirty-six and demonstrably capable of teaching medical students, this is a course of action Dr. Baichwal is, understandably, reluctant to take.

Krishna Baichwal is not a rarity. Dr. Apkar Aynaciyan is a forty-four-year-old Turk who seems similarly well qualified. He graduated in medicine from Istanbul University, spent four years studying internal medicine in the United States (where he could

sit the qualifying exams if he could get U. S. citizenship) and holds the certificate of the U. S. Educational Council for Foreign Medical Graduates. The ECFMG certificate is one which both the American Medical Association and the U. S. Association of American Medical Colleges believe is "evidence that the recipient (has) medical knowledge comparable to that expected of graduates of approved medical schools in the U. S. and Canada." Dr. Aynaciyan is a fellow in gastroenterology at Toronto Western Hospital but he cannot, under Ontario regulations, qualify to practise on his own.

An "unqualified" Egyptian

Dr. Rasheed Afifi and his wife Mary Papantony are both doctors; he a surgeon, she an anaesthetist. Both were trained in Egypt and have three post-graduate work in the U. S. They cannot practise in Ontario.

Nobody knows exactly how many other foreign-trained doctors there are in Canada today who find themselves in the same circumstances. But in Ontario alone, where the provincial College of Physicians and Surgeons takes a tougher line than most, there are at least a hundred such people — perhaps as many as three hundred. They are permitted to work as hospital residents, medical researchers or medical teachers. But they are not allowed — and perhaps never will be allowed — even to try the exams every doctor must pass to go into private practice.

Such an arbitrary ruling would be distressing enough to the doctors in-

volved if they felt it was being imposed equally on all nationals. But the policy which the Ontario college laid down last May actually spells out what one Turkish doctor describes as "a sort of ethnic discrimination." One passage of the policy statement says bluntly that "graduates of medical colleges in India and Pakistan [are not] accepted for full registration . . ." And the college's list of seventeen countries whose doctors may be eligible for the qualifying exams does not contain a single nation (except the U. S.) outside Europe.

An "anti-college" club

This policy ruling has so angered and frustrated a group of foreign doctors in Ontario that they have formed a loosely knit organization called the Foreign Medical Graduates' Committee. It is dedicated to "convincing the College it should not be so stubborn and arbitrary." Its spokesman is Dr. Suresh Anand, a thirty-three-year-old bachelor who got his training in Lucknow and the United States and now works as an intern in the emergency ward at Wellesley Hospital, Toronto. Dr. Anand says he knows of at least a hundred foreign doctors, most of them non-Europeans, whom the Ontario college refuses to accept as candidates for the qualifying exams. Among them are Turks, Italians, Filipinos, Egyptians, Frenchmen, Dutchmen, Indians, Pakistanis, Japanese, Chinese (from Red China), Formosans and Latin Americans.

"All any of us want is for the college to treat each of our cases on its individual merits," says Dr. Anand. All other provinces, he says, do this. In Nova Scotia, for instance, a doctor from anywhere in the Commonwealth can hang out his shingle if his training is recognized by the General Medical Council of the U. K. as qualification for practice in Britain.

This high opinion of the British council's judgment is not shared, evidently, by Dr. Laurence Wilson, the Ontario College's president, or by its registrar, who insists on remaining anonymous. Dr. Wilson has defended the college policy in letters to the newspapers. And the registrar says many medical schools in India are so ill-equipped with teaching hospital beds and have such a high ratio of students to teachers that they produce graduates trained only to pass exams,

"not practise medicine as we expect it to be practised in Ontario."

"Nonsense," says Dr. Baichwal, the cardiovascular specialist who trained in Bombay. "They set about evaluating India's seventy or so medical schools by writing to thirty of them and asking for details of their establishments. When they got six replies, they used that information as the basis of the decision that no Indian doctor was fit to practise in Ontario."

Dr. Baichwal has a letter from a college official saying they did, indeed, receive only six replies.

The college's reluctance to see foreign doctors fully registered would be easier to explain if there were a surplus of doctors in Canada. But, as the Hall Royal Commission on Health Services warned, a severe shortage of physicians seems a real possibility within a few years. Dr. Glenn Sawyer, general secretary of the Ontario Medical Association, says Ontario is already short of doctors. He knows of ninety openings for doctors in Ontario, while only sixteen doctors are registered with him as job-seekers. Other surveys show there are about thirty small communities that are seriously short of doctors — or have no doctors at all.

They'd work in small towns

Spokesmen for the medical college insist that the shortage of doctors is an irrelevant issue. As evidence they cite the ten-year record of foreign doctors, most of them Europeans, who have been allowed to go into practice. More than half of these, the college points out, set up practice in Toronto, not in small communities where the shortage exists. But Dr. Anand says: "I think there is little doubt that most of the hundred or so foreign graduates in touch with our committee would be prepared to work where directed for specified periods of time as a condition of being granted a place on the general-practice list."

And he has personal reasons to scoff at the college's claims that foreign doctors, while denied private practice, can work safely enough as residents or interns because they are under constant supervision. An emergency-ward intern himself, Dr. Anand rarely has a supervisor with him when he treats patients with symptoms (lung congestion, for instance) that can

Here's a little gallery of foreign-trained doctors who aren't allowed even to try making the grade in Ontario.

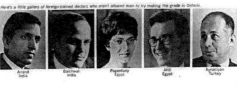

Anand, India   Baichwal, India   Papantony, Egypt   Afifi, Egypt   Aynaciyan, Turkey

Figure 5.4 "Foreign Doctors Who 'Aren't Good Enough,'" 1965
Unaware that the licensing of doctors was a provincial constitutional jurisdiction in Canada, many immigrant doctors were dismayed and confused by the inconsistent treatment they and their conationals received in different provinces. *Maclean's* magazine, amongst others, reported on the alleged discrimination against "Asian Doctors" in the Province of Ontario in the mid-1960s. Here five doctors from Egypt and India lead the charge against the College of Physicians and Surgeons of Ontario.

maintained that "Race, colour, creed and other discriminatory attributes have been of no concern [in their decision]; the only consideration … is the qualifications of the applicant."[55] In a manner that had parallels to the deaccreditation of South Asian medical schools in the British NHS, the Ontario college identified a drop in the quality of Indian and Pakistani medical education (due to the rapid expansion of medical schools) as a reason for new restrictions.[56] In his outgoing address in June 1966, the

CPSO president was "critical of the manner in which postgraduate training may be offered to these [foreign-trained] graduates and question[ed] whether this may not be done to meet service needs in the hospital or its research departments."[57] Ultimately, the doctors asked the Ontario Human Rights Commission to intervene.[58]

Although Egyptian and Filipino doctors figured prominently in the new regulations, the Ontario College admitted that the largest number of the more than 1,000 applications for registration from foreign-trained doctors each year were originally trained in India and Pakistan.[59] That same month, *The Times of India* and Regina *Leader-Post* reported that the college would be considering the applications of two of the physicians leading the protests.[60] In August 1965, the college permitted more than 150 foreign-trained doctors to write qualifying exams but barred a further sixty on grounds of unsatisfactory medical training.[61] To refute the allegations of racism, the college highlighted its acceptance of applications "from Indians, Africans and Chinese from accepted foreign schools" and rejection of some applications "from English, US and even Canadian graduates from medical schools in Europe or Asia which failed to meet college standards."[62] The college reminded complainants that they could practice in some other provinces and claimed they had been "informed they would be unable to obtain licenses for full practice in Ontario when their names were entered on the educational register."[63] Reportedly, by 1966, "many of the Asian doctors [were] leaving Ontario to practice elsewhere."[64] A "violent debate" erupted at Queen's Park, where MPP Stephen Lewis charged the college with discrimination "and demanded a public inquiry."[65] In addition to prompting the Ontario College to hire a public relations consultant,[66] the controversy compelled Ontario to engage in a major reconsideration of how it evaluated graduates from foreign medical schools.

FLEEING FORMOSA

Cold War conflicts erupted around the globe, providing the political backdrop to the exodus of hundreds of doctors who would find their way to Canada. The island of Taiwan was certainly no exception. Taiwan remained under Japanese colonial rule from 1895 until Japan's surrender in

1945, which introduced Kuomintang Nationalist rule over the island. During the Second World War, the 1943 Cairo Declaration between the Allied powers established an agreement that specified that "all the territories Japan [had] stolen from the Chinese, such as Manchuria, Formosa … shall be restored to the RoC [Republic of China]."[67] As a consequence, following the surrender of Japan in August 1945, Taiwan was "returned" to China, after decades of separation from the mainland. And yet with China itself imploding into civil war – between the Kuomintang (led by Chiang Kai Shek) and the Communist Forces (led by Mao Tse Tung) – Taiwan increasingly became a haven for the retreating Kuomintang forces. As Mao's Chinese Communist Party expanded and consolidated their power on the mainland, Chiang Kai Shek and his Kuomintang troops looked to Taiwan as an interim base where they hoped to regroup.

From the late 1940s, Taiwan experienced an increasingly challenging economic situation. In addition to Kuomintang soldiers, crowds of mainlanders looking to escape Communist rule were migrating to the island.[68] By 1949, Taiwan was experiencing heightened rates of crime, shortages of food and housing, as well as hyperinflation.[69] While the Kuomintang was initially welcomed (at least, in comparison to the Japanese government), the first few years under Chiang's leadership fuelled opposition and calls for Taiwanese independence. Along with the expanding population of mainlanders, there was a growing attitude amongst the Taiwanese that the Kuomintang government was simply another "foreign power" abusing their position. After a series of popular uprisings in 1947, the Kuomintang instituted martial law in Taiwan, placing the island in a permanent state of emergency for four decades. During the ensuing period of martial law, public rallies were prohibited in addition to the suspension of various civil rights including freedoms of speech, the press, and political assembly.[70]

Given the polarization of the Cold War, it was unsurprising that Taiwan would be identified as a geostrategic placeholder, straddling the South and East China Seas. By the early 1950s, American politicians were invested in ensuring that Taiwan not fall under the influence of mainland China, as the United States sought to contain the spread of communism in East and Southeast Asia. Americans preferred Kuomintang nationalist rule – no matter how oppressive – to Mao's Communism and sent American troops and ships to the Taiwan Strait to protect the island from potential invasion. The constant presence of military troops and looming

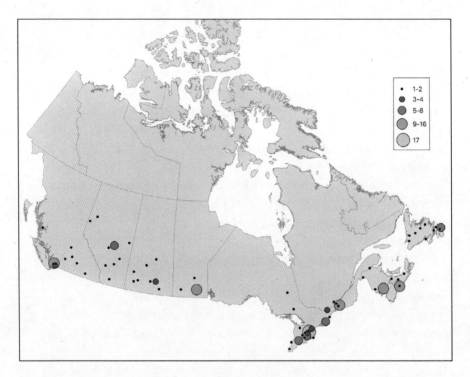

Figure 5.5 Taiwanese-trained doctors in Canada, 1961–76

threat of invasion ensured Taiwan was still controlled by foreign leaders, despite its growing economic prosperity. Taiwan remained a strategically valuable, if also volatile, asset for the Americans, as the United States became embroiled in other East and Southeast Asian conflicts, including the Korean War – in which Canada participated in a United Nations-led intervention – and the Vietnam War – in which Canada remained neutral.

Throughout the 1950s, Taiwan experienced rapid economic growth such that by 1963 the unemployment rate had fallen to a meagre 5.2 per cent.[71] Prosperity brought new investments in higher education. From 1954 to 1968, the nationalist government dedicated 13 per cent of its total budget to education and increased the length of compulsory schooling from six to nine years.[72] The higher education sector in Taiwan trebled from twenty-seven institutions in 1961 to ninety-one by the end of the decade.[73] The United States played a key role in this expansion. At the conclusion

Table 5.3

Countries of Southeast and East Asia that had graduated fifty or more CMD-listed doctors, by place of undergraduate medical training, as listed in the 1976 *Canadian Medical Directory*

Philippines	211	Hong Kong	105
Taiwan	**170**	Korea	77
China (Rep)	109		

Source: *Canadian Medical Directory, 1976*. "Others" include Japan (thirty), Vietnam (ten), Thailand (nine), Malaysia (three), and Indonesia (three).

of the Korean War (1953) the American government committed fifteen years of funding into research infrastructure and bursaries for Chinese students, as one of many measures to stem the tide of Communism and prevent young educated professionals of the wider Chinese diaspora from "returning" to the People's Republic. As a result, an estimated 40 per cent of medical school placements in Taiwan were reserved for non-Taiwanese Chinese students of the wider Chinese diaspora who were, indirectly, funded by the American government. In particular, under financial aid from the United States, the government changed the medical school curriculum from a German-style curriculum established under Japanese colonial rule to an American-style credit system. The numbers of medical graduates increased rapidly; for example, Taiwan National University admitted fifty-eight people in 1946 and around one hundred to 110 in the late 1950s.[74] Taiwanese universities achieved greater levels of prestige, and many students used their education to seek opportunities and postgraduate training abroad, most often in the United States, Canada, and Australia.

Lily Cheung was one such medical trainee. Born in Southern China in 1936, her family relocated repeatedly as the Japanese invasion spread wider across mainland China. Her parents – both teachers – would move with their students to safer locations further south as the situation deteriorated in 1937 and 1938. "I moved six or seven times in eight years," she recalls, as the family relocated to Xiamen and then left mainland China for the Philippines and then ultimately for Indonesia. After the conclusion of the war, her brother returned to communist China but her father insisted that she

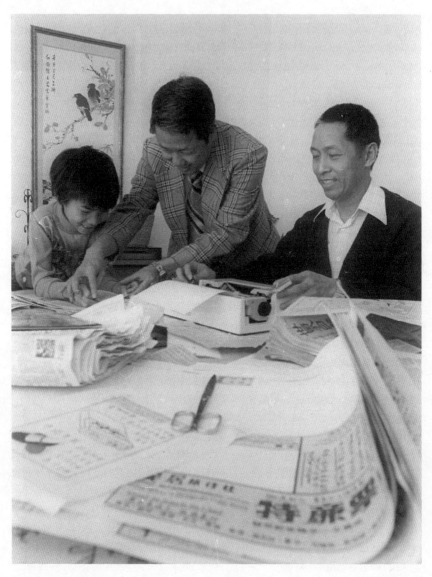

Figure 5.6 Dr Yantay Tsai (right)
Outside of Ontario, many provinces were only too eager to see the settlement of doctors who had been trained in the far reaches of the former British empire. Taiwanese- and Hong Kong–trained doctors, such as Dr Yantay Tsai and his wife Dr Rozane Tsai, would ultimately settle in the province of Manitoba. Many Taiwanese doctors had been educated through American bursaries as part of a Cold War initiative to prevent the island from falling under the control of Communist China.

accept an American bursary and study medicine in Taipei at the National Taiwan University. There she met her future husband, another non-Taiwanese Chinese student who was one year ahead in his studies. When asked why she and her husband left the island upon graduation she stated flatly, "I was not Taiwanese … I was stateless." She followed her husband, who had sent several letters of interest to American and Canadian hospitals. The first one he received was from Saskatoon, which is where the couple settled temporarily before moving to another prairie city.[75]

The decision to emigrate for doctors like Cheung reflected both professional opportunities and also deteriorating political conditions on the island. Despite the economic progress of the postwar period, the Kuomintang maintained a practice of intimidating political opponents critical of the government. During the period of martial law, sometimes called the "white terror," it is estimated that Kuomintang forces executed upwards of 5,000 people and imprisoned a further 80,000.[76] Within a climate of constant scrutiny, students critical of the government were subject to surveillance and potential political imprisonment. For those Taiwanese-born students studying abroad, the Kuomintang would sometimes threaten or interrogate students' relatives or deny students' re-entry to the island.[77] As a consequence, countries such as the United States and Canada offered economic opportunities and an environment free from unrelenting surveillance. Moreover, with the liberalization of immigration policies in North America, a period of unprecedented migration of East and South Asians to the United States and Canada began in the mid-1960s. These factors combined to create a professional brain drain, where many students abroad remained in their new host countries and new medical graduates – particularly those of the wider Chinese diaspora who studied in Taiwan but did not consider themselves Taiwanese – embraced opportunities to emigrate permanently.[78] A 1970s report, looking back at the 1965 medical graduates of the National University of Taiwan, for example, concluded that almost two-thirds of that student cohort remained abroad in the United States, Canada, the United Kingdom, and Japan.[79]

Taken as a cohort, just fewer than 200 Taiwanese-trained doctors settled in Canada for the period under study, graduating from the National University of Taiwan and the National Defence Medical Centre. Their geospatial distribution across Canada was quite remarkable, with a particular representation in rural prairie farming towns such as Castor (Alberta),

Hodgson (Manitoba), and Gull Lake (Saskatchewan) and an unusual number practicing in Newfoundland. There were about one-half-dozen Taiwanese-trained surgeons and physicians in the principal cities of Canada. Specialties spanned the medical and surgical disciplines, with a significant number of radiologists and paediatricians in the cohort. Although 80 per cent of these doctors who appeared in the 1971 CMD reappear in the 1976 edition, of the four select countries of training under investigation in this chapter they had the highest rate of relocation, mainly to Ontario and British Columbia. This is particularly true of surgeons, who left the provinces of Nova Scotia and Manitoba, provinces to which they had first immigrated and where they had begun practice in Canada.

PAKISTAN AFTER PARTITION

The year 1968 witnessed popular protests across the globe. While the situation in Czechoslovakia made international news, perhaps the most famous and widely covered were the student uprisings in Paris and the race riots in Chicago. However, mass student and worker demonstrations also erupted in disparate locations around the world. In Pakistan, for example, popular outrage with government corruption and military rule led to months-long strikes and street protests that turned bloody, forcing the president General Ayub Khan to relinquish power. The year 1968 was not supposed to have gone this way for General Khan. The military dictatorship he headed was gearing up to celebrate his first decade in power and, to his mind, ten years of economic advances. This so-called "decade of development" witnessed an explicit attempt to modernize the otherwise poor and agriculturally based country. Initiatives included a Green Revolution, government-sponsored industrial development that led to rapid urbanization, and social legislation for women's rights.[80]

Pakistan had begun life in 1947 as a poor, largely agrarian, and federated society of five provinces, each a distinct ethnolinguistic nation that gave birth to the country's name itself.[81] The situation remained unstable, as tensions fluctuated over differential access to jobs and power, contributing to reoccurring ethnic violence.[82] Meanwhile the redrawing of British India had led to unprecedented and at times violent migrations, social unrest, and political instability as whole states – the Punjab and Kashmir in par-

Table 5.4

Five countries of South Asia, by place of undergraduate medical training, as listed in the 1976 *Canadian Medical Directory*

India	682	Sri Lanka	14
Pakistan	**140**	Burma	13
Bangladesh*	33		

Source: *Canadian Medical Directory*, 1976. In this table, "national designations" must be understood within the changing national boundaries of Partition and post-Partition India.[1]

1 During Partition (in 1947) and the creation of the states of India and Pakistan (and East Bengal affiliated to Pakistan), millions of people voluntarily migrated or were forcibly displaced across the new national borders. Some of the doctors who ended up in Canada had begun medical school in pre-Partition British India. Others may have moved between medical schools due to interethnic and interreligious violence. In addition, Bangladesh obtained its independence from Pakistan in 1971 in the midst of a bloody civil war.

ticular – were divided between so-called Muslim- and Hindu-dominated regions.[83] It has been estimated that from 1947 to the late 1960s somewhere between twelve and thirteen million Hindus, Muslims, and Sikhs crossed the border as refugees seeking to rebuild their lives on the "right" side of the new divide. But migration upset existing social orders, for the outflow of non-Muslims to India drained many regions of middle-class professionals and administrators, while the inflow of Muslims from India into Pakistan complicated the ethnocultural balance. Although a lot of focus has been on the western border between India and Pakistan, there was also a pronounced migration of refugees in the east. While (west) Pakistan was nearly emptied of non-Muslims, more non-Muslims stayed than left in the separated dominion of what was then known as East Pakistan, a truncated geographical area that more or less coincided with the old boundaries of East Bengal.[84]

After Partition, Pakistan was thus disadvantaged by being segmented into two geographical units; India, by contrast, retained most of the central institutions of the former British Raj as well as major ports and industrial centres. A power vacuum followed the death of independence leader Muhammad Ali Jinnah, and Pakistan witnessed seven changes of government and the rise of military officers as key political figures.[85] Money poured into defence and the army (enhanced, like Taiwan, by support from the United States), which consolidated power within the public administration. The country's experiment with democracy, however, ended in 1958 when a coup installed a military dictatorship.[86] General Ayub Khan, the former commander in chief of the army, took power in 1958. During this time, the official government line promoted "liberal Islamic values," which translated into, amongst other things, a tolerance of various sects and religions.[87]

Pakistan, however, remained a nation divided, with most of the riches and industrial growth occurring in the west at the expense of the east. A cultural movement in East Pakistan succeeded in establishing Bengali as an official language (alongside Urdu) in 1954, but this did little to dissuade the sense in the east that the elite in Islamabad were interested in pursuing only their own interests.[88] Over time, many East Pakistanis felt that "a new form of colonial rule had replaced British imperialism."[89] As Davis Lewis explains, "The West Pakistan elite had monopolised most of the key positions in the new state of Pakistan, from banking and administration to business and banking ... and also dominated the armed forces."[90] Bengali presence remained minimal in the army and bureaucracy.[91] East Pakistani leaders became convinced of the need for greater autonomy.[92] As in many parts of the world, an autonomy movement grew in strength by the late 1960s.

Economic policy and development priorities accelerated the growing inequality between East and West Pakistan.[93] While East Pakistan had the majority of the population, it received only one-quarter of budget allocations. Per capita income fell in the east while it increased in the west,[94] and by the late 1960s incomes were 50 per cent higher in West Pakistan.[95] While the state expanded higher education it "was largely indifferent to mass education," doing little to improve the statistics of 1961, which indicated that 82 per cent of the East Pakistan population was illiterate and 80 per cent of rural villages lacked primary schools.[96] Policies also favoured military and business classes, and the military gained enormous economic power while martial law "weakened the political elite and civil society."[97] The 1960s, then, had actually resulted in concentrating wealth amongst about two-dozen influential families, all West Pakistanis, who reputedly

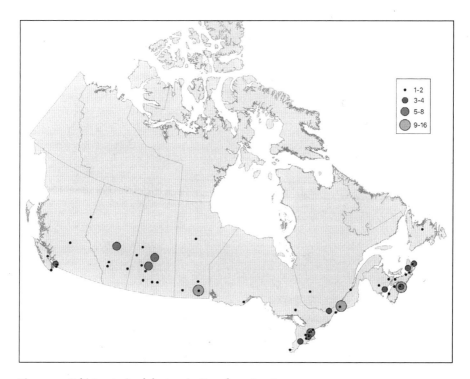

Figure 5.7 Pakistan-trained doctors in Canada, 1961–76

controlled two-thirds of all industrial assets and four-fifths of all bank assets.[98] The growing Bengali resentment in East Pakistan fuelled an opposition movement that embraced a program for self-government, growing into a mass struggle for independence in the final years of the 1960s. In the 1970 national elections East Pakistanis virtually all voted for the pros-overeigntist Awami League, thus controlling 167 of 313 seats in the National Assembly. The government attempted "to suppress Bengali nationalists by force," triggering a civil war that killed an estimated one million people and prompted migration of ten times that number.[99] The war gave birth to Bangladesh (formerly East Pakistan) but only after dragging (West) Pakistan and India into their third major post-Partition war, in 1971.

It was at this time that 140 Pakistan-trained[100] doctors settled in Canada. Their appearance as Muslim medical practitioners was somewhat novel. There were only two such doctors in 1961 and thirteen in 1966; by

1976 they were ten times as many, dotted across the country (see table 5.4) in almost every province and with a particularly surprising presence in Winnipeg.[101] There were also a dozen medical practitioners from Pakistan in the Halifax–Dartmouth area and in Montreal but very little presence in Toronto, Calgary, or Vancouver. There were surprisingly clusters in Prince Albert (Saskatchewan), the Sydney-Glace Bay area (Nova Scotia), and solo practitioners in small towns from Dawson Creek (British Columbia) to Grand Falls (Newfoundland). Most had originally graduated from medical schools at the University of Karachi or Punjab University in the years 1957–65, with smaller numbers from Lahore and Sind. As alluded to in an earlier chapter, a certain proportion of them had already left for advanced training in Britain when the racial backlash in that country combined with the deteriorating situation back home made remigration to Canada in the late 1960s a desirable professional option. As mentioned above, however, their reception was uneven, with their presence in the Maritimes and Prairie provinces in part a reflection of ongoing professional barriers and discrimination in Ontario and Quebec.

DIVERTED BY THE DRAFT

Canada, of course, was not the only option open to English-speaking medical practitioners choosing to emigrate or remigrate during the tumultuous years of the late 1960s. In fact, the United States, where the most technologically advanced research and clinical practice seemed to be taking place, had become the destination of choice for many globally minded practitioners. The United States, however, had been itself polarized by its entanglement and growing military presence in former French Indochina. Over time, the civil war in Vietnam became a proxy battle of the major superpowers, with the United States propping up the southern republic's leadership in Saigon and the Chinese (and to a lesser extent, the Soviets) backing Hanoi. As the 1960s wore on the Americans dedicated more and more troops to the conflict, eventually supplementing the regular forces with drafted young men. The United States Military Selective Service Act of 1967 stated that every male citizen over the age of eighteen years six months and under twenty-six years was liable for training and service in the armed forces. These draft protocols faced strong criticism, however, as accounts of higher draft rates of people of colour drew much public attention.[102] Nixon's "lottery system" in 1969 sought to end the perception of this inequality as well as cease the uncertainty men faced for the seven years between the ages of nineteen and twenty-six. Regardless of the process of randomization that a lottery entailed, there were a myriad of ways that people were able to avoid the draft. Those who tended to learn the tricks or had the means to dodge the draft through education tended to be the children of better-educated and wealthier families.[103]

While the randomized selection of able-bodied men would provide enough troops to fit the army's combat needs, highly skilled occupations – such as medicine – required another form of draft. Brigadier General Thomas J. Wheelan Jr, special assistant to the army surgeon general, warned that if the army was without a method other than the general lottery they would not have the means by which to acquire the necessary medical specialists.[104] As a result, despite the changes to the general draft selection in 1969, the medical draft of 1950, otherwise known as the "doctor draft," continued during the Vietnam era.[105] This federal statute inducted members of the medical profession into military service for assignment to the medical corps as commissioned officers. Under the Doctor's Draft Act doctors were given commissions commensurate with their age, ability, and experience.[106] The act required twenty-four months consecutive service unless the doctor, dentist, or allied health specialist was prematurely discharged or released.[107] The creditable occupations for fulfilling this obligation was service in one of the seven uniformed services consisting of the army, navy, marine corps, air force, coast guard, public health service, and working in the Indian health services or the environmental science services administration. Others might fulfil their requirements by conducting clinical research at the National Institute of Health in Bethesda, Maryland.[108] This substitute service was known in the United States as the Berry Plan.

Oral interviews of foreign-trained doctors indicate that many non-American nationals were motivated by the Vietnam turmoil to settle in Canada despite their professional preference to relocate to or remain in the United States. Dr Nemec, an Eastern European postgraduate trainee, remembers clearly that "I had to register [for the draft], it was compulsory and I got a classification, I don't remember now what it was, a letter and a number, classified as such and such and so I called them cause I said

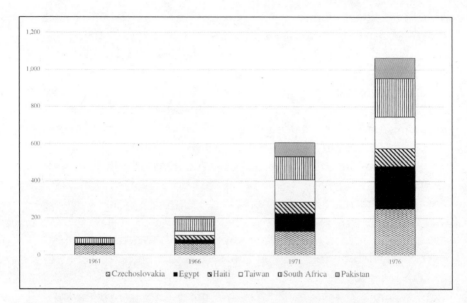

Figure 5.8 Immigrant doctors in Canada, select countries, 1961–76

what does this mean?" He at first did not understand how he could have possibly been drafted because he "thought … I was not a US citizen so how can you be drafted if you are not a US citizen?" He was told by the recruiter that there was little to worry about as he was probably "too old" to actually be drafted and that it was his impression that "not many US doctors were drafted." He felt that most of the great medical research was done in cities such as New York, Chicago, and Washington yet he did not want to sacrifice his family's quality of life for his own research opportunities. Although critical of Canada's transition towards socialized medicine, he resigned himself to moving north of the border. He reflected that he was not alone. Due to Vietnam, he recalled, "people were leaving."[109]

Dr Nemec's rhetorical question – How could I be drafted if I am not a US citizen? –raises an important component of the history of physician migration to Canada. According to US law, a person did not have to be a citizen of the United States to be eligible for the American doctor draft. The Military Selective Service Act of 1967 stated not only that every male citizen over the age of eighteen years six months and under twenty-six years was liable for training and service in the armed forces of the United

States but that, additionally, the same obligation applied to *all male non-citizens* of the same ages *who had been resident in the country for a year or more*.[110] In the case of physicians, dentists, and certain allied specialists, the upper age limit was raised to thirty-five for all those who had received an educational deferment.[111] The possibility of being drafted if one wished to stay in the United States after postgraduate studies as a doctor was a serious consideration. Such issues caused stress in the medical community among nonnationals. Another Czech doctor remembers his family fleeing the Warsaw Pact invasion of 1968. When his father and brothers arrived at the US embassy in Vienna, the immigration agent, assuming they were trenchant anticommunists, insisted that they commit to service in Vietnam before validating their applications. So put off were they by this that they decided to try their luck at the Canadian embassy.[112]

As word circulated in medical circles that foreign-trained doctors could be drafted for Vietnam, a number of defensive articles appeared in contemporary journals downplaying the effect of the doctors' draft in the hope that it would not dissuade doctors from immigrating to the United States. Dr Anthony Hall of the Department of Medicine of the University of Washington in Seattle, for example, wrote in the *British Medical Journal* that the draft was not actually as bad as it seemed. In response to a critical article written the previous year, he insisted that the author "has reminded us foreign physicians in the USA (with an immigrant rather than a visitor's visa) … are liable to be drafted for military service. This should not deter any potential immigrant. By most accounts military service can be a worth-while experience (life is what you make it!)." Hall insisted that foreign physicians were, in practice, rarely drafted; that even if they were technically drafted, it was unlikely that they would be posted overseas; and even if they were overseas there are plenty of places other than Vietnam. For good measure, he offered his observation that "The only doctor I know who has served in Vietnam … enjoyed the experience."[113]

Despite these upbeat assurances, Vietnam redirected scores of physicians to Canada and other countries who might otherwise have chosen the United States. Dr Taylor, a man born and raised in South Africa by British parents, returned to England for postgraduate medical training. When faced with the prospect of pursuing further training in the USA (as was the advice of some of his colleagues in England), he rather chose Canada primarily because of the Vietnam War. He did not, he readily insisted, "have any anti-American feelings ... but it was the time of Vietnam and I really disapproved strongly about [the] war."[114] "I had no sympathy for [the Vietnam War]," he continued, "and as for the domino theory which was what it would be, I thought it was just silly, it was beyond stupid ... And to lose how many men and countless civilians and I think it is a terrible mistake that the states made and I didn't want to be a part of it."[115] One of his good friends and former lab partners at Oxford had established himself in Canada and helped him imagine having a life in a country which he had not yet even visited. A Hungarian doctor was motivated to move to Canada for similar reasons. This physician never actually lived in the United States but considered it for a short time. "[W]ith the Vietnam War going on I didn't want to end up in the army," he admitted. One of his friends who had "graduated earlier, a fellow Hungarian, six months after he arrived in the United States he was drafted and was sent to Vietnam as a physician [and] he was serving on a ship in you know somewhere in Vietnam, so that wasn't very attractive." He knew that he could facilitate the acquisition of "[American] citizenship because [of] serving in the army, but no, no, no if you are a landed immigrant or whatever they will call and you would end up there before the year is over" and US citizenship was not worth the deployment. Ultimately, he decided that Canada would be a much better home for him and his young family.[116]

The Vietnam War ended in the spring of 1975. It is thus instructive to see how many foreign-trained doctors may have been biding their time in Canada before moving south. A rough proxy for the degree to which doctors settled permanently (or semipermanently) in their first place of residence and practice can be gleaned by comparing decanal cohorts from the CMDs under study. Using data from the select six countries, one finds that approximately 80 per cent of doctors in the 1966 cohort could be found in the *Canadian Medical Directory* ten years later in 1976, with a low of 74 per cent for the South Africans and a high of 84 per cent for the Taiwan-trained medics. The "missing" doctors could reflect return to their countries of training, to a third country, such as the United States, or reflect those who ceased to practice due to illness, retirement, or death. Nevertheless, the 80 per cent retention of these doctors within Canada offers a corrective to contemporary commentary that sometimes implies that foreign-trained doctors were merely opportunistic, relocating to

Canada temporarily as a steppingstone to the United States. According to CMD data, it was much more likely for foreign-trained doctors to relocate within Canada than to move again to a third country.

CONCLUSIONS

The period 1961 to 1976 fundamentally reconfigured the medical workforce in Canada. During the hearings on the Royal Commission on Health Services, Canadian medical leaders lamented the loss of Canadian medical graduates to the United States, which they estimated to be in the range of the equivalent of the total annual number of graduates of McGill University and the University of Toronto combined.[117] For the Canadian Medical Association and its provincial counterparts, this spelled doom and disaster for the future of any federally sponsored system of universal health insurance. And yet, a combination of hardening attitudes in Britain, changes to Canada's own immigration system, the emergence of the Vietnam War, and political upheaval around the world led to the recruitment and retention of thousands of doctors who were more than content to relocate to Canada. The medical workforce expanded at a faster rate than the general population.

By the time that provinces passed their enabling legislation pursuant to the Medical Care Act, certain ones – such as Newfoundland and Saskatchewan – had more foreign-trained doctors than graduates of Canadian medical schools.[118] These provinces also saw the ratios of residents to doctors converge with that of more prosperous provinces of the country. Others – such as Prince Edward Island and Quebec (particularly off the island of Montreal) – would have comparatively lower numbers of foreign-trained doctors. The total number of doctors increased dramatically, but the maldistribution of doctors did not appear to have changed fundamentally, at least on a national level, by the early 1970s. Contemporary studies began to emerge that claimed foreign medical graduates appeared to populate rural areas, small towns, and larger suburban/urban centres at more or less the same proportion as Canadian-trained graduates.[119] Only the three Prairie provinces appear to have been somewhat successful in recruiting *and retaining* foreign-trained doctors to smaller towns in greater proportions than

Canadian graduates. Chapters 7 and 8 take a closer look at the debates about maldistribution, the growing use of incentives, and how this relates to the problems servicing rural and remote areas including the regional industrial centres and emerging resource towns of Canada's new north. The next chapter addresses the growing recognition of the impact of physician migration on the countries left behind.

Chapter Six

The Brain Drain

Jonathan Murphy[1] admitted that he still tries to avoid entering his country of birth. Born and raised in the USA, he left America to begin his undergraduate medical studies in Dublin, since he considered himself "Irish American" and had relatives still living in the republic. He returned to Syracuse, New York as a medical intern but found himself in the middle of a polarizing national crisis over the escalating Vietnam War in the late 1960s. He had been active in the antiwar movement in Ireland and became quite involved on campus back at Syracuse, admitting that his position "wasn't very healthy." Ultimately, he received his draft notice. Deeply opposed to American military involvement in Southeast Asia, he found little bureaucratic trouble crossing the border into Canada. Unlike Australia and New Zealand, Canada had remained neutral during the conflict. He worked first as a junior medical staff in Montreal – arranged by some former classmates – and then in Newfoundland before finally settling in the Toronto area in response to an opportunity at a teaching hospital.[2]

In retrospect, he was content with his decision to leave the United States; he found Canadians "kinder and calmer ... and in general, it was just a very comfortable place."[3] The decision to dodge the draft, however, continued to affect his life long after he crossed the border. As happened to many of his compatriots who chose to flee to Canada, a grand jury trial indicted him as a felon *in absentia* for draft evasion and bail jumping. His outstanding warrants did not seem to pose a problem for medical licensure and practice in Canada, but he had reason to be nervous for some time to come about his status as a fugitive doctor. He claims that when he was a medical resident in Montreal, "the Mounties [the Royal Canadian Mounted Police] called several times, just to check that [he] was legally in Canada." Meanwhile, his family members in the United States were, according to him, "hounded by the FBI for about five years" after his departure. When he moved to Ontario and began work at his new hospital in Toronto, the Ontario College of Physicians and Surgeons (OCPS) requested his presence and informed him in person that he "'should be very careful.'" He guessed that perhaps the RCMP had contacted people at his hospital, yet his colleagues and the OCPS remained tight-lipped as to where they received their information. Even after President Jimmy Carter granted a general amnesty in 1977, which eliminated the draft dodging felony in the United States, the immigrant doctor avoided going south of the border, for fear of being arrested.[4]

Murphy was a small part of a larger story of the wave of Americans departing northward to avoid involvement and indirect support of American military intervention in Vietnam. Indeed, the migration of an estimated 125,000 Americans between 1966 and 1976 is well known in both countries.[5] For the purposes of this book, however, Murphy's story introduces the interconnectedness of Canadian medical immigration to broader geopolitical events of the post-WWII era. In this case, an American doctor left for moral and practical reasons: he opposed American involvement in Southeast Asia and undoubtedly did not want to die in his twenties or be placed in a situation where he was patching up other young men so that they could return to the fighting and be killed themselves. As mentioned in the previous chapter, the Vietnam War had a measurable impact on the net inflow and outflow of doctors and nurses. For a brief period of time, the century-long drain of medical minds, from Canada to the United States, reversed itself at the close of the 1960s.

In this respect, individual stories – sometimes mundane, other times marvellous – morph into a large story of global interconnectedness. Geopolitical events – the Hungarian uprising, the ascendancy of Duvalier in Haiti, the bloody Sri Lankan civil war, the expulsion of Asians from Uganda, the Troubles in Northern Ireland, the tragedy of Apartheid – all informed, directly or indirectly, the flow of doctors into Canada during the early years of Medicare. This chapter illuminates the intersection of personal choice, political upheaval, and global health care ethics. In the case of Murphy, it is unlikely that an American, partly trained in Ireland and then moving to Canada, had any appreciable impact on health care delivery in the most powerful nation in the world, which at the time boasted more than 300,000 doctors. By contrast, the aggregate decisions of hundreds of Indian, Pakistani, Ugandan, Haitian, and South African doctors immigrating to richer, industrialized countries did indeed have tangible effects on their countries of origins. As early as 1966–67, Canadian reporters were beginning to sense the broader impact of what was increasingly referred to as a medical brain drain. Citing a United Nations internal report John Hess, writing for the *Globe and Mail*, alerted readers that "Young physicians, nurses, scientists, engineers and teachers are abandoning poor countries for richer ones in growing numbers ... these people, needed in their homelands, are emigrating from the undeveloped countries, and from both these areas to North America."[6] This represents a "cruel doctor drain," commented the *Globe and Mail* during Canada's centenary year.[7]

DOCTORS ON THE MOVE

By the end of the 1960s, it was becoming clear, to those who were inclined to look, that thousands of doctors, nurses, and medical research scientists were on the move, transferring their education and skills – what economists termed "human capital" – between countries in a manner that was dizzying and difficult to quantify. Growing international recognition of this transnational phenomenon was nevertheless gaining attention at the highest levels. The World Health Organization estimated that in 1972 more than 140,000 of the world's physicians and 170,000 of the world's nurses were found in countries other than their native ones, and one half of these were living in the United States, the United Kingdom, and Canada.[8] With the emergence of immigration protocols focusing on highly skilled persons, however, anxieties over the brain drain became multidirectional and not simply focussed on the movement of "manpower" from the "developed" to the "developing" world, to use terms commonly deployed at the time. Britain and Canada, for example, both wealthy, English-speaking,[9] industrialized countries, were identified as both in the top ten countries receiving foreign-trained doctors *and* the top ten countries losing doctors to elsewhere. In this context, it was easy for political leaders to become inward looking in their conception of the competition for highly skilled labour, to perceive it as akin to a larger social Darwinistic competition between nation-states for "global talent."

Canada constituted an important node in this web of international migration; however, it was hardly alone in terms of filling gaps in health services by inducing foreign-trained medical practitioners to immigrate. Britain, as mentioned earlier in this book, had quietly accepted hundreds of Indian and Pakistani doctors to staff the National Health Service in the 1950s, as British-born "NHS refugees" left for North America. Some of these South Asian physicians would themselves remigrate to Canada and the United States. Meanwhile, the United States began receiving thousands of doctors and nurses from around the world from the mid-1960s to the early 1970s. By the mid-1970s, the US was home to a staggering 63,000 foreign-trained medical graduates, prompting the Bureau of Health Manpower, Education Division to comment how the rate of foreign medical graduates entering the country "has increased at a faster rate than domestic production ... [and that d]eveloping countries, particularly in the Far East, have become the principal sources of supply."[10] Their presence in the American system formed the basis of an important study on "alien doctors" and a concurrent debate about the desirability or not of foreign-trained doctors in the American health care system.[11]

The remigration of doctors inhibited a clear understanding of the magnitude of the problem at the time. However, researchers in the global north began to slowly piece together some of the broader trends and hint at the moral and ethical dimensions of health care migration. For example, health economist Rashi Fein argued in 1967 that it was the responsibility of the United States as a leading world power to encourage the thousands of foreign medical graduates already in America to return to their native lands following their advanced training. Of course, foreign-trained physicians could not be forced to return to their home countries. As Fein opined somewhat unhelpfully, "Immigration policy is complex and involves moral issues."[12] Fein's writings reflected the ambivalent feelings about America's increasing reliance on foreign-trained doctors, practitioners who posed a "risk" because they were "generally not as well trained."[13] Two years later, a 1969 monograph published by Harvard University's Margulies and Bloch presented a critical review of the subject of foreign medical graduate migration to the United States. They focused on the problem of foreign doctors who came to the United States for advanced training then failed to return to their home countries. The authors went so far as to state that the United States had in fact done

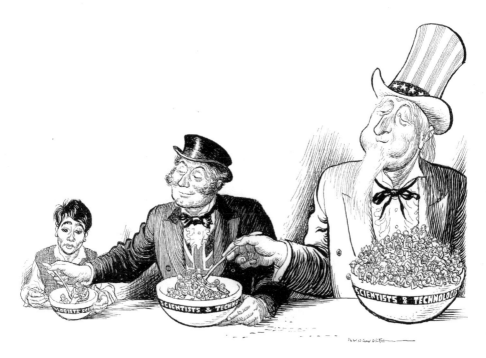

Figure 6.1 "To Him That Hath"
The drift of what was then termed "highly skilled manpower" from poorer to richer
countries did not go unnoticed by economists and policy makers interested in a field
that was then known as "development studies." The phenomenon – popularly known
as the brain drain – went beyond medical doctors and included research scientists,
engineers, and nurses. Here, the famous British syndicated cartoon *Punch* depicts
richer countries literally feeding off of the meals of poorer ones.

many international medical graduates (and their host countries) a favour
by providing them with advanced clinical experience and a familiarity
with First World technology that could be taken back with them to their
"less developed" countries. Like Fein, they recommended that programs
should be implemented whereby foreign medical graduates were encouraged to return to their countries of origin.[14]

In Canada, medical journals began to discuss the ambiguous situation
of foreign medical residents in Canadian university training programs
and the ambivalence of the Canadian medical profession toward the new
influx of foreign-trained physicians who were becoming their colleagues.

As early as 1966, A.D. Kelly, the general secretary of the Canadian Medical Association believed that such doctors had a moral obligation to return to their native countries. Yet he observed that many non-Canadian medical residents and fellows often proved reluctant to go back to "where they are needed."[15] The next year, at the new York University outside of Toronto, Lord Bowden, the dean of technology of the University of Manchester, made waves in Canada by criticizing the new immigration era which encouraged young, highly skilled professionals to emigrate from the Caribbean and South Asian to Britain and then from Britain to Canada and the United States. He blamed the space race and massive technological investment in the United States for starting off a chain reaction of migration of science and health sciences professionals.[16] During the same month, the federal deputy minister of manpower and immigration, Tom Kent, during a speech in Edmonton admitted that the new points system for immigration, being introduced in 1967, might very well "increase the gap between wealthier and poorer nations." By "recruiting skilled immigrants there is a danger," he acknowledged, "that we may attract people who the poorer nations can ill afford to lose."[17] As political commentators began to digest the new changes to immigration, the *Globe and Mail* would follow-up with an editorial in September of 1967 lamenting the brain drain that was building, questioning "What can be done to contain, if not reverse, the flow of doctors from needy countries?"[18]

In 1970, two further studies appeared which examined the international migration of skilled labour. One, headed by F.J. Van Hoek of the Institute of Social Studies (The Hague, Netherlands) recognized that scientific and technological developmentshad caused a gradual shift in emphasis from "labour-based" to "science-based" capital formation, which meant that there was an increasing demand for skilled and highly educated workers – especially engineers, scientists, and health care personnel – in the richer nations. Although it was exceedingly difficult to accurately measure the impact of physician emigration from developing countries simply because of the lack of statistical data, Van Hoek concluded, as Bowden had three years earlier, that the loss of physicians had inevitable detrimental effects on the development process. Van Hoek vaguely called for a "better educational policy in relation to manpower needs" in both the global north and south.[19] As Bloch and Margulies presciently concluded, "Although the poor will not become richer through better use of indigenous brain power alone, without it their prospects are very bleak indeed."[20]

A second study, in 1970, was authored by the "Committee on the International Migration of Talent" (CIMT), a team of economists and university professors from the United States with representatives from the International Bank for Reconstruction and Development, the Institute of International Education, the American Association for the Advancement of Science, and Education and World Affairs, a New York-based organization that oversaw cooperative initiatives between various American universities and countries in the industrializing world. Findings were presented from a two-year study, supported by the Rockefeller Foundation, that attempted to explain, region by region, the impact of the international migration of "highly-trained people." By this time, the term brain drain had become common journalistic shorthand for the transnational migration of highly trained professionals. However, the committee commented, somewhat defensively, that the popular use of this term seemed to "communicate an act of international wrongdoing."[21] Speaking more positively about the "supply of talent" in other countries, the CIMT study suggested that the impact of health human resource migration was not so much of a problem in countries like India – one of the leading so-called "donor countries" at the time – where, they believed, the annual output of that country's education system was sufficient to replace those physicians leaving for other parts of the world. However, in African nations, such as Tanzania and Kenya, which did not have as strong an educational system in place, the authors concluded that the depletion of health human resources was a much more serious matter. Like Van Hoek's work, the CIMT study lamented the lack of proper statistical information available for measuring the true impact of professional migration on these parts of the world.[22]

One of the most acute observers of the decision of doctors to migrate to so-called first world countries was Oscar Gish, a European-trained health economist based in the United States. His work attempted to tell part of the story from the foreign medical graduates' perspective, while at the same time investigating the economic impact of physician emigration on poorer countries. Between 1971 and 1977 he published three important monographs. In *Doctor Migration and World Health*, Gish thoroughly

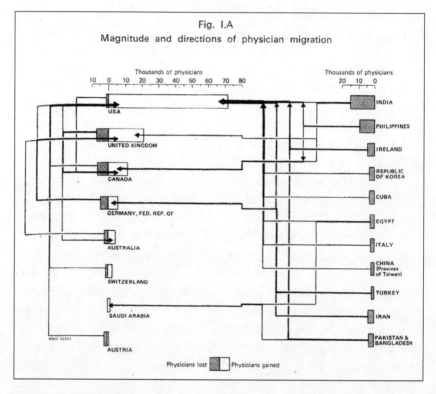

Figure 6.2 The Brain Drain
The complicated flow of doctors between poorer and industrialized countries, and between industrialized countries, proceeded at a dizzying pace. Contemporary observers
found it very difficult to determine precise numbers of those permanently settling
elsewhere or to represent the flow of professionals in any understandable manner. This
chart, from the World Health Organization, illustrates the complicated directionality.

examined each developing country in the context of its health care, providing a picture of the nuanced circumstances that contributed to a health
care worker's decision to leave his or her home country. His in-depth case
study of Ceylon (Sri Lanka), for example, was especially poignant in its
demonstration of the complexity of political, social, and economic factors
that left, in his opinion, some medical graduates no other alternative but
to leave their native country in search of better opportunities.[23] Gish
brought attention to the fact that the migration of health care personnel
had largely been ignored by economists and other scholars in order to

concentrate on other skilled groups, namely engineers and scientists. Whereas the study by the Committee on the International Migration of Talent described earlier made an attempt to explain the migration of many different types of skilled labour, Gish recognized that the complicated dynamics of health care services required separate (country by country and even region by region) scrutiny. For example, the CIMT study had suggested that India's annual educational output was large enough to supply talented professionals for both home and abroad. By erroneously clumping scientists, engineers, and medical personnel into one category they had glazed over the disparity of health care personnel between rural and urban areas. While this rural–urban divide was less of an issue for engineers and scientists (because there was not as large a demand for these professionals in rural areas), Gish observed that the rural–urban divide in health care services could not be solved by simply increasing the number of graduates a country produced annually.[24]

Gish's work provided strong empirical basis for the eventual findings of the landmark World Health Organization studies of the mid-1970s. He observed that there was considerable movement of physicians *between and among* industrialized countries – particularly Canada, Britain, and the United States – and a certain circulation of practitioners in the English-speaking Commonwealth. However, Gish also recognized that the general flow of foreign-born doctors exiting the global south was overwhelmingly towards more economically advantaged countries. Like Van Hoek's monograph of 1970, Gish suggested that the responsibility for this transnational migration (and the responsibility for diverting it) lay with the industrialised countries, like Canada, that preferred to use "high-level manpower" from "less-developed countries" because of the cost savings and efficiencies of doing so: the "fewer difficulties encountered if employment has to be terminated in the event of a decrease in demand or financial austerity."[25]

As the international literature on physician and nurse migration began to grow, the World Health Organization entered the fray, with major reports from 1972 onwards on the findings of a multinational study of physician and nurse migration. They were comprehensive studies (these reports were also consolidations of earlier findings over the preceding decade) in the understanding of the complex international movement of health care workers. The final report, which combined the findings of the previous three, was published in book form in 1979 as *Physician and Nurse Migration* under the lead authorship of Alfonso Mejía. Together, these reports were the first widely recognized work (the more obscure Gish and Van Hoek aside) to appreciate the complicated nature of international physician flow.[26]

The WHO's estimates were sobering. The industrializing countries of the world (except the People's Republic of China, for which no accurate data on population or physician numbers was available at the time) contained two-thirds of the world's population and possessed only a quarter of the world's physicians. Moreover, nearly 90 per cent of the world's migrant physicians were absorbed by the wealthiest nations. Predictably, the poorest countries were recognized as the big losers in the international flow of physicians. The WHO put to rest claims made in the late 1960s by Fein, Margulies, and Bloch, who asserted that additional training in "technologically advanced countries" such as the United States or Canada was beneficial for their native countries. According to the WHO, even if most foreign-born physicians did return home, physicians were not likely to benefit their home countries with their new-found skills and experience simply because of the disparity in health infrastructures and the technology gap between the so-called developed and developing nations.[27]

THE "DONOR" COUNTRIES

Understandably, countries that occupied the highest rungs on the list of "donor" countries had begun to complain bitterly about the medical brain drain to wealthier nations. Within this literature, the Indian medical community emerged as one of the most vocal critics. This was understandable: Indian doctors had become the largest group of diasporic doctors in the world. One report suggested that, by the mid-1970s, one in every two Indian-trained doctors were working outside the country. As mentioned in previous chapters, Indian doctors were staffing the British National Health Service in unprecedented numbers by the early 1960s. Using the UK's own General Medical Council data, the *Journal of the Indian Medical Association* (*JIMA*) estimated that there were approximately 1,600 Indian doctors in training courses in Britain in 1962, "of whom 400 had been there for more than five years."[28] Within Canada, there were just over 700 Indian-trained doctors in the country by 1976, making Indian doctors the second largest national group of foreign practitioners in Canada behind the British.[29]

The emigration of Indian doctors after Partition did not go unnoticed by the medical community back home, though there was considerable confusion as to its amplitude, its permanence, and its underlying causes. The *JIMA* began to track what appeared to be the rising number of Indian physicians residing in the United Kingdom from the mid-1950s. They reported with alarm not just the absolute numbers of Indian doctors training and working in other countries but also, perhaps more disturbingly, the intention of about half to settle permanently abroad. Within these emerging debates, Canada was singled out for particular criticism. The *Times of India* reported that the concern had reached political circles with the Indian minister of commerce, on a trade visit to Ottawa during 1967, complaining about the rising emigration of "Indian doctors and other professionally skilled people" to Canada and other "advanced" countries. He argued that the "'brain drain' cannot be reduced … unless the developed countries also co-operate … instead of welcoming them en masse as at present."[30]

Ironically, some of the problems of physician migration had been exacerbated by the very bilateral programs that were supposed to increase capacity in developing countries. For example, the United States had been active in reconstruction programs in Western Europe in the postwar period and had taken part in bilateral or regional development programs. The Fulbright Act of 1946 provided educational assistance to students in the "developing world" with specialized skills, while the Smith-Mundt Act of 1948 created an exchange visa program that gave professionals the chance to train in the United States.[31] Doctors were one of the largest groups of skilled workers on such exchange visas, the stated purpose of which was bilateral knowledge transfer rather than permanent resettlement.[32] The United States was also an early participant (and the only non-Commonwealth member) of the Colombo Plan for Co-operative Economic Development in South and Southeast Asia, a multilateral development plan established in 1950. The Colombo Plan facilitated the temporary exchange of scientists and technical workers, including health

care practitioners, within South Asia and from South Asian countries to
Britain, North America, and Australasia.[33] Too often, these graduate students and fellows were simply not returning home. Reflecting on the ethical dimensions of the movement of health care practitioners from India
to the industrialized north, one American researcher observed that "The
loss of large numbers of physicians is something developing countries
cannot really afford. Each physician represents an 18 to 20-year educational investment by both the individual and the country."[34]

Concern over the growing problem of this Indian brain drain prompted
international foundations and governments to fund comprehensive
studies of the problem. In response to the early recognition of the loss of
doctors (and also engineers) to wealthier nations, the Ford Foundation
provided financial support for the Indian government to create the Institute of Applied Manpower Research (IAMR) in Delhi, which was founded
in 1962.[35] The IAMR issued reports and surveys of regional and occupational labour and in 1965 introduced its own *Manpower Journal*.[36] One of
its first reports was tellingly entitled *Migration of Indian Engineers, Scientists and Physicians to the United States* (1968) and was followed by two
studies on Indian physicians and scientists residing temporarily in the
United States.[37] The so-called "Stock Study" reported on the characteristics of Indian physicians in the United States, relying predominantly on
American Medical Association data; the equivalent study for scientists
used data from the National Register of the National Science Foundation.[38]

The problem, unsurprisingly, was that there was no systematic tracking
of the *emigration* of Indian physicians and scientists from India. Nevertheless, the group undertook an unusual and rather painstaking study of
passports issued to "highly-educated" Indians from 1960 to 1967. The second phase of the study was an attempt to locate the migrants abroad and
evaluate their movements and intentions. In 1970, the institute published
the *"Brain Drain" Study*, which concluded that

The percentage of gross outflow to total outturn [*sic*] is indeed
striking in the case of Engineers; and more so, in the case of Medical Doctors. In the case of Engineers, the gross outflow was equal,
on average, to about one-fifth of the total outturn [domestic production from Engineering Schools]; and in the case of Medical

Doctors it was, on average, more than one-fourth of the total out-turn. The percentages of gross outflow to the total outturn in 1966 and 1967 are much higher than the average percentages over the eight-year period in the case of both categories and suggest the possibility of a sharply increasing trend in the outflow of Engineers and Medical Doctors.[39]

The analysis showed that, for the period 1960–67, engineers were the largest single group of trained professionals granted passports for long-term departures (44 per cent), followed by doctors (24 per cent). Indeed, passports had been issued to 27 per cent of the 38,709 doctors who graduated in India during the period under study. The outflow of nurses, teachers, veterinary scientists, and postgraduate scientists was significant but comparatively less severe.[40] As the study conceded, the methodology was somewhat suspect: not all passport holders necessarily went abroad, and some did return. Using data from the Indian section of the National Register, it was estimated that more than half of scientific and technical personnel reported returning to India during that time. Medical doctors had an estimated 58 per cent rate of return (6,153 vs 4,455 remaining abroad).[41] The study called for further investigation of the outflow of doctors and an attempt to produce a "qualitative profile of Indians abroad."[42] Nevertheless, many Indian commentators were rueful in the face of addressing the country's public health needs while hundreds of doctors were leaving for the West: "It is interesting to note," lamented one commentator, as he sensed the transnational domino effect of physician migration, "that doctors from low income countries are migrating to high income countries and as our doctors are migrating to England about 400 English doctors are annually leaving their home to set up practice in countries like United States, Canada, and Australia."[43]

The solution, however, was less than straightforward. This same commentator suggested a type of compulsory "national service" for those who wanted, ultimately, to study abroad. More radically, he even mused that passports could be withheld from Indian practitioners who would not "give an undertaking to return home."[44] However, the author acknowledged that this would be largely unworkable and ineffective, since most of those migrating were specialists and research scientists and the most pressing need in India was for general practitioners working in the villages. Despite this observation, for twelve months starting November 1964 it does appear that the Ministry of External Affairs in India imposed some restrictions on the extension of passport facilities to doctors, dentists, surgeons, and nurses. However, for reasons that are unclear, the measure appears to have been only temporary: the annual number of passports issued to medical doctors dropped from 1,186 in 1964 to 992 in 1965 before rebounding to 2,064 in 1966.[45]

A more inventive measure was to attempt to prevent Indian physicians from taking the foreign medical graduate examination required to practice or pursue graduate studies in the United States. When India passed a law against this exam in 1970, 500 Indian doctors travelled to Sri Lanka and joined 400 Sri Lankan physicians taking the exam.[46] The following year, the examination was banned in Sri Lanka for the same reason. Subsequently, 1,100 Indian physicians applied to the Education Council for Medical Graduate Examinations organized by the Malaysian American Commission. Only 500 were able to successfully make the trip to Kuala Lumpur.[47] In this cat-and-mouse game, the Indian government was at a distinct disadvantage. Reciprocal agreements between Britain's General Medical Council and most Canadian provinces,[48] and between Canadian provinces and many American states, facilitated the licensing of Indian-trained physicians in North America, particularly those who had already gained experience and residency in the United Kingdom.[49] Thus, Indian-trained physicians would migrate to Britain for postgraduate or fellowship training, work for a few years in the British hospital system, become qualified and registered under the General Medical Council of Britain, and then use this accreditation to migrate to a Canadian province or an American state in need of doctors. Faced with an almost impossible situation to regulate, the Indian government introduced incentives to attempt to entice scientists, technologists, and physicians to return home.[50] To ease the transition back, the government provided returning physicians with guaranteed temporary work with the Union Public Service Commission and offered "special aid" to those establishing clinics, especially in rural areas.[51] It appears to have yielded some results. From 1958–67 just under 800 doctors had apparently returned home to work.[52]

DICTATORS AND DOCTORS

Far removed from the outmigration of Indian doctors from the subcontinent, upheavals in the French Caribbean also directly affected physician migration to North America during this period. The same year as the Hospital Insurance and Diagnostic Services Act (1957) set the stage for universal health insurance in Canada, Haiti witnessed the ascension of a new president, Francois (Papa Doc) Duvalier. Duvalier was born into Haiti's elite class in Port-au-Prince fifty years earlier, completing his medical training at the University of Haiti School of Medicine. Duvalier demonstrated diverse interests in academic research, becoming a published ethnologist and, eventually, a member of a small group who wrote the influential political journal *Les Griots*. The group was embarrassed by the American occupation of Haiti from 1915 to 1934 and furious with their upper-class peers for accepting the state of affairs without protest or resistance.[53] Through his growing activism, Duvalier became drawn more and more to political life. He served as minister of health under transition presidencies of the 1950s. After being elected in 1957 he began consolidating his power and eliminating opponents. In 1964 he named himself "President for Life."[54]

Duvalier's regime turned violent and brutal. After the formalization of his dictatorship, Papa Doc and his son Jean-Claude presided over three decades of "vicious repression, martial law, violence and political assassinations."[55] A secret militia not only intimidated citizens but killed tens of thousands in state-sponsored violence. Despite his own medical training and membership in the Haitian professional middle class, Duvalier targeted elite families, educated professionals, and university students. Perhaps his anger towards them for remaining silent during the American occupation was a starting point for his resentment. On a more strategic level, however, educated Haitians were more likely to be anti-Duvalierists, and his political opponents were largely drawn from these elites.[56] Clearing the country of influential individuals thus allowed Duvalier to strengthen his control over the population. As a consequence, engineers, scientists, and doctors began to stream out of the country by the end of the 1960s. They would be followed by tens of thousands of poor Haitians.[57] As Sean Mills has observed, these Haitians would form an important Caribbean diaspora in Montreal during a tumultuous time in the political history of Quebec itself.[58]

Quebec became a natural destination for many of these French-speaking migrant medical practitioners. The Haitian middle class would have had multiple generational connections with Quebec society due to the longstanding work of French Canadian missionaries on the island.[59] The presence of these doctors can be seen clearly in the entries of the Canadian medical directories of the time. There were approximately one hundred Haitian-trained doctors[60] in the 1971 and 1976 editions, almost of all whom were listed as resident in Montreal and, more unusually, Joliette. In the late 1960s, there were rumoured to be as many as 150 Haitian doctors, not all of whom were fully licensed. It was an oft-cited statistic, verging on urban myth, that by the early 1970s there were more Haitian doctors in Montreal than in all of Haiti itself.

Haiti's small medical community dated from a national medical school that had first began granting degrees in 1870. Over the course of the first half of the twentieth century, many physicians completed their medical training (or engaged in postgraduate training) in France. There thereby emerged a distancing between the middle-class western-oriented medical practitioners and the poor population, 95 per cent of whom were struggling in poverty. Indeed, the "westernized" medical elite was regarded with resentment and a degree of suspicion by the general population, who felt that they catered to a small cadre of wealthy foreigners during and after the American Marine occupation of the island.[61] While Duvalier first targeted the elites, his rule became increasingly more oppressive to Haitians of all socioeconomic backgrounds. In this way, the skilled and professional Haitian émigrés were soon joined in the 1970s by a second, larger migration of poorer, Creole-speaking families. Interestingly, the tensions and mistrust of the general population towards the elite French-speaking medical professionals re-emerged in Montreal where Haitian medical practitioners of colour were doubly marginalized – from the Québécois and anglophone medical establishment as well as from their newly arrived compatriots.

The targeting of Haitian professionals by Duvalier arose from a complicated mix of political calculation, class tensions as well as racialization of Haitian society (since a good part of the Haitian elite were labelled *mulatto*).[62] Indeed, Duvalier used *noirisme* (a type of racial pride and

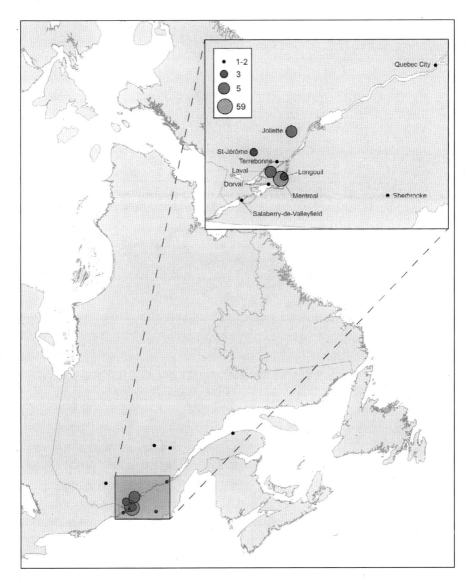

Figure 6.3 Haitian-trained doctors in Quebec, 1961–76

nationalism) to recognize Haiti's African roots and engender resentment amongst the Creole-speaking working class towards the mixed-race, French-speaking elite families. One sees parallels in another racially justified (if politically calculating) forced migration – namely the expulsion of "Asians" from Uganda in 1971–72. Idi Amin, who had seized power in January 1971, engaging in a bloody purge of opponents that would rival the brutality of Duvalier. By 1972, having consolidated power, Amin moved to isolate and expropriate the properties of 80,000 Asian Ugandans. These families – predominantly ethnic Indians many of whom had been born in the country – included numbers of professionals who would flee to Britain, Canada, and the United States as their property and businesses were expropriated in Amin's "Africanization" project of ethnic cleansing. At least a dozen doctors, all trained at Makerere University[63] (Kampala), would appear on the Canadian registers as medical practitioners (mostly in the greater Toronto area) by 1976.

OUT OF AFRICA

Perhaps the archetype of physician migration to escape political repression lay in the case of South African physicians who, by the end of the twentieth century, would replace Indians as the most significant group of migratory global physicians. Understandably, much of the literature on the history of South African medicine in the second half of the twentieth century has been framed by the long shadow cast by Apartheid.[64] By the 1950s, nonwhite ethnocultural groups were assigned to residential areas and ethnically based "homelands" or Bantustans. By 1970 this process had had dramatic demographic effects, with nearly seven million "Africans" being resettled.[65] Hospital and medical training in post-WWII South Africa reflected the shocking inequalities of the country itself. The health care system was fragmented among a multitude of departments of health and welfare for the Bantustans as well as municipal and provincial authorities.[66] By contrast, membership in private health insurance schemes was restricted to the white population.[67] There was a stark urban–rural divide in the availability of primary care; moreover, the medical labour force manifested a gross maldistribution of doctors.[68] While 40 per cent of the population lived in the Bantustans, they were served by only 3 per cent of the country's doctors.[69] As Anne Digby has observed, "The fractured spaces of apartheid South Africa meant that whilst a third-world standard of health care was more generally experienced in overpopulated rural Bantustans, the Republic maintained 'high tech' hospitals of first-world standard" in the urban centres.[70]

Medical training was also not immune to the changing fortunes of Apartheid. By the early 1950s there were five principal medical schools in South Africa: (1) the University of Witwatersrand (Johannesburg); (2) the University of Cape Town; (3) Pretoria University; (4) the University of Stellenbosch; and (5) the University of Natal (Durban). The medical traditions of each school were framed by language, tradition, race, and religion. The universities of Cape Town and Witwatersrand were "English" insofar as they featured a British-style medical curriculum with English-language instruction. They were open to women medical students and, until 1959, a small number (about a dozen) of Indian and black African students. Jews made up approximately one-third of the student population of these "open" universities. By contrast, Pretoria University and the University of Stellenbosch were considered to be "Afrikaans," both by language of instruction and political orientation. "African" and "Coloured" medical candidates, two dominant racial classifications of the time, were shut out of these institutions and instead found their options increasingly narrowed to the University of Natal, the unofficial "nonwhite" training ground for medical practitioners in the country.[71] A small minority of nonwhite medical candidates might find training outside of the country – in neighbouring countries (if African) or in India (if Indo South African). But this presumed the means and opportunity to do so and graduates risked nonrecognition of credentials when they returned to South Africa.

The racial segregation of medical education in South Africa was by the 1950s deeply entrenched and becoming increasingly polarized and polarizing. From 1959 onwards, blacks admitted to the "English" medical schools "had to make an individual application to get ministerial consent" to attend.[72] For those nonwhite medical students who did attend the "open" universities, the quality of their education was compromised by segregated clinical and pathological experience as well as limited internship opportunities.[73] Black doctors faced further obstacles after graduation and were expected to serve their own racial groups, mostly in rural

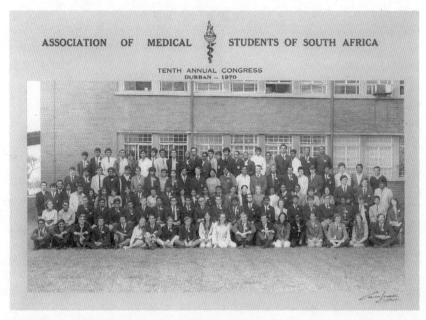

Figure 6.4 Association of Medical Students of South Africa, 1970
The turmoil of the late 1960s created situations in which young doctors eagerly left their
countries of origin for the perceived stability of Canada. This photograph of the Association of Medical Students of South Africa meeting in Durban, 1970, occurred in the second last year that an integrated multiracial association was permitted under Apartheid.
Several of the South African doctors pictured here would end up settling in Canada.
No fewer than three South African grads would eventually become deans of Canadian
medical schools.

areas and the Bantustans. Many were required, by virtue of government
scholarships, to take up public positions where they faced further discrimination and professional restrictions both in terms of low salaries
and poor conditions of service.[74] Private practice offered somewhat better
prospects and many black doctors worked as general practitioners, albeit
restricted by the permit system, Group Areas Act, and with unequal access
to hospitals.[75]

Like New Zealand, there was a longstanding tradition of English-
speaking South African doctors completing an undergraduate degree at
home and then going abroad after completing their internships for postgraduate and/or fellowship training.[76] Some of these graduating doctors,

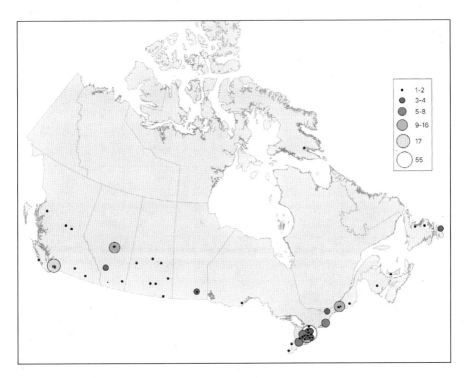

Figure 6.5 South African–trained doctors in Canada, 1961–76

of course, had family connections in other countries such as Britain; others had been supervised as undergraduates by British-trained medical faculty who no doubt provided encouragement and professional connections. Going to the famous British teaching hospitals for the status and experience had a certain cachet, if a family could afford it. As a consequence, some South African medical graduates found themselves in Britain amongst a diverse set of "colonials" – Indians, New Zealanders, Australians, Canadians – travelling to Britain for postgraduate training in the 1950s. However, as Britain lost its lustre in the postwar period, South Africans increasingly looked to the United States and Canada. Some even went abroad for brief electives, prior to their graduation, in order to seek out possibilities. As one South African interviewee recalled, "during our medical school training we had a 3-month block of an elective period and a large number [of students], I would say about, at least 50% or 60% … went abroad with the specific intention of making some sort of connection in North America."[77]

The doctors who permanently left South Africa in the 1960s and 1970s were small in number, as compared to the large numbers who would migrate in the 1990s.[78] Most of these so-called "pre-Soweto" emigrants were English-speaking and Jewish, coming from families who had fled Lithuania at the turn of the twentieth century, desperately escaping the Eastern European pogroms. Following the Sharpeville massacre of 1961 many of these Jewish South Africans felt that the "writing was on the wall." As the government's Apartheid policy tightened, the doctor trainees felt caught between the Afrikaans government and the black majority, being trusted by neither. As one recalled, "I guess growing up in South Africa, we always knew that there were problems. My anticipation was that there would be a violent revolution in South Africa. I always felt uncomfortable living in that environment. I felt that I wanted to move from the country. So, right initially, I saw medicine as a vehicle to move out – as an international passport to move out of the country."[79] As the situation in South Africa became increasingly tense, many used their medical degrees as such "international passports" to leave the country for Canada, United States, Australia, and Britain on a semipermanent basis. Most would not return. For some, the irony of remigration to escape persecution, as their grandparents had done at the dawn of the twentieth century, was part of a larger transgenerational narrative. As one ruefully remarked, "When the trouble gets bad enough, we Jews need to be first on the boats to leave."[80]

MULTIPLE AND COMPETING BRAIN DRAINS

By the middle of the 1970s the concept and broad contours of the brain drain had manifested themselves across the globe. But apart from academic reports, the occasional political rebuke, and a series of position papers from the World Health Organization, the problem did not coalesce into any major international initiatives or policy response from the "recipient" countries. This can be attributed to a number of factors. The first complicating factor was the unpredictable movement of the physicians themselves. While plenty of statistical information was available regarding the inflow of migrating physicians to wealthy countries, the emigration records of developing countries (or still less, from countries suffering civil war and dictatorships) were fragmented, if they existed at all. Social scientists had to piece together the larger puzzle by working backwards from data generated by the wealthier nations. In addition, this poorly understood drain of resources was often assumed by scholars to be only temporary. It was frequently assumed that many foreign-born or -trained physicians who had migrated would eventually return home following a period of additional or "advanced" training, certain to come back when political unrest had died down in their countries of origin.[81] The reality was that most of these physicians settled abroad permanently or migrated to other countries in the wealthy Commonwealth and global north.

Complicating matters, as Gish first demonstrated, was the phenomenon of certain developed countries – like Britain and Canada – being in the then top nations as both donor *and* recipient countries owing to their status as countries used as stepping stones to elsewhere. In these cases, nations simultaneously received physicians from abroad while they themselves were losing health human resources to medical migration. Indeed, a 1968 report prepared by the United States and submitted to the Organisation for Economic Co-operation and Development (OECD) identified Canada as the principal "country of transit" towards America for research scientists during the first half of the 1960s. Though these research scientists, in contrast to the doctors, were predominantly from Northern Europe.[82] Both Britain and Canada considered themselves to be suffering from their own brain drain of doctors and research scientists, thus contributing to a global competition for highly skilled professionals that had increasingly high stakes.[83]

There were also a small number of countries that began *supporting* the migration of physicians either for geopolitical or economic reasons. Fidel Castro, for example, embarked on a self-conscious policy of training physicians for export, particularly to Latin America, a "medical internationalism" designed to showcase the positive outcomes of his socialist politics.[84] As mentioned earlier in this book, Ireland reconciled itself to the fact that many physicians would leave for elsewhere by generating a capacity to graduate more doctors than the country could absorb. Exporting physicians to the world became a source of almost national pride.[85] Finally, in a manner analogous to its support of nurse and caregiver migration, the Philippines appears to have encouraged the out-migration of physicians (and, on a much larger scale, nurses and homecare workers) in order to facilitate the flow of hundreds of millions of dollars of remittances.[86] Private medical colleges – particularly for the training of nonnationals – began to multiply in the Caribbean. Within this context of globalization, a new cohort of "international" doctors – intending to move transnationally – became established.

Finally, there seems to have been an implicit understanding that it was ultimately the individual physician's choice to leave his or her home country. This ethic of personal mobility removed moral culpability from developed countries and shielded them from accusations of "stealing" or "poaching" medical personnel. As health economist to the World Health Organization Alfonso Mejia put it, "Learned men (and women) have always travelled abroad seeking a more congenial intellectual milieu to realise their full potential."[87] Framed like this, the physician's decision to migrate was understood to be a very *personal* calculation based upon a unique set of factors for each individual, the prevention or prohibition of which would itself be both impossible and unethical in its own right. How could the postwar "Western world" embrace refugees and economic migrants but deny the right of educated individuals to better their own personal situations? Oscar Gish described both sides of the moral dilemma for the physician migrating from developing countries in his discussion of the term brain drain itself: "The term itself conjures up images of highly sophisticated men (and women) who choose to work in countries other than those in which they were born. Because of such images feelings of great loss may be held by countries being 'drained of brains'. On the other hand ... spirited defences of the free movement of great men (and women) are made in the name of freedom as well as in the interest of maximizing the output of world science and/or economic output."[88] Thus even those who were coming to understand the magnitude of the problem recoiled from suggesting interventionist measures to stop it or, alternately, measures of compensation. There appeared to be a conceptual chasm: how could thousands of defensible individual moral decisions constitute one large collective ethical problem?

The conceptual leap – from an individualistic orientation which framed ethical issues within the doctor–patient relationship to a conception of ethics that began to think of collective rights and identify problems of *global* social justice – simply did not gain traction in the period under study for this book. Bioethics as a discipline was, for the longest time, rooted in moral dilemmas arising from the increasing use of medical technologies. As a discipline, it was thus preoccupied with clinical-ethical issues such as informed consent. The term "global health" – with all its ambiguity and emphasis on interconnectedness – began to be used regularly in health sciences literature only in the 1990s.[89] The transnational migration of health workers clearly falls within this "global" realm of thinking and outside the traditional discourses of bioethics that dominated the 1970s. It is unsurprising, then, that countries, like the United States, Canada, and Great Britain, replete with other potential issues of historical compensation and reparations that were going unattended (slavery in the United States; the treatment of Indigenous peoples in Canada; the multiple impacts of colonialism in Britain), would pay scant attention to creating policy remedies in response to the self-evident economic gains of physician migration.

BLOODSHED AND BELONGING

Although the impact on "donor countries" did not figure prominently in mainstream national policy discussions before the 1990s, that is not to say that the moral framework of migration – of leaving one's country and its patients – did not emerge repeatedly in the personal reflections of physicians interviewed for this book. Quite the contrary, the lament of loss and regret – the self-reflection and, at times, self-questioning – run deep in the oral interviews of physicians who left countries in turmoil for opportunities in Canada. This was nowhere more pronounced than in the case of South African doctors. As one expat recalled, "[W]e also thought one day that this [Apartheid] is going to come to an end and there is going to be tremendous bloodshed."[90] Many agreed with her that few South African doctors fleeing the country could have anticipated the release of Nelson Mandela and a nonviolent transition to black majority rule by the ANC. Other South African-trained doctors openly expressed regret or how they were troubled by their own decision to leave South Africa and not to assist more actively in the worsening health care situation of the 1990s as Southern Africa became overwhelmed by the chaos and tragedy of the AIDS epidemic. Considering their own affluence and success in Canada with the plight of those who remained despite the troubles and challenges of the transition of South Africa out of Apartheid generated no small amount of guilt. Many could not help but reflect on the relatively nonurgent cases they dealt with on a daily basis in Canada while the South African system lurched from crisis to crisis. As one South African doctor recalled in a mixture of self-effacing humour laced with regret,

> So I went back last year to give some talks at University of Cape Town and a guy came up to me afterwards and said "Hey, we were in the same class together!" He introduced himself and I said, "I remember the name, I don't remember the face," because this is a long time back. I said, "What do you do?" He said, "I went to London to do some training and I missed South Africa so much that I went back and I bought a farm in the top northwest corner of the Transvaal …" He said, "And I have a private practice in paediatrics and I have a farm and I make some money. That money pays for a school for the kids in the area because they have terrible education and it pays for [an NGO] which runs the school and free AIDS treatment centre." I said, "Shit, you make me feel guilty!"[91]

In a similar way, oral histories with elderly, mostly retired South Asian doctors, some of whom lived through the trauma of Partition in 1947 during their youth, elicited a complicated and layered reflection on their life's trajectories. Most would say their successful careers and their opportunity to raise a family in Canada was "lucky in retrospect."[92] Few expected to settle permanently in Canada; most having left for England for what they had originally thought would be a relatively short period of time for advanced training. Some, however, were forthcoming about life's regrets and the sense of taking an "easier" path to Canada rather than returning to help build up the health system in their native countries. One Indian woman doctor remembers bargaining with God: if he got her into medical school, she would return to India and dedicate her life to a rural village. While "originally you expected to go back … all that idealism was there. But then I didn't do it because I got married and came here [to Canada]."[93] She spoke openly about how she failed to keep her "side of the deal." Her husband, also a doctor, was similarly torn on this issue.

"Materialism gets into your blood," he acknowledged somewhat ruefully about the success and wealth he accrued as a surgeon in North America. "Not everyone can be a Gandhi."[94]

CONCLUSIONS

The postwar history of immigration to Canada has often been framed as a larger narrative towards a "race blind" system based on "merit," a first and progressive step towards a pluralistic, multicultural society. There is much to be said for this interpretation. After 1967, Canada became the destination for hundreds of thousands of immigrants from countries that had been largely denied entry for much of the twentieth century. However, the points system that accompanied the early years of Medicare also facilitated, indeed encouraged, the rapid relocation of highly skilled health care practitioners that had been trained elsewhere. Canada, like Britain, began to ramp up the recruitment of doctors and nurses, particularly to solve the problem of the maldistribution of health care personnel in their respective countries. In this new era of national competition for highly skilled immigrants, Canada, it was thought, could not afford to stand on the sidelines.

It would be unfair to say that nothing was proposed or initiated to counter the loss of health care practitioners to Canada. Some universities embarked on outreach training projects in niche areas. For example, as early as 1966 the University of Toronto, with the financial support of the Department of External Aid, engaged in a mental health project in the West Indies sending Canadian-trained psychiatrists, psychologists, and social workers to Trinidad and Tobago to build local capacity.[95] Other Canadian medical schools and some powerful hospitals also engaged in similar bilateral agreements, often inspired by foreign-trained practitioners who had resettled in Canada but remained deeply cognizant of problems "back at home." Certain newspapers – even the *Globe and Mail* – encouraged Canadian institutions to help abroad. Following the clarion call of John F. Kennedy several years earlier, the editors even briefly proposed a "medical Peace Corps."[96] Nonetheless, these measures were often limited to small, and often time-limited, bilateral training agreements that scarcely addressed the magnitude of the transnational movement towards the industrialized West.

While the liberalization of medical immigration requirements was spurred by population growth, the implementation of Medicare, and the concomitant shortage of doctors felt across the country, this "shortage" did not magically disappear once the immigration taps were opened and foreign-trained physicians flooded in. Previous chapters have pointed out how important the medical diasporas and Canada's "brain gain" were in terms of the overall accessibility of physicians and the need to expand the medical school system to train more doctors. As we will see in the next two chapters, they were also perceived to be important to rural and remote health care, although the willingness of policymakers to take the needs of "sparsely settled regions" into account when adjusting the levers of medical immigration, varied widely.

Chapter Seven

Satisfying Rural Health Needs

As a medical student, Paul Minc remembers being deeply inspired by the stories told and written by Sir Wilfred Grenfell and his famous medical mission to the deep-sea fishers along the northern Newfoundland and the Labrador coasts.[1] Grenfell was an alumnus of Royal London Hospital, the same school where Paul Minc had trained. His stories left such an impression that a young and newly minted Dr Minc set off for Canada almost immediately upon graduation. Initially, he left to answer an advertisement for physicians to work in rural Newfoundland and Labrador as part of a new Cottage Hospital Medical Service. This program was established by the midcentury government of Joey Smallwood to serve outport communities along the vast coastal reaches of the new Canadian province,[2] and Minc found this type of medical work suited him. After spending several years as a cottage hospital doctor, he moved to Nova Scotia's Bay of Fundy region in 1959 and became resident physician to the fishing villages of Long Island and Brier Island. Occasionally, he would get called to treat visiting fishermen from Grand Manan, as well as tanker fishermen returning from the George's Banks off the coast of Maine. He relocated in 1965 to a practice in Sault Ste Marie in Ontario, and then in 1981 he moved again to a rural dairying area close to Trenton in the eastern part of the province. There he stayed until a final move to Guelph in 2004. Occupying five family practices over a half century in Canada, Dr Paul Minc looked back with contentment on his active professional life. But echoing other British-trained physicians represented in this book, he complained that he originally left for Canada because "the NHS did not provide the opportunity to practice full care medicine that we had been trained for, whereas in Canada it was possible to obtain the facilities to provide good care."[3]

For such physicians, the decision to pursue rural and remote health care preceded the decision to emigrate. Once licensed to practice in Canada, physicians willing or even desiring to work in nonurban areas found ample scope for practice across the far-flung geographies of Canada. These might include small Atlantic fishing islands and outports, eastern Ontario dairying communities, as well as reservations in Canada's north. Despite such opportunities, Dr Minc's Canadian story is remarkable for its transience. While most other physicians interviewed for this project moved practices twice or sometimes three times before settling into a long-term arrangement, Paul Minc moved five times, each time to fill a different kind of service need in a different part of rural Canada. Did physicians like him find the facilities to "provide good care" in every new stop on the way?

For foreign-trained physicians intent on general practice in rural and remote areas, the opportunities were many because the need was great. This chapter surveys the use of foreign-trained physicians to service such communities across the country, blending policy analyses with on-the-ground accounts of service challenges. The staggering diversity of "rural" life in Canada complicates this story significantly. And the approaches to managing care in rural areas, including the difficulty of recruiting and retaining health practitioners, could vary by region and be influenced by social class, gender, ethnicity, and race. From the 1950s to the 1970s, we see the problem evolve in the minds of Canadians from a systemic problem of servicing "sparsely-settled areas" to one that saw service access by geography as a more "localized" problem that should be best addressed by bolstering community resources and enhancing provincial supports to attract physicians to a certain area. Briefs brought before the Hall Commission situated the geographic disparities of physician distribution in terms of overall access to newly licensed doctors, both from medical schools and through immigration. Calls to action focused on managing supply for the entire system. By the 1970s, however, supply management had created expensive and "overdoctored" populations, largely in the wealthy urban areas of the country. In order to manage costs, measures to increase supply of physicians through education and immigration were abandoned at the expense of "underdoctored" populations, usually located in more rural and poorer provinces. Policymakers with an expertise in rural health care, mostly from the Prairie provinces, protested but in vain. The perceived problem of "overdoctoring" dominated public policy discourse to the degree that federal government economists began to claim that, among their own ranks, "everyone hates an immigrant physician."[4]

DOCTOR DISTRIBUTION AND RURAL HEALTH

Meeting the incipient demand for doctor care was high on the list of priorities for Emmett Hall and his Royal Commission on Health Services (1961–64). As they travelled across the country, they heard briefs that underscored a deep anxiety about physician access. Physician organizations and community groups presented briefs that voiced a variety of concerns about the problems inherent in servicing rural and remote communities. But the health services among the provinces also diverged in their prioritization of ways to address the need. Not only had health services – whether organized by provincial governments, local municipalities, or voluntary organizations – evolved differently among the jurisdictions, there were significant regional variations of what "rural and remote" communities looked like and who lived in them. This variation among provinces and regions made it extremely difficult to plan and enact a Canada-wide strategy for rural and remote health care or even for provinces to work together to address this common problem. Unsurprisingly, there was also little consensus on what role foreign-trained physicians might play, or what role they could play, in alleviating the special pressures on rural and remote care.

Some of the strongest community briefs on rural health care and related concerns came from agrarian parts of Canada like Saskatchewan. Nonetheless, "rural" life in Saskatchewan was fundamentally different from "rural" life in Prince Edward Island, and the distribution of physicians reflected this. Of the 908 physicians in Saskatchewan in 1961, 282 (31 per cent) practiced in rural areas, and of those rural-based clinicians twelve were in government service, held research or administrative positions, or were practicing a specialty.[5] Compared to Prince Edward Island, forty-four (49 per cent) of the ninety physicians in the province held practices in the rural and small towns, and only two of those were specialists.[6]

Social norms influenced health care access, and subsequent expectations on doctors were deeply embedded in local culture. This exacerbated statistical differences in the rural–urban physician distribution. With almost half of their membership in small town private practice, the Medical Society of Prince Edward Island[7] did not think residents suffered from lack of physician access, estimating that "no resident of this province lives farther than fifteen miles from medical services"[8] and the geographic distribution of hospital beds in the scattered community hospitals was "satisfactory."[9] But local custom required general practitioners to travel and make house calls in order to draw and hold a practice. While many had office hours and looked after patients in the small rural hospitals, more time was spent in arduous travel. The very first problem the Medical Society raised was the workload of rural physicians, practitioners they described as "overburdened" and "carrying an excessive work load."[10] Prince Edward Island was not an easy or desirable location for new physicians (of seventy-five PEI-born medical graduates in the previous decade, only forty-four had registered in PEI),[11] even though the Department of Health had provided support by making laboratory and x-ray diagnostic facilities available to all physicians, as well as tuberculosis, cancer, and mental health diagnostic clinics.[12]

Small community hospitals over these decades supported a wide range of surgical facilities in order to attract specialists to their areas. O'Leary, a small village on the western rural end of the province serving a rural population in Prince County of approximately 4,000, was home to a general hospital that had offered a wide range of surgical services since the interwar period. With the physician shortage of the late 1960s, surgical and obstetrical patients were moved to nearby Alberton (population 1,100) or twenty kilometres away to the larger town of Summerside (12,000). Over 1973–74, however, the small community welcomed two physicians, a married couple who not only established a collaborative practice but started their family in the community. Dr Terrance and Dr Prem Verma, with their respective training in general surgery and obstetrics/gynaecology and anaesthesiology, effectively restored the full range of clinical services to the western end of the Island.[13] Both were experienced doctors. Terrance Verma trained in Burma but pursued surgical training in the UK and qualified as a member of the Royal College of Surgeons of England and the Royal College of Surgeons of Edinburgh. He originally came to Canada in 1973 to work as a resident at the Isaac Walton Killam Children's Hospital in Halifax but relocated to O'Leary a year later. Prem Verma took her medical degree at the University of Indore, India and had an active practice in India for many years before coming to Canada with her husband. She took specialist training in anaesthesiology while in Halifax and added that to their joint rural practice when the couple eventually relocated across the Northumberland Strait.

Calling for studies to alleviate health services demands and attract more clinicians like the Vermas, the PEI Medical Society focused on bringing the structure of amenities available to rural practitioners in line with urban doctors. Key among these was improving communication and transportation, training and utilizing more paramedical services, and "[e]stablishing a pattern of practice whereby the responsibility of bringing the patient to the physician rests upon the family or community."[14] When pressed for details about why most Island physicians were overworked, Dr Clarence Coady admitted that most were likely taking on too much medical work themselves instead of involving nursing services and other health professionals. But to manage some of the winter travel conditions, he suggested "helicopters, [and] snowmobiles when travelling conditions are difficult ... modern means of communications might assist the physicians here, such as walkie-talkie."[15] He and other members of the society also agreed that mechanisms for "attracting physicians to low income rural areas"[16] would also benefit the province. While some communities had already provided housing and office facilities to recruit resident physicians, this was beyond the means of some impoverished areas. "We will endorse any measures which may be undertaken," they stated, "to promote the supply of medical personnel to the rural areas where need exists."[17]

By contrast, house calls were rare in the Prairie province and the burden of travel largely fell on the prairie patient. This was influenced by the distribution of physician services. In Saskatchewan the physician per population was 1:990 in 1961, but this ranged from 1:760 in Regina to 1:1906 in Yorkton to 1:3130 in the northern reaches of the province. Most rural physicians in a Saskatchewan private practice worked almost exclusively out of a county hospital system, which meant the service was more institutionalized, even in rural areas. Indeed, rural health outreach tended to take the form of targeted programs. Perhaps more than most other provinces, the Saskatchewan government had made very generous attempts to offset the disparity of opportunity in rural and urban areas, including air ambulance services, travelling clinics that brought general medical but also dental and specialist care to the countryside, public health nursing services, and a "scattering of outpost hospitals and institutions of one kind or another."[18] And yet, the distribution and social organization of physician services as part of a rural hospital system meant a lot of travel for farm families. For this reason, the "farmer on the farm is at a disadvantage to the urban dweller in availability of health care services," the farmer's union of the Saskatchewan Wheat Pool wrote in their Royal Commission brief, "Not only does the farmer have to travel longer distances to get to health centres but sometimes he experiences inconveniences in acquiring treatment once he does reach the urban centre merely because he is from the country ... longer wait times to see a physician on arrival."[19]

The problem of serving "sparsely settled areas" also plagued wealthier provinces with large aggregate physician populations. The Ontario Public Health Association reported that "some of the more remote areas of the Province ... do not have sufficient medical service ... And hospital care is not so readily available in the more sparsely populated areas." This resulted in pernicious public health problems in rural parts of the province, like higher rates of infant mortality.[20] Professional organizations responded by calling for subsidies for private practices. And such calls were not limited to general practice. The province's dentists also called on government action in the form of tuition subsidies to incentivize rural dental practices and called on local communities to encourage dentists to locate in their area by offering free facilities.[21] In very underserved areas, the province could consider providing mobile dentistry service, salaried by the government.[22]

The OMA was opposed to a single-payer plan and was defensive about the shortcomings of the provincial system. Indeed, the provincial medical association was loathe to suggest incentivizing rural medical practices or interference in the medical economics of rural areas. "First in regard to availability of medical care," they wrote in their brief, "we would state our opinion that in Ontario medical care is at present available to all citizens having only regard to geographic circumstances."[23] Spokesperson Dr Bruce-Lockhart argued that the province did not have a shortage overall, only problems of distribution and shortages in certain fields such as mental health.[24] "Ideally, we would like to have the doctor with the right training in the right place at the right time to render required services," the OMA acknowledged in their submission, arguing that "[t]his visualizes not only a proper geographical distribution but also an appropriate balance between the number of specialists and general practitioners as well as among the various specialties."[25] Ultimately, the provincial association believed that any Ontarian who sought medical services would be able to obtain them, even if some might have to travel farther than others. The OMA representative Bruce-Lockhart wrote argued that Ontario patients were well served: "with modern means of transport they are probably closer on a time basis than in any period of our history."[26]

Nonetheless, the association promised to undertake a special study to "seek information" about rural physician access.[27] Studying this problem was challenging because of the variables influencing the location of private practices in such a large provincial jurisdiction. The OMA observed that educational and recreational facilities were superior in urban and suburban areas, and new physicians were attracted to "the calibre of the house and office available" as well as "the diagnostic, consultative and hospital facilities." Younger graduates were used to hospitals, and most "junior intern and specialist training programs, are of necessity located in the larger cities." This was why a disproportionate number of doctors start practice in these larger centres. But there were also structural disincentives, including "too large a work load but one not sufficiently large to warrant a partner." The difficulty getting time off, and hence a lack of opportunity for postgraduate training, made rural practice "a less than satisfying experience" for new physicians graduating at midcentury.[28]

MEDICAL (IN)MIGRATION: OPEN BORDERS AND "CLOSED SHOPS"

The mobility of physicians over the span of a career factored into discussions about rural health care, even as physician mobility became a hot policy topic. Young foreign medical graduates were already well utilized throughout the Canadian system, including rural areas, by the 1950s. Between 1951 and 1954, 708 immigrant physicians came to Canada, and the majority of them were between the ages of twenty-five and forty-four.[29] But the doctor shortage precipitated by the advent of Medicare meant even urban areas had difficulty satisfying physicians in such a competitive environment for their services. Physician mobility accelerated in this period; many medical societies across the country began to worry openly about losing physicians to opportunities in other provinces and south of the border.

Back in Ontario, in an attempt to understand the dynamics behind physician location, the OMA surveyed classes of first-year medical students in Ontario Universities in the 1950–51 term. The survey included questions about present and future personnel requirements. Of new graduates, "47% came from the five largest cities, and 35% from the remainder of the province. Only 27% are now practising in the large cities, and only 25% in other areas of the province ... Of the remaining 47% more than half are practising outside the province (chiefly overseas, in the United States, and in British Columbia), and 23% are not licensed to practise in Ontario [drop-outs or registered elsewhere]."[30]

Next, the OMA surveyed physicians in practice. In the lead-up to the Royal Commission hearings it had sent a questionnaire to fifty-seven branch societies, received twenty-three back, and tabulated sixteen for the Hall Commission. From these results, the OMA concluded that the problem of underserviced areas lay with the communities themselves: "The large cities contribute more students to medical schools than they get back in the form of graduates. The same is true but to a lesser degree, of the smaller centres."[31] While the numbers of surgeons was healthy, Ontario needed to plan for shortages in several specialties and, of course, "persuading [doctors] to practice in the smaller centres," which included Sudbury, a city experiencing significant wait times for a hospital bed.[32]

From these results, the OMA claimed to lose many recent graduates to salaried positions in the United States, anywhere from 13 per cent to 30 per cent of Ontario's medical school graduates over the 1960s. In fact, they claimed, "the annual loss of Canadian-born and educated physicians to the United States as immigrants is ... roughly the equivalent of the total annual graduating class of University of Toronto and McGill combined."[33] While income for "self-employed physicians" in private practice in Canada and the United States were comparable as of 1961 census, salaried positions in the United States were better compensated. According to the OMA, these were significantly higher, as much as 50 per cent to 75 per cent as compared to Canadian positions. Citing "[m]uch correspondence and interviews with Canadian-educated physicians in the United States," the OMA was of the opinion that many new graduates would prefer to return to Canada, but low income dissuaded them.[34] Ultimately, the primary reason why rural and remote areas of Ontario struggled to find practitioners was recruitment. "The province-wide trend to urbanization which is reflected in the large proportion of medical students coming from large centres and showing little inclination to practice in the smaller communities, the majority of graduates of foreign medical schools have stayed in the larger cities where there are more of their fellow countrymen."[35]

Other provinces also saw a regional reliance on foreign-trained physicians and, sometimes, credentialing new doctors created tensions between provincial governments and local medical societies. In the 1950s, the Alberta government threatened to take over the licensing of medical doctors from the provincial medical society. The government was keen to break what they described as a "virtual closed shop" of medical practice and grant licenses to postwar displaced persons who came to Canada with medical degrees.[36] Alberta would join Saskatchewan, Manitoba, Nova Scotia, Prince Edward Island, and Newfoundland and guarantee reciprocal registration privileges to British-trained doctors licensed with general Medical Council of Great Britain (GMC) and the medical licensing authorities in Alberta and Saskatchewan. Elsewhere, even with a GMC qualification, a new graduate sometimes needed to pass a License of the Medical Council of Canada (LMCC) examination.[37]

New Brunswick was the only one of the poorer provinces in Canada who kept a very tight control on their medical marketplace despite long-standing problems underservicing rural areas, especially the francophone north.[38] The distribution of doctors and health services could vary widely, and such areas had come to rely on outpost nursing stations for their health care needs since the 1920s.[39] Along with British Columbia, Ontario, and Quebec, the province did not automatically recognize the licenses of foreign-trained physicians, even those registered with the GMC. At the same time, the jurisdiction was very reliant on external institutions to supply the province with physicians; like Prince Edward Island, the province had no local medical school and relied on graduates from elsewhere, principally Dalhousie and (later) Memorial, to provide new doctors.[40] Credentialing was the sole prerogative of the Medical Council of the provincial College of Physicians and Surgeons, a body that preferred to grant new graduates and recruits a two-year transitional "enabling certificate"

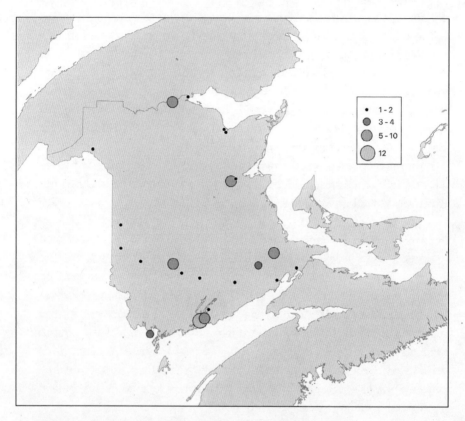

Figure 7.1 Map of foreign-trained doctors in New Brunswick, 1961

before allowing a prospective doctor to sit the LMCC exam and enter into a New Brunswick practice. As shown in previous chapters, it should come as no surprise that this was one of the Canadian provinces to benefit least from the midcentury surge of foreign-trained physicians. But it did, ultimately, benefit along with the rest of Canadian jurisdictions. In this context, how was the distribution of physicians affected by medical immigration in such a province? And did the medical immigration benefit rural and underserviced areas?

In 1961, just over 14 per cent of the registered physicians in New Brunswick declared medical degrees from outside Canada.[41] Of these sixty-two doctors that we know to be foreign-trained, 26 per cent (sixteen) received undergraduate medical training in the United Kingdom, with approxi-

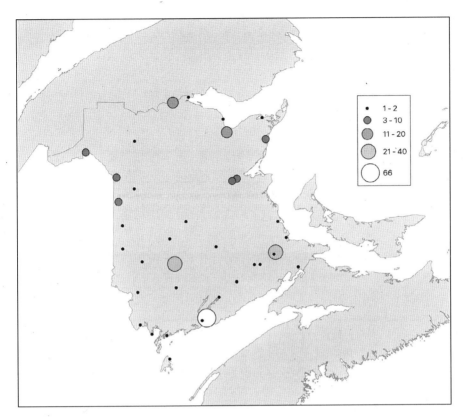

Figure 7.2 Map of foreign-trained doctors in New Brunswick, 1976

mately another 20 per cent from countries belonging to the Commonwealth (seven physicians from Ireland, two from South Africa, and three
from Australia). Twenty-one physicians (just less than 35 per cent) came
from other European nations, while only about 8 per cent (five physicians) were American-trained. This cohort includes a single immigrant
doctor trained in India and another trained in Jamaica. The diversity of
European physicians is striking. A healthy contingent of ten doctors hailed
from Eastern Europe: Estonia (four), Hungary (four), Czechoslovakia
(two). And another twelve come from an assortment of western European
nations: Netherlands (one), Italy (three), Switzerland (one), Austria (two),
Germany (two), Denmark (one), France (one) and Yugoslavia (one). Those
from Eastern Europe, almost to a person, graduated from medical schools

before 1945, suggesting that they emigrated as a result of displacements caused by the Second World War. The doctors from the former western European states, on the other hand, were more likely to have been recent graduates, with degrees from the 1950s.

When considering place of practice, foreign-trained physicians can be divided as a group between those with Anglo-American and Commonwealth training and the rest. Thirteen physicians with foreign credentials from continental Europe worked in the Provincial Hospital for Veterans in Lancaster, New Brunswick. This is where we find three of the four physicians from Estonia and eleven others from both Eastern and Western Europe. A similar situation existed in the tuberculosis sanatoria in the province. Three European-trained physicians were attendant physicians at the Jordan Sanatorium in The Glades and another three at the tuberculosis hospital in Saint John. Those from the UK or Commonwealth countries, on the other hand, tended to end up in private practices, which may or may not have a hospital affiliation. These were distributed rather evenly throughout the rural and urban sites of New Brunswick, from St John (twelve), Fredericton (eight), and Moncton (nine) to the Acadian north shore in Campbellton (five), Vallee Lourdes (one), Ste Basil (one), and Dalhousie (two). Overall, the distribution of foreign-trained physicians through New Brunswick in 1961 illustrate that 52 per cent (thirty-seven) were in the metropolitan areas of the province (including Lancaster) and 48 per cent (twenty-four) in the small towns and rural areas (including those who worked in the technically rural environment of the Jordan Sanatorium).

By 1976, the number and proportion of foreign-trained physicians in New Brunswick had grown to 241 doctors, now comprising almost a third (29 per cent) of the 741 registered members of the medical profession in the province.[42] Patterns of hospital building become even more evident, while there are some significant changes to the rural–urban split. Physicians generally clustered closer to the general hospitals, which were evolving into regional health centres. More than half (51 per cent) of foreign-trained physicians were located in nonurban areas of the province, a higher proportion than we observed for 1961. But the institutionalization trend accelerated. This means that while Saint John (sixty-three), Fredericton (twenty-five), and Moncton (thirty-five) continued to benefit from concentrated clusters of doctors with foreign medical degrees, we see smaller but still significant clusters in towns emerging as regional health centres, such as Bathurst (fifteen) and Campbellton (eighteen). Additionally, physicians with foreign credentials were finding their way to new areas of the province, like the northwest county of Madawaska. Traditionally served by graduates of McGill and Laval, the francophone communities of Grand Falls (three), Edmundston (nine), and Chatham (six) now seemed to equally rely on foreign-trained physicians to staff their local clinics and community hospitals.

GIVE US YOUR BRITISH DOCTORS

Not only were foreign-trained medical graduates welcomed into tightly controlled provincial systems, they were increasingly recruited by representatives of the Canadian Medical Association, representatives who often attempted to guide such physicians into rural service. In 1957 the general secretary of the CMA, A.D. Kelly, penned a recruitment article for the *British Medical Journal*. "Canada," he declared to the new graduates of British medical schools, "is well along the road of transformation from an agricultural to an industrial economy, with the consequent trend towards urbanization."[43] This made the country a prime destination for British physicians who were intent on relocating either temporarily or permanently. And though emigration was a prospect not to be taken lightly, there was space to explore medical careers off the urban beaten path.[44] "Opportunities arise most frequently," he explained to *BMJ* readers, "in the more sparsely settled rural areas and in the new communities which open up as the natural resources are progressively developed," he explained. Such regions, like New Brunswick's small hospital centres of Campbellton, Dalhousie, and Bathurst and the rural areas like Tracadie, Bath, and Petit-Rocher. While considering family interests, Kelly encouraged the young British doctors reading the journal to consider these options. "A well-qualified general practitioner who is prepared to accept the rigorous conditions and the scant amenities of such locations can establish himself in practice," he ended, especially if they demonstrate "a high degree of resourcefulness and training."[45]

Other articles rejected this rosy picture of rural Canadian medical prospects. A subsequent *BMJ* editorial evaluated careers in Canadian rural public health with a great degree of circumspection. Compared to Britain, BMJ editors explained, public health administration in Canada was woefully underfunded. Even though many provinces had established rural health units to cover the population in outlying areas, "closer study reveals that many of these outlying units are understaffed or staffed by general practitioners who are working on a part-time basis." Indeed, they warned, "[t]he local medical officer of health in Canada does not enjoy the respect that his professional colleagues accord to clinical consultants and specialists."[46] Newfoundland, New Brunswick, and Nova Scotia were "under-doctored" provinces, along with the Yukon and Northwest Territories. And, while they agreed with Kelly's recruitment pitch several years earlier that many provinces had reciprocity with the British Medical Register, other provinces, they noted, such as Quebec and British Columbia, "present obstacles to the British immigrant doctor in the form of residential requirements or very high fees."[47]

Private practice, on the other hand, held more promise. General practitioners wishing to move to Canada and practice in outlying areas had the prospect to do so. Nonetheless, new graduates were encouraged to consider differences in scope of practice and interprofessional relations. Immigrant physicians "should remember that domiciliary midwives are almost unknown outside Newfoundland, and that it is difficult to build a good general practice in most parts of Canada to-day unless one is competent to one's own obstetrics." Still, it was not necessary to buy out a local resident doctor. Service scarcity being what it was, the average British graduate could "simply to put up one's plate" and get started. The group practice model was uncommon in Canada, even in the larger urban centres, but established practitioners sometimes hired assistants and junior partners. For the new graduate from Britain determined to emigrate, "Either form of association would be invaluable in learning Canadian ways," and in terms of finding such an opportunity they noted, "the Canadian Medical Association ... or its Provincial Divisions would be helpful in finding such a position."[48] As discussed in chapter 2, most of the British professionals' editorials from midcentury worried about losing physicians to other jurisdictions in the British Commonwealth.[49] Indeed, in the 1950s one author complained that "our medical manpower loss over a nine-year period is equivalent to the total GP and specialist services of the cities of Manchester, Leeds, Liverpool, Sheffield, and Bristol combined."[50]

The trend continued into the first half of the 1970s. As discussed in a previous chapter, British commentators did not consider Canada a land of unlimited opportunity later in the decade.[51] But the opportunities that still existed tended to present in rural and remote locations. Along with research fellowships and residency training opportunities, the possibility to "experience the rigors and pleasures of practice in a remote community" were one of the chief "pleasures and advantages" of emigration.[52] They may offer adventure and excitement in remote or unusual places or where a given practice might be "more humdrum" but definitely well paid when compared to salaries in Britain: "The very fact that they may be in Yellowknife or Thunder Bay rather than Tunbridge Wells or Glasgow makes them more interesting."[53] As one 1977 report astutely observed, "the restrictions on where individual doctors may practice are less than those under the National Health Service ... the opportunities for local misalignment of supply and demand are considerable."[54] Local shortages in rural areas provided ample and ongoing possibilities, in other words, for British-trained graduates over the better part of three decades.

OVERDOCTORING AND UNDERDOCTORING:
"LOCALIZING" THE PROBLEM

By the mid-1970s, professors in the University of Manitoba's Faculty of Medicine observed that the public discussion about the doctor shortage had "come full circle."[55] With the sudden realization that there may be too many physicians within Canada's borders, a debate took shape around the issue of rural and remote health care. One side argued that a physician oversupply would be good for underservices communities, effectively "pushing" doctors to outlying regions and "perhaps even encouraging emigration to where medicos are needed instead of draining them from those places."[56] But, on the other hand, some government planners worried the glut would merely cause physicians to "overdoctor" some populations and areas and, as a result, overbill the new Medicare system. The points awarded immigrating physicians were gradually retracted and the flow of doctors came to a sudden halt.

We have shown how concerns about maldistribution were increasingly voiced from central Canada, and from Ottawa, earlier in the decade. But a more detailed nuanced examination of this issue, which by the 1970s became a regional debate, sheds more light on the specific concerns of rural and remote physician access. Those who advanced arguments premised on the "maldistribution" problem ultimately shifted the national conversation about rural and remote health care in ways that absolved the federal government in particular, and the mostly urban/southern legislators of larger provinces by extension, from taking any real action. In this last section of this chapter we critically revisit these policy debates from this perspective.

Political economist Freda Hawkins noted that Canada admitted 987 physicians and surgeons, fifty-five dentists, 749 medical and dental technicians, and 1,538 other professionals in the health services field in 1971–72, many, she observed, "from developing countries." While the federal government was satisfied "that the supply of doctors is perfectly adequate," she lamented that physicians were nonetheless still "badly distributed."[57] For instance, more than half the immigrants that came to Canada in 1973 went to Ontario and most of those to urban parts of the province.[58] By 1972, the federal government had inaugurated a medical service inventory as part of the Health Manpower Directorate organized under the Department of National Health and Welfare. This directorate would analyse the inventory in order to better predict the national need for more physicians. In the early 1970s, this included select specialties such as internists, neurologists, and obstetricians, but it also included general practitioners. The inventory analysts soon saw signs of oversupply of all kinds of practitioners in British Columbia and Ontario, and as a result, by 1973, the messaging about physician access from the federal government began to shift. Director General of Health Manpower W.S. Hacon began to press for target physician population ratios for Canada. One year later, in a conference of provincial health ministers, the "impending physician surplus" emerged as an official political problem. The possibility of restricting the immigration of foreign medical graduates was a hot button issue and an increasingly publicized concern; as a consequence, the occupational points awarded to physicians applying for Canadian immigration were removed from the regulations of the Manpower and Immigration Act.

One of the federal policymakers leading this change was Robert G. Evans, the political scientist at the University of British Columbia who has featured prominently in previous chapters. Evans observed the troubling signs that the physician "stock" was growing more quickly than the Canadian population.[59] Examining the data on the maldistribution problem, and working within that framework, he claimed the foreign-trained physicians were simply not going into areas where there was a critical need for more doctors. Indeed, he compared census data to physician registration data, looked at the number of general practitioners and specialists, and broke these categories down further by place of training. His results suggested that, in most Canadian provinces, foreign-trained medical graduates were more likely than Canadian-trained physicians to enter specialty practices than general practices.

But other research pointed out important exceptions to this trend. One is the case of New Brunswick, above. In Manitoba and Alberta, between 1968 and 1974, foreign graduates were more likely than Canadian graduates to enter general practice. Thus, there were many critics of this position, especially in the Canadian west, including Noralou Noos and her colleagues in the Faculty of Medicine at the University of Manitoba. Back in Manitoba, the struggle to recruit and retain physicians to rural and remote areas continued. Noos and her colleagues lamented the ineffectiveness of national health insurance for automatically alleviating a country's physician distribution problems, writing how "It is sometimes assumed that universal medical coverage will enable the poor and rural residents to buy more medical services and hence attract more physicians to the underdoctored areas ... However, Canada's experience demonstrates that while universal coverage gives the underdoctored areas more money to spend on health services, it provides the same benefits to the overdoctored areas, and little fundamental shift in the distribution of physicians takes place."[60]

While data from across the country was difficult to acquire for a national analysis, there was ample evidence that in Manitoba, Alberta, and Saskatchewan the fall of population–physician ratios was more rapid in the rural areas than in urban areas. This can be seen as a desirable redistribution. This was due to population shifts from rural to urban areas as well as to physician movement. In Ontario, the province with one of the greatest increases in physician supply, the gap between the relatively underdoctored north and the potentially overdoctored south actually widened over 1961–71. Moreover, while about half of recent Canadian graduates entering general practice were locating outside metropolitan areas, these graduates were disproportionately choosing nonmetropolitan

areas in British Columbia and Ontario. This exacerbated the interprovincial distribution problem at the same time as it may have been alleviating urban–rural inequities.[61]

Prairie critics were not alone. Even in provinces like Ontario there was
no consensus on the reasons behind and the solution to the maldistribution problem. Rural health experts worried about "turning off the taps"
of immigration. In this wealthy and largely well-serviced jurisdiction, a
lack of rural and remote health service was evidence that immigrant physicians needed more love than Evans's research might suggest. In 1972, for
instance, two clinicians at McMaster University, William Spaulding and
Walter Spitzer, examined the distribution of physicians across Ontario.
While certainly some areas like Kingston had a population to physician
ratio of 1:296, most parts of southern nonmetropolitan areas of Ontario
had a much wider ratio of 1:1722, comparable or even worse than the ratios
in Canada's poorest provinces like Newfoundland and New Brunswick.[62]
Indeed, the province of Ontario had, over the early 1970s, implemented a
program of incentive grants and contracts that attracted 255 physicians to
practice in 157 rural and isolated communities. Such researchers claimed
that if a physician could access a new medical facility, the chance of them
staying when the incentive ran out was more than 80 per cent.[63]

Still, the province of Ontario looked to the restrictions to physician
movement imposed by British Columbia and considered taking similar
measures. As discussed further in chapter 9, British Columbia adopted
specific measures to halt the licensing of foreign medical graduates unless
they were relocating to "underdoctored areas."[64] This was understandably
controversial, and the Human Rights Commission was beginning to question the legality of such arrangements. The impact on the equitable distribution of physicians would be profound and "the prairie provinces and
the Maritimes will be forced," they wrote, "to become even more dependent upon foreign trained physicians and/or turn to other mechanisms for
retaining their own graduates and providing services to the rural areas"
such as incentives and compulsory service.[65] By the mid-1970s, policy analysts began to claim that service access problems could be addressed by
increasing "less highly trained" personnel, principally nurse practitioners
and new types of nursing assistants, writing "The solution to local shortages and inadequacies will not be found simply by increasing the overall

supply of health manpower ... [focusing on] the poor economic, poor social, poor work and poor professional environments."[66]

The solution to the physician distribution problem increasingly turned the attention of policymakers and researchers to local solutions. From its 1972 inception, the Health Manpower Directorate tried to understand the factors that might influence physicians to move into "special work areas"[67] including rural and remote locations across the country. The directorate's policy position was that with reported gains in the overall number of physicians in the country Canada need no longer rely on foreign-trained physicians. "Provincial licensing authorities," one federal researcher suggested, "could perhaps assist by granting conditional licenses to immigrants and others from outside the province requiring them to work in underserviced areas for certain periods of time."[68] It was not just a matter of the appropriate numbers but also the right mix and implementing the best incentives to draw doctors into rural and remote health care.

Many provinces began to encourage communities to build clinics and offer other incentives to attract doctors, putting schemes in place to make it financially lucrative for newly graduated (or in the case of IMGS, newly licensed and arrived) practitioners to locate in rural and remote areas. Others focused on improving the public health infrastructure that had drawn criticism from commentators in Britain. Ontario's Underserviced Area Program, for example, dated from 1969, and other provinces were using some form of direct economic incentive by the early 1980s. In these systems, doctors were paid extra to practice in rural "special work areas."[69] Hoping to focus on younger (and thus presumably more mobile) practitioners, five provinces[70] had also implemented loan forgiveness programs by this period.[71] Saskatchewan set up ambulatory care and dental care programs in underserviced areas, and physicians relocating to some parts of northern Ontario were guaranteed a minimum annual income. In addition, Ontario had a summer medical student employment program, implemented a program to subsidize students for a return of service in underserved communities, and arranged with universities to organize health services or clinics in underserved areas. By the late 1970s, New Brunswick offered cash resettlement grants to dentists and was considering extending that to doctors. And Newfoundland enrolled "health manpower" into government service and arranged for new medical graduates and the newly licensed physicians that still came in from abroad to work in underserviced areas as provincial employees.[72]

CONCLUSIONS

Social scientists, medical economists, rural health advocates, and policy-makers debated whether these strategies had had a positive effect on the geographies of health care or would improve physician access in the future. While some dismissed them as having "only minimal effect in attracting physicians to these areas,"[73] others more generously concluded that it was "more effective than previous research has indicated" and better than doing nothing at all.[74] All agreed that such incentives and improvements were insufficient to solve the problem entirely. Despite the shifting discourses among provincial ministers of health, many in rural areas continued to speak of a doctor shortage throughout the 1980s. The public too often conflated access with supply and continued to characterize the longstanding maldistribution of physicians as a "shortage."[75] But this is likely because there were so many persistent "local shortages." The macrolevers of power would not be pulled for the interests of sparsely settled areas of Canada. In fact, the whole conversation about supply and demand had shifted to focus on provincial and local agency.

With these intractable challenges, federal government authorities in effect passed the problem of physician access entirely off to their provincial counterparts. It was the provinces, not the federal government, who were in the best position to manage health care accessibility, and to do so internally, reliant on the graduates of Canadian medical schools and the various incentives and improvements that could be offered to entice them to a rural practice. As the next chapter points out, however, provinces were selective themselves about which rural and remote communities they would support in physician recruitment and retention efforts. Local mechanisms used in this recruitment were increasingly, for better and for worse, private and public forms of group practice.

Chapter Eight

Doctors for the New North and Old Industry

With the ultimate goal of setting up a general practice in "some nice place" in Britain, John Carter considered his options as a newly minted MD. He remembered thinking that without the strategic backing of a senior practitioner in the National Health Service (NHS) his immediate prospects in the British system were unpromising.[1] He also remembered thinking how pleasant it would be to "do a bit of travelling" before he settled down. Short of cash, he and his wife began perusing contract positions abroad, as were commonly advertised in the *British Medical Journal*. He was particularly drawn to one in a remote industrial town in Canada. They were offering what seemed to him "a remarkable amount of money": $19,000 per year. He applied, sight unseen. He was a bit naive, he admits in retrospect, but the plan was to simply earn a lot of money for twelve months, embark on some travelling with his young family, and then return to England to re-evaluate his options for the future.[2]

Arriving in a northern Canadian industrial town "in the dark in February,"[3] the doctor and his family were at first greeted kindly by his new employer. However, Carter quickly got a sense that something was awry. The first night, they were invited to stay with one of the two senior physicians of the practice, at which point the British émigré doctor observed, "the number of times the phone r[a]ng. It rang, and rang, and rang. And he [the senior doctor] would, he wasn't, he didn't go anywhere, but he kept saying, 'Send so-and-so out,' 'Send so-and-so out,' 'Send so-and-so out.' And, the next day we moved into a house that he'd rented for us. And we met the team."[4]

The team, as he was to discover, consisted of three young physicians, all of whom were also immigrant doctors who had also answered the call in various British medical periodicals. Like John Carter, they had arrived in recent months.[5] As a recent arrival, the immigrant doctor soon came to understand that he had landed in a particular type of "industrial practice." As he cleverly summarized, "It was industrial in a number of senses ... it was in the [resource] area, and it was industrial in the sense that it was all about maximizing the number of people that could be seen, and, quite frankly, making the most money that could be made from those people. It was before ... Medicare – so people had to have private insurance or else they paid cash. It was only just before that came in actually ... he [the senior doctor] employed as many young assistant doctors as he could get."[6] With the two other immigrant physicians, both of whom hailed from South Asia, the team found themselves overwhelmed in their service of the huge practice and its multiple medical needs. "[B]asically," our respondent recalled, "we ran like hell."[7] Looking back on his first clinical experience in Canada, Carter felt deeply uncomfortable recounting some of the professional duties he was asked to pursue by the senior doctors in the group, so much so that he insisted on anonymity both of his name and the location of where he worked.

This British doctor's experiences raise many questions about the place of foreign-trained physicians within the expanding and varied Canadian economies for medical practice at midcentury. His experience highlights the special circumstances of foreign-trained physicians in group practices, especially the high-volume group practices of Canada's industrial towns and cities, communities that drove the economy of mid- to late-century Canada. As economic historians have well demonstrated, industrial towns supported Canadian industrial expansion from the late nineteenth century while resource towns became critically important to the postwar economic boom in Canada. Foreign-trained physicians were prime targets for recruitment to support such growing but usually underserviced municipalities. Surveying experiences with group practices at several locations across Canada, this chapter contextualizes this British doctor's life events within the broader phenomenon of group practices in Canada. In contrast to industrial towns, foreign-trained physicians found more opportunities in towns attached to the rapidly growing resource sector, two of which are included here. Examining the social history of immigrant doctors who arrived at different points in the expansion of industrial sectors and the development of new resource towns provides a novel perspective on the practice of medicine in Canada's older industrial zones as well as the "new north." It also permits us to better understand how industry, government, and the resource communities themselves worked to create the new infrastructure necessary to recruit (if not retain) health care practitioners.

INTRODUCING GROUP PRACTICE

The vagaries of place and local medical economics make the history of group practice, and the history of foreign-trained doctors in these arrangements, remarkably complex. As American historian Donald Madison has shown, private group practices were very common in the United State before the managed care revolution entrenched Health Management Organizations (HMOs) as the main regulatory force in American physicians' lives in the 1990s.[8] No Canadian history scholars have systematically examined the prevalence of the model on this side of the border, but evidence suggests Canadian physicians were intrigued by the promise of private group practice. The benefits and drawbacks of group practice were often discussed in the pages of the *Canadian Medical Association Journal* (CMAJ).[9] In 1954, for instance, the CMAJ asked Philadelphia medical economist C. Rufus Rorem to explain the benefits of this new type of collaborative medical organization to Canadian physicians. Rorem, a key architect of Blue Shield and Blue Cross, was a proponent of medical practice in a liberal, competitive, fee-for-service environment.[10] He and other medical economists of his day recognized that the costs of care provision could be offset in a shared work environment.[11] Private group practice was widely adopted in the western states and provinces and tended to be more common in the smaller cities and larger towns of North America, yet the analyst saw the potential for the model in almost every region and sector that involved private practice medicine.[12] Rorem acknowledged there were challenges negotiating the terms of professional collaboration and financial remuneration but saw the adoption of a hierarchical model as the solution to both successful recruitment and succession within the practice.

The hierarchy offered many benefits to the physicians at the top. Rorem's idea of group practice was modelled on a corporate structure that gave considerable power to long-standing investor physicians. These senior physicians would, ideally, recruit and cultivate relations with those junior physicians they found "temperamentally and professionally" suitable to bring into a position of greater empowerment in the practice in due time. Loosely inspired by the Mayo Clinic in Rochester, Minnesota, the model assumed the practice operated in an open medical marketplace, designed and implemented in a private fee-for service environment, in support of a private clinic. Rorem plied his model in Canada in the mid-1950s, a decade and half before universal health care. It was not envisioned to work in a single-payer system that underwrote public hospital care, and even before Medicare was implemented this model was not without its detractors in Canada. Many medical societies resisted the trend, seeing it as unfair competition to the "independent practitioner." And, as Rorem himself pointed out, many of the professional and economic advantages of group practice in a private clinic were available to individual practitioners through an affiliation with public community hospitals.[13] But, especially in western Canada, an increasing number of CMAJ commentators believed that group practice worked just as well, if not better, alongside prepaid systems.[14]

In Canada, public group practice – community health care clinics that employed many physicians in affiliation with the services and technologies of a publicly funded institution – seemed to be more common than private. Revised versions of American-style group practice proved most easily workable in Canada where prepaid plans were common and group practices seemed an efficient way to service industry-sponsored health plans for employees.[15] Such arrangements existed alongside community health centres that were community-owned and operated, sometimes organized through labour unions. These forms of medical practice, described in some detail below, persisted after the implementation of free hospital and diagnostic services in 1957 and the adoption of Medicare among Canadian provinces. But the challenge that group practice posed to physician autonomy was not limited to those organized on a prepayment model. In 1972, for instance, a landmark court case in Ontario outlawed the practice of using restrictive covenants on junior physicians in group practices in that province. An immigrant physician from Hungary, hired as medical assistant in a St Catharine's practice, challenged attempts to stop him from establishing his own practice in the same city, possibly in service to some of the same clientele. While this doctor had been an employee in the previous arrangement, and had signed a noncompetition contract, the On-tario court ruled that he had a right to continue to practice in the city.[16]

For this reason, the 1960s doctor shortage was of potential concern, not just to Canadian patients but also for private group practices intent on re-cruiting and retaining a workforce of junior physicians as well as group practices organized by industrial workers under the auspices of commu-nity health centres. According to *CMAJ* reporter and writer Milan Korcok, at the inaugural meeting of the World Congress on Group Practice held in Canada in 1970 a pressing concern was sourcing a supply of new phys-icians to bring into group practice arrangements of all kinds.[17] Many new graduates of Canadian medical schools were attracted by the idea of col-laborative medical practice. A survey of new graduates taken in the mid-1970s reported that 21 per cent of new graduates "hung out a shingle" in solo practice, 57 per cent entered a group practice of some kind, while only 22 per cent became salaried physicians in a number of different areas, mainly public health.[18] But the rates of turnover at the junior levels in group practice prompted many physicians to support and engage in re-cruitment from abroad. The British foreign-trained physician who "ran like hell" for his employer credited his patron with a smooth, almost "cur-sory," evaluation of his credentials when he and his family went through their initial application to immigrate in 1968. "I suppose this doc I worked for ... smoothed out some of the bumps," he observed. "He said, 'I need the doctor.' So, he had some influence, I expect, at the college."[19]

RECRUITING FOREIGN-TRAINED PHYSICIANS

The desire to recruit and retain foreign-trained junior physicians seemed to play a role in shaping group practices. It makes sense that senior members of group practices might go abroad to recruit physicians for group practices since most foreign-trained physicians who arrived in Ca-nada at the time would have been used to working in medical hierarchies within the British medical system. And such physicians seemed keen to emigrate. British-trained physicians accounted for one quarter to one third of all newly licensed foreign-trained physicians each year.[20] Many were drawn by the desire to travel, as well as the salaries. These physicians were, relative to the day, very well paid.[21] The British MD in our opening paragraphs said that the annual salary of $19,000 was the reason he came to Canada without asking proper "questions" in advance. Many physicians in Canada actively resisted taking on salaried positions by the 1960s, so recruitment from abroad might well have presented the only option for the senior physicians of this practice to recruit assistants on such terms.[22] These push and pull factors helped create a climate where the National Health Service became a hub or "labour exchange" that facilitated the ultimate migration of foreign-trained doctors to Canada.[23] While it is generally understood that these new doctors were recruited to underserviced areas and hung out shingles as independent practitioners in rural and remote regions of Canada, this immigrant cohort also played a critical role serving industrial areas.

The proportion of foreign-trained physicians in the medical complement of industrial and resource towns in Canada could vary widely. For the purposes of this chapter, industrial towns are defined as municipalities and regions with a secondary manufacturing sector, which may or may not also be located approximate to a resource extraction site. Resource towns, by contrast, are communities that have sometimes been referred to as "instant towns," or "single-industry communities."[24] Both industrial and resource towns might be dominated by one single corporate enterprise, becoming "company towns" in the process. But industrial towns tended to benefit from more infrastructural investment; they exist not just to extract resources but had factories present that added some value to the resource and provided a more well-rounded complement of primary and secondary industry. While many in Canada's Great Lakes region started to decline by the early 1970s, the resource town economic boom lasted longer and, in many ways, continues to drive the Canadian economy into the twenty-first century.[25]

Resource towns, which also have a long history in Canada, have often suffered greater economic precarity because of fluctuating global prices for the resource commodity. In the late nineteenth and early twentieth centuries, resource towns were largely unplanned, had few services, and a transient population that came and went according to the vagaries of boom or bust economic cycles.[26] Cobalt, Ontario, for instance, was already Canada's largest producer of silver in 1908 but remained a "poor man's mining camp" over most of the first sixty years of its existence.[27] By contrast, Thompson, Manitoba, was a carefully planned town with schools and a hospital and professional building for physicians ready for the first flood of miners to arrive in the late 1950s. In table 8.1, below we document the complement of foreign-trained physicians in several resource towns and cities across the country, comparing the physician populations in 1961 and 1976.

This sample of industrial and resource cities and towns across several provinces in 1961 and 1976 leaves out Prince Edward Island, the smallest province whose economy was not transformed by industrial expansion as much as it was by the growing service sector and the burgeoning tourist trade. The survey from the remaining nine provinces, however, shows an overall increase in the reliance on foreign-trained physicians in every province except Quebec. In Canada's largest French-speaking province, physician immigration remained an urban phenomenon and was largely limited to the city of Montreal. Elsewhere, the role of foreign-trained physicians in community expansion is clear. Some variation is observable by industry/resource type, and the degree of reliance on foreign-trained doctors seems also to be influenced by the wealth of each jurisdiction, and the geographic location played a role in the degree of and type of physician immigration, but all such communities across English-speaking Canada relied on the medical services of foreign-trained physicians by the mid-1970s.

This trend is observable among established industrial towns, where an expansion to approximately one-third of the physician population is common. Such communities likely already had foreign-trained physicians on site by 1961 but saw a robust expansion over these years. In 1961, for instance, the combined region of Sydney, North Sydney, and Sydney Mines, Cape Breton, home to coal mining and steel production, had fifty-five physicians, 22 per cent of who had foreign credentials. By 1976, the overall number of doctors in town had risen to 111, and 32 per cent of this complement were foreign-trained. In Sault Ste Marie, where Algoma Steel was the primary employer, the overall number of physicians increased approximately three-fold, from forty-one doctors in 1956 to 119 doctors in 1976. Here, the proportion of foreign-trained physicians doubled, going from 15 per cent to 30 per cent of the overall complement. Both were long-standing communities with established resource and industrial economies dating back to the late nineteenth and early twentieth centuries. These increases are significant but not as dramatic as the increases observable in

Table 8.1

Foreign-trained physicians per total population of physicians, select Canadian industrial and resource cities/towns, 1961, 1976

City/town	1961		1976		Proportional change
Prince George, BC	3/18	(17%)	32/87	(37%)	+20%
Port Alberni, BC	4/16	(25%)	10/22	(46%)	+21%
Kitimat, BC	0/5	(0%)	9/22	(41%)	+41%
Red Deer, AB	9/26	(36%)	27/73	(37%)	+1%
Fort McMurray, AB	0/2	(0%)	3/9	(30%)	+30%
Uranium City, SK	0/1[1]	(0%)	5/5	(100%)	+100%
Lanigan, SK	0/2	(0%)	2/2	(100%)	+100%
Flin Flon, MB	0/4	(0%)	5/10	(50%)	+50%
Thompson, MB	1/3	(30%)	16/24	(67%)	+37%
Snow Lake, MB	1/1	(100%)	2/2	(100%)	+/-0%
Cobalt, ON	0/1	(0%)	0/1	(0%)	+/-0%
Collingwood, ON	0/6	(0%)	4/25	(16%)	+16%
Hearst, ON	2/5	(40%)	6/10	(60%)	+20%
Sault Ste Marie, ON	6/41	(15%)	36/119	(30%)	+15%
Timmins, ON	1/23	(4%)	12/43	(28%)	+24%
Murdochville, QC	0/1	(0%)	0/2	(0%)	+/-0%
Asbestos, QC	0/5	(0%)	0/15	(0%)	+/-0%
Abitibi/Noranda, QC	1/16	(6%)	3/36	(8%)	+2%
Thetford Mines, QC	1/15	(7%)	2/25	(4%)	-3%
Baie Comeau, QC	0/6	(0%)	0/11	(0%)	+/-0%
Corner Brook, NL	13/20	(65%)	29/40	(73%)	+7%
Grand Falls, NL	3/8	(0%)	16/30	(53%)	+53%
Labrador City, NL	No doctors listed		2/7	(29%)	+29%
Bathurst, NB	1/14	(7%)	15/32	(47%)	+40%
Sydney (+area), NS	12/55	(22%)	36/111	(32%)	+10%
Glace Bay, NS	3/15	(20%)	13/20	(65%)	+45%

Source: *Canadian Medical Directories*, 1961, 1976.

1 Physician has no graduation data and is listed as the district coroner.

more rural and remote areas of the country where regional poverty levels remained high relative to the rest of Canada.

Some of these areas were on Canada's Atlantic coast. Bathurst, New Brunswick established iron mines by the first decade of the twentieth century. These operations were eclipsed by pulp and paper mills, which dominated the local economy until the 1950s, when several large deposits of lead and zinc were discovered in the southern parts of the Bathurst area. Over the late 1950s and early 1960s mining gradually replaced pulp and paper as the major industry in the area. Economic growth expanded the need for physician services, and, as chapter 7 has shown, Bathurst became a regional hub for the communities of the Bay of Chaleur region. As the medical population doubled from fourteen to thirty-two doctors from 1961 to 1976, the foreign-trained complement went from a single physician to almost half the medical population of the area by 1976. While Cobalt was too chaotic a silver boomtown to have more than one registered physician in the area, the valuable coal in Glace Bay made it a viable economic region until the end of the twentieth century. Glace Bay was a strong union town by the interwar period, both retaining its importance as a site of the Atlantic fishery and because of coal expansion, and was among the largest and fastest-growing municipalities in 1940s Nova Scotia. While the long-standing Dominion Coal Company withdrew in 1967, the publicly owned Cape Breton Development Corporation remained open until the 1980s. Nonetheless, Glace Bay could not service its population with local physicians, and its reliance on foreign-trained physicians rose from 20 per cent in 1961 to 65 per cent in 1976, a proportion far greater than the nearby region of Sydney/North Sydney/Sydney Mines described above. This reliance is matched by Corner Brook in western Newfoundland. An urban municipality dominated by pulp and paper, its longstanding reliance on foreign-trained physicians, at 65 per cent of the medical population in 1961, rose to 73 per cent by 1976. Western Newfoundland, as with Newfoundland more generally, could not service its population without a constant and steady stream of foreign-trained physicians for most of the postwar period.

In western Canada the international recruitment of physicians might have already been underway. Red Deer and Fort McMurray were two Alberta communities that saw an economic and population boom due to

expansion in the oil and gas sector. But Red Deer's fortunes had been rising since oil was discovered in the region in the 1940s, and so while the
city's physician population doubled, the proportion of foreign-trained
physicians held steady at around 36–37 per cent. The community of Fort
McMurray saw a later, 1960s expansion into what would become the lucrative oil sands project at the turn of the twentieth century. Located in a
more remote northeastern part of Alberta, "Fort Mac" residents on the
front end of this later boom saw their physician population increase from
a mere two Canadian-trained clinicians in 1961 to nine doctors in 1976,
three of whom had foreign credentials: a smaller number, certainly, but a
similar proportion. On the other side of the Rocky Mountains, Kitimat
saw an expansion in kind; the five resident physicians in 1961 all had
Canadian credentials, and there were no foreign-trained physicians serving the rapidly expanding hydroelectric sector and the growing number
of workers at the Rio Tinto aluminium smelter. But by 1976, right around
the time when the economy diversified to pulp and paper, just under half
of the twenty-two doctors who served the northern town were trained
outside of Canada.[28]

   This suggests that new municipalities on the geographic fringes of the
resource expansion phenomenon, tended to see more dramatic increases
overall. With the aforementioned exception of Quebec, resource sectors
in English-speaking parts of Canada could feel a clinician resource pinch
on par with the precarity of western Newfoundland. Prince Rupert in
British Columbia and Thompson in north-central Manitoba were two
relatively new resource towns, and these fast-growing areas seemed to rely
more on immigrant physicians as a health workforce. If the nickel town
of Thompson drew on foreign-trained physicians for more than 60 per
cent of its resident registered physicians by 1976, the pulp and paper town
of Prince Rupert was not far behind at close to 40 per cent.[29] Once again,
this suggests that the faster the resource economy was growing, and the
more remote the respective town or city, the greater the number of foreign-trained physicians. Expansion and relative remoteness created both
need and, therefore, also opportunity. This is especially the case in the
smaller but underserved resource towns of Saskatchewan. The heavy
metals and minerals extracted by mine workers of Uranium City and
Lanigan, Saskatchewan were of vital importance for Canada's energy and
agricultural sectors, respectively. But the residents would have had no

resident physician services at all if it were not for the small but critical complement of British, Scottish, and Indian-trained doctors who set up practices there by 1976.

THE PRACTICES OF PAYING FOR MEDICAL CARE

In many ways, a resource town's reliance on new cohorts of foreign-trained physicians might be related to the structures of medical practice and forms of payment. For instance, Sydney and Sault Ste Marie were home to powerful labour unions that sponsored prepaid health care schemes for many years before Medicare. Case studies reveal a significant level of interest at midcentury in labour-sponsored health care schemes. In industrial Cape Breton, the "check-off" system was a well-established program.[30] But it was not the only such program in the country.

An early clinic organized with salaried physicians paid on a capitation basis was established in 1963 by Algoma steelworkers in the northern Ontario community of Sault Ste Marie. The Sault Ste Marie Community Health Centre (CHC), which operated in collaboration with the federal government of Canada and with the sponsorship of the World Health Organization, was among the first of its kind in North America. A remarkable success in many ways, the CHC was popular with patients, most of them steelworkers, who paid a subscription rate in return for care at the group practice. The program's success, especially in the early years after opening, put pressure on clinic organizers to recruit and expand the physician complement.[31]

David McNair, a British radiologist, spent the better part of his professional life in "the Sault." His decision to make a go of it in the industrial town came after two years working as a GP in Muskoka in the mid-1960s and later, when he returned with postgraduate training in radiology in the early 1970s, working in a junior position for an Ottawa group practice. His career decisions highlight the ways foreign-trained doctors negotiated the group practice hierarchies. It is clear that even taking junior positions allowed many foreign-trained physicians to raise capital for their own offices more quickly than they might have elsewhere, such as in the UK. With relatively few resources, but often abundant ambition, the group practices that successfully attracted such physicians for the long term tended to be located in regions where population growth and medical professional turnover went hand in hand. This meant a swift rise to partner and equal pay.

The Ottawa practice was a mixed clinic and hospital practice, and the immigrant doctor split his time between a downtown practice on Metcalfe Street and travel to several hospitals in Perth, Renfrew, and Smith's Falls. After two years he decided to leave when his employers told him "it was going to be a long time before I achieved parity with partners in the practice … about eight years." There was little demand in 1976 for radiologists, so the offer from Sault Ste Marie was very welcome. Touring the city in June of that year, he and his wife liked the possibilities that presented to them: "It was a very good move job-wise and we thought it was a good place to bring up children. We were pleased with the schools and we enjoyed the lifestyle." The pair also liked the size of the city, which boasted a population of 85,000 at the time, and managed the geographic isolation by driving down occasionally to southern Ontario. His pay exceeded his income in Ottawa and his growing family "settled in quite quickly." His family enjoyed "outdoorsy" activities and made good use of the nearby national parks. Although his wife experienced some homesickness, he never did. There was a lot going on in the medical world of Sault Ste Marie, and it seemed to keep the immigrant doctor quite occupied.[32]

As Jonathan Lomas has pointed out, the professional and economic advantages that the CHC offered physicians "was not entirely congruent with the values instilled in most of them during their training."[33] Many physicians chafed at the identification as "employees of the steelworkers." Unsurprisingly, McNair's affiliation changed over the course of his decades in the steel town, and his memories of life in the town describe a medical community divided. The physicians in the Sault, he remembered, were "divided between downtown and uptown." The "downtown" physicians all belonged to the community health centre and worked on a capitation basis. After twenty years doing radiology at one of the two city hospitals, he and a colleague set up a private clinic "uptown." And while he remembered "a bit of tension," as a hospital-affiliated specialist he avoided most of it. Of the two hospitals in the city, the Plummer Hospital where he worked had additional services and better technology than the General Hospital for most of his career. For instance, he recalled being in demand because of the ultrasound training he had done in Scotland in the 1970s; indeed, he opened an ultrasound department six months after his arrival and found himself very busy. As a result, the "downtown" physicians referred maternity patients to radiology services in the Plummer at the same rate as the "uptown" physicians. Although, in general, McNair recalled "The two groups never really mixed."[34]

Although "it was an interesting time politically," with the medical community split one might have expected the tensions to spill over into private life. Nonetheless, the radiologist and his wife enjoyed a wide circle of friends. Foreign-trained physicians dominated some of specialties like radiology, "particularly when we arrived," he said. Many came and went from the radiology community, and he remembered sharing the radiology work with physicians from the UK but also South Africa, a few from Australia and the United States, and occasionally physicians from the global south: India, Egypt, and other countries in Africa. But by far the largest number came from the UK, and he and his wife got to know many of them quite well. "You tended to mix socially with the same people," he explained, "people with the same experience as yourself: immigrants." His group practice, its international complement and recruitment strategy, and the place it played in the medical marketplace of the city, alleviated any competition and, hence, any unpleasantness.[35]

By contrast, the group practices in general medicine tended to lie at the fault line. There were three private medical buildings in "uptown," and those general practices were run mostly by Canadian-trained physicians. Indeed, most of the foreign-trained doctors in Sault Ste Marie were recruited for the community health centre. At the centre a new physician "could walk straight into a practice, with no expenses," McNair explained, "and you didn't have to worry about secretaries, so it was attractive for immigrant doctors." Because he had so many friends among foreign-trained physicians at the centre, McNair avoided the worst of "the feud." He also maintained good relations with the radiologists who worked out of the general hospital. Until they acquired a CT scanner in the 1980s, it was a very low-key practice and did not pull too many patients from his practice at the Plummer.[36]

And he advanced more quickly in Sault Ste Marie as compared to Ottawa. In the northern town "as soon as you get the Canadian fellowship [LMCC], you get equal pay," he remembered. This meant he was a full partner in his clinical practice after only two years. He and his colleagues maintained it until the mid-1990s. Then, after approximately a decade in private practice, a "bridge" he appreciated for the independence it afforded him, they joined the community health centre.[37] In the final years of its operation, health policy researchers debated whether the health centre would survive, given the challenges and competition from local independent practitioners.[38] But by McNair's testimony, the centre adapted to a pluralistic environment. It eventually took over all the private general practices, the private specialist clinics, and most of the outpatient services in the city. Additionally, as a radiologist McNair found he could receive pay on a fee-for-service basis. This transition to fee-for-service was already underway. By 1966 The CHC had replaced mandatory payment on a capitation system with a more flexible, voluntary system that allowed for some members to operate on a fee-for-service basis. The strict patient sharing system also relaxed, and by the late 1960s the CHC had ensured patients faced no bureaucratic hurdles to free choice of physician in the practice.[39]

The situation in Sault Ste Marie is instructive for many reasons. It highlights how attractive group practices could be for immigrant physicians with few resources, so much so that even if they had private practice options, payment on a capitation basis was tolerable at least in the short term. But it highlights the inability of programs like the CHC to retain practitioners, particularly specialists, in the long term. McNair's preferred time horizon to join a practice was three years, and to keep physicians like him in affiliation, strict rules on capitation payment had to be relaxed to accommodate the desire for a more open and liberal practice model.

THOMPSON, THE MUSKEG METROPOLIS

Manitoba was home to many "resource towns" developed in the postwar era to both exert Canadian sovereignty in the north and, of course, extract the rich natural resources of the province. Amongst these new communities, Thompson, Manitoba, located in the granite, geographic heart of Canada, offered wealth and opportunity for many. Over the 1960s and 1970s The International Nickel Company (INCO) worked with the Manitoba government to create a model flagship resource town. In this "miracle town of the north,"[40] INCO paid for the construction of a private hospital, among other services, and naturally this attracted physicians.[41]

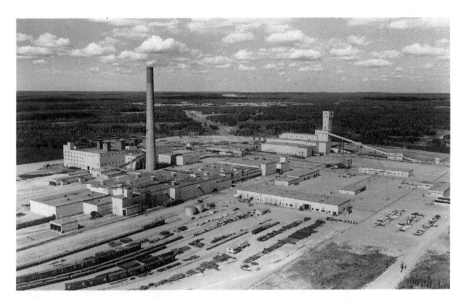

Figure 8.1 Thompson, Manitoba
The Canadian economy was booming in the 1950s and 1960s, establishing the country as having one of the highest standards of living in the world. Much of the economic boom was due to the growth of resource extraction which quite literally created entirely new communities, like Thompson, Manitoba. Here, the photograph of this industrial town reflects both the economic energy and the geographic isolation of these communities which had to search for novel ways of attracting medical practitioners.

During the period sometimes described as the "government era" of community planning of resource management, Thompson was part of "a phenomenal expansion of the resource sector."[42] Indeed, the creation of Thompson was an attempt by the province to share in the benefits of the Second National Policy, which Janine Brodie explains was "an amalgam of several distinct policy initiatives, which together constituted a model for economic growth and development."[43]

Resource development was equated with general economic growth at midcentury. When base metals were discovered in the province of Manitoba in 1956, the Cold War economy was inflating the value of this new resource.[44] American stockpiling of strategic minerals under the Resources for Freedom program of 1952 promised prosperity for many parts of the country. Of the twenty-two "strategic" resources listed by the program's first report, thirteen were found in Canada.[45] As a result, the Canadian economy drifted into the American economic sphere, a trend supported by federal policies encouraging American corporate investment, largely in Canada's natural resource sector. These supported the "new industrialism" built around the extraction and refining of coal and iron, pulp and paper, hydroelectricity, and, of course, the industrial mining of minerals like nickel.[46] Indeed, nickel was one of the most desired metals expected to increase in demand as a result of stockpiling between 1950 and 1975.[47] This makes the creation of Thompson a prime example of "province building" in the postwar economy.[48]

The possibilities of this continental resource capitalism encouraged provincial governments to actively seek out investment from large corporations like INCO.[49] Government and the International Nickel Company of Canada entered into an agreement in 1956, which resulted in the creation of the town site of Thompson and the local government district of Mystery Lake; within this arrangement, the parties agreed that the district would be established for mining, milling, smelting, and refining; Inco Ltd. further assented to annual payments in lieu of municipal, district, school district, and other local government taxes and rates. The company committed to spend $10 million in the first two years on water and sewer systems, roads, sidewalks, schools, and municipal buildings. The site and city was developed by urban planner Carl Nesbitt, who worked with the metropolitan planning commission in the capital city of Winnipeg.[50] The planner was responsible for erecting the "nickel curtain," creating a zone that forbade visitors around the Mystery Lake district while development and construction was underway.[51]

Doctors were also a service to be planned; they enabled the extraction of "resources for freedom" by caring for the workers and their families. INCO's investment included a sixty-bed hospital and a "professional building" to house physicians' offices (the expectation was that these would be deeded to the town eventually). Physicians at the Thompson clinic would pay rent to the municipality of Thompson, though all would have admitting privileges at the nearby hospital. Only the physician who provided health care to the construction crews went behind the nickel curtain, and this practitioner stayed on as the senior physician in the Thompson Medical Clinic located in the aforementioned "professional building." This would be the site of a group practice affiliated with the local Thompson hospital, ready to serve the first wave of miners who arrived in 1959.

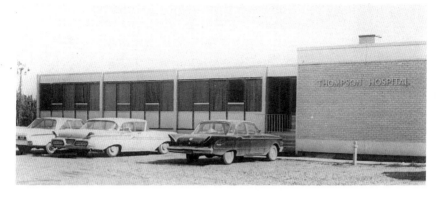

Figure 8.2 New Hospital, Thompson, Manitoba.
Large multinational companies like the International Nickel Company (INCO) engaged
in joint projects with respective provincial governments to build and staff local community health centres. At first, doctors were hired and paid as "company doctors" or
organized into group practices, some of which became dependant on cheap medical
labour of new immigrant doctors. Later, with the onset of Medicare, medical practices
transformed and distanced themselves from the oversight of the large corporations.
In either case, recruiting and, more importantly, retaining doctors in remote locations
proved to be a challenge.

Thompson sprung up from a population of about 800 Indigenous
people in the Nelson House reserve,[52] to a mining operation that expanded the community to a population of 24,00 by 1959. That year, the
first school opened and families began arriving.[53] At its ten-year anniversary, the town had grown to 12,000 residents, though originally designed
for 8,000.[54] In 1967, INCO expanded operations and a second boom[55] made
Thompson the second-largest nickel development in the world after Sudbury, and the population peaked at 24,000 in 1970.[56] During this second
boom, community leaders worried about social development, including
physician access, keeping abreast of economic expansion.[57] "It is very important to us that we develop a good community in which to live," said
local lawyer Donald Cameron in the *Winnipeg Tribune*.[58] Newspaper reports estimated that "for every man working in the mine, there are about
1.6 needed to provide services: merchants, teachers, police, firemen, *doctors*, lawyers, mechanics, caterers, and the like [emphasis added]." This
new resource town was initially serviced by local, western Canadian-

trained doctors, but these are soon joined by new graduates of the Scottish medical system. In 1962, Donald Campbell, a 1960 graduate of Glasgow medical school, responded to an ad for two junior doctors. He did not stay, leaving for Newfoundland only a couple of years later. Indeed, all the newer graduates on the CMD register tended to move on fairly quickly. Most years, the roster of physicians in Thompson saw quite a few come and go – more than thirty-nine physicians registered in Thompson from 1960 to 1976,[59] and the average length of practice was four to five years.[60]

Like other industrial and resource towns, Thompson benefitted from the migration of disgruntled registrars and consultants from the NHS looking for better options. But despite the arrival (and departure) of doctors like Campbell in the 1960s, such arrivals were only a precursor to a second boom, precipitated by the advent of universal health insurance and the dramatic increase of nickel production, and hence the population, at Thompson. By 1970, the proportion of foreign-trained doctors skyrocketed, and the physician complement diversified to include a large cohort of practitioners who received their first medical degree from schools in Ireland, Egypt, and the countries of the "Indian subcontinent."

PRACTICING IN THE NEW NICKEL BELT

As the 1960s wore on, the clinical group practices in the northern mining town begin to multiply and the original Thompson clinic was supplemented by group practices in two new locations. The Burntwood Medical Clinic had been was founded over 1969–70 by two relatively young Canadian-trained physicians who wanted to work separately from the Thompson clinic that had previously dominated the medical marketplace. In addition to the new clinic at Burntwood, another clinic called Southwood Medical added to the landscape of physician practices. Eventually, the Thompson clinic facility was repurposed into a medical resource centre, with radiology services and other diagnostic facilities. The two new clinical group practices integrated quickly with the local Thompson hospital as well as the broader service of regional fly-in First Nations reserves. Under this new structure, the newly configured group practices were formed and staffed by new recruits who came after the second boom.

Surajit Ghosh and Lachlan McIntosh both sought out Canadian practices because they had married Canadian nurses who wanted to leave the UK so as to be closer to their families. Both were practicing in Britain at the time and responded to advertisements in the *British Medical Journal*. Ghosh was more established; he had spent close to fifteen years in Britain after supplementing his Kolkata medical degree with postgraduate training in internal medicine, while McIntosh was a relatively new Scottish medical graduate. Once Ghosh and his wife established the fact that they would be immigrating to Canada, Thompson "seemed as good an option as any" under their consideration at the time. While McIntosh did not talk about salaries, Ghosh did because the difference from what he was paid in the NHS system was astounding to him, both at the time and in retrospect. While he was paid the equivalent of $150 per month in the UK as a consultant, the Thompson practice offered him considerably more. "[My wife and I] had an interview, the Canadian embassy, in Birmingham," he recalled, "and they said 'okay, to immigrate.' And there's no problem getting a job." As he considered his options, he received a phone call from Thompson and a Burntwood representative simply asked him when he was available to start. "We'll give you two thousand dollars every month ... What a difference, eh? At that time," he marvelled.[61]

Ghosh remembered Thompson had an air of abundance. The resource town was new and "there was incentive [in] coming ... there was plenty of work. People from all over came to make money." And the remuneration changed for both physicians over the course of their time in Thompson. "I went in as an employee, being employed by the group." Ghosh explained. "They called it Burntwood Clinic ... there were seven other doctors and as soon as I could, in 1972, I took the exam for FRCP [internal medicine] and I was now being paid like a consultant and so then, when I found that I could make enough to pay the overhead, I said I'll just work on my own. I was in the clinic, but ... I was not working for them ... I billed the government like everyone else."[62] Becoming a partner and gaining the respect of his Canadian colleagues was also important for McIntosh, who opted to take the extra accreditation for the College of Family Medicine so he could "prove" himself to local physicians.[63]

The structure of the practice combined general practitioners and specialists. Ghosh described it as having "two obstetricians, they had three surgeons, they had three general practitioners." He was the sole internist in the group and also the oldest among the medics at the age of thirty-four.[64] But the practice evolved organically to meeting the needs of the particular community to which they were recruited. Since both Ghosh and McIntosh stayed for more than just a few years, this required them to diversify their skillsets to serving the young working class population. McIntosh and most others in the practice generally treated accidents, which were part of life in the mine. He recalled his interest in the industrial work: "I went down the mine out of interest to see what my patients were doing or I went into the smelter to see what they did and into the refinery to see what they did. I remember what in the mine they call 'loose' – the rocks give way, crushing two people and I got called to go and see and confirm they were dead. And then, with the mining manager, [I] went to the house of the family of the person that died, which was partly public relations but also good medicine."[65]

Community integrated practice, or what McIntosh referred to as "good medicine," required diversifying skillsets to accommodate the specific needs of the practice, and so, in Ghosh's case, he "ended up doing a lot of pediatrics, cause I had a specialist degree [in internal medicine] from England."[66] McIntosh had his heart set on family medicine, but even he tailored his skillset to meet the needs of Thompson's growing population. In Thompson "specialists came and went very quickly, usually, so there were always gaps in the medical coverage. So you may suddenly be doing a lot of internal medicine and running the critical care unit – equally well, you delivered lots of babies, but that meant you were also doing a lot of neonatal work."[67] Both physicians also spent a good deal of time managing sexually transmitted diseases, which both doctors thought were quite common – indeed Ghosh remarked that he'd "never seen so much gonorrhea" as in Thompson – and, in some communities, families were large due to a lack of education or lack of access to birth control.[68] McIntosh "started working for the alcoholism and drug abuse so they had many patient treatment centres." The culture, he remembered, leant itself to "hard-drinking."[69] Ghosh agreed, noting with a laugh that there were "not many heart attacks, the only heart attack I saw was the hospital administrator."

The doctors also cultivated the ability to practice general emergency medicine in circumstances where resources were limited. In the early 1970s, the medical clinics took on government contracts to provide physician services to regional First Nations reserves and practice medicine on a fly-in basis. McIntosh explained, "Thompson was a medial hub for northeast Manitoba so First Nations people were coming in for acute medical care as well." While they came to the group practice in small numbers, they comprised well over half of the hospital patients. And physicians flew out as well. "For a while I flew out to various reserves or Metis communities – drove to one Metis community [Wabowden] – but didn't do that for more than two or three years."[70] Indeed, the Burntwood Medical Clinic was contracted with Indian Health Services, who McIntosh remembered "were always trying to get people to service outlying areas … and I spent some time, once every week or two weeks, flying for a day into a more remote community – mostly a place called South Indian lake." At these locations, they were consultants to the nurse practitioners that were already working in these communities. "They were bringing in the people they were looking after and wanted a physician to look at."[71] Ghosh also remembered, "our clinic had seven doctors so we took turns to go so it came to your turn [to fly up to reserves and] once a month that you go: Wabowden, Nelson House, Cross Lake." Ghosh recalled going out "on a small plane to reservations and I would do, I did deliver babies, pulled tooth [*sic*] out, lots of dysentery, nephritis, meningitis, children's disease, dehydration."[72] Staying with the nurses overnight, in their homes, allowed him to evaluate their capacities first hand. "Some of them were brilliant," he said admiringly and, like him, were largely foreign-trained, hailing from British nursing schools. "They could diagnose nephritis looking at x-rays, do a lumbar puncture, diagnose meningitis."[73] The service provided in the fly-in communities stood out for McIntosh as well. He explained, "You get to do things you don't get to do in southern Canada."[74] There, the physicians often attended to life and death situations, resuscitating people who had got lost in the bush: "Kids were coming in from Indian reserves very sick and needing a lot of resuscitation – mostly with chest infections and gastroenteric infections. And if the snow was flying, you couldn't get them out to Winnipeg so you were left having to look after them yourself. So, you were working as an internist when you were only a GP. It was exciting and also very tiring."[75] Except for this oblique reference, McIntosh was taciturn about the mental and emotional challenges of such a practice. Ghosh, on the other hand, was more direct. He found the variety and challenges very interesting from a medical perspective, but the emotional toll was great. "The native Indians," he said, "their standard of living is so poor, not running water, not enough heat, and cold and by the lake. Constant misery, that's what I used to think."[76]

The fortunes of these northern communities rose and fell over those decades. In the early 1970s, INCO scaled back production as the era of "stockpiling" came to an end, and the US market for minerals cooled. Hospitals in Thompson saw several acrimonious strikes by nurses and then support staff in the late 1970s and 1980s. Thompson survives as a nickel town, although on a smaller scale. Though it remains a community of just more than 13,000 residents, it is no longer called a "miracle town." Many of the physicians recruited to serve the population during the boom years moved on in the late 1970s or early 1980s, often to practices elsewhere in western Canada, especially British Columbia. McIntosh ended up in Chilliwack and Ghosh in Trail. McIntosh left because the demands on his time were untenable. His daughter knew him only as "Bye-Bye," he was out on call and at the hospital so much.[77] Ghosh was a little more circumspect and cited his wife's desire to be closer to her family.[78] But, for a time, this resource town was a small-scale, but critically important, labour exchange for foreign-trained physicians. The terms of the labour exchange, like the economic fortunes of the north, were in flux.

The first-person accounts from three physicians who came through Thompson in the 1960s and 1970s reveal an evolution in the group practices and the experiences of the immigrant physicians. Campbell came during the early years of the first nickel boom, and his discontent with being the "junior doctor" suggests a hierarchy that was fixed and ultimately untenable: he "would not be happy" working in such a structure for long. He does not mention problems with remuneration; it was just the structure of the practice that undermined the Thompson clinic's ability to keep him for longer than a couple of years. For later physicians, those who came after the implementation of Medicare, the medical landscape had shifted. The democratization of group practices in the late 1960s played an important role in retaining physicians during this period of resource town creation and health system expansion. These later physicians tended to stay much longer than a couple of years; indeed, they persisted up to a decade in the nickel town. Surajit Ghosh and Lachlan McIntosh were both explicitly happy with their starting salaries, which were far higher than the remuneration either could have expected in Britain. But it was more important to both that they could achieve parity with their Canadian-trained colleagues quickly, to bill as consultants, and practice as full partners, at least after passing their Royal College exams and securing Canadian credentials. Both appreciated the interesting pediatric and neonatal work that would otherwise not fall under the purview of either a geriatric-focused internist or general practitioner; the group practices were not so structured that either physician felt constrained professionally. Both found a great deal of satisfaction with the demands of fly-in medicine to the reserves and Metis communities. The life-saving work was as exhausting as it was engaging, but despite its stressors it enabled both to feel like they were making a significant difference in the lives of Indigenous communities in the north, at least until they'd had enough of the small planes or the living conditions of Canada's First Nations.

CONCLUSIONS

The experiences of foreign-trained physicians highlight both opportunities and inequities emerging in the Canadian medical marketplace at mid-century. Many resource towns struggled to recruit and retain doctors, and some came to rely on foreign-trained physicians to keep the social fabric in resource towns and surrounding areas from fraying. For this to work, a social restructuring of physicians' health care practices from hierarchical to collaborative group practice models was required. In some places like Thompson, Manitoba foreign-trained physicians seemed to comprise an unusually large complement of the local medical workforce. But it is clear throughout Canada that foreign-trained physicians provided important services to flagship communities of Canada's "new north." Industrial growth generally, but resource expansion specifically, heightened the demand for physician services across the country. Managing the supply of physicians was critical to servicing such towns, preoccupying both local and provincial authorities. Opportunities opened the door for new graduates and many foreign-trained physicians, so many of the latter that, through much of the country, the newer resource towns would become very "international" communities of physicians. The health of communities that supported both the old industries and the resource towns would have been compromised, like Medicare itself would have been compromised, without the availability of immigrant physicians.

Chapter Nine

Too Many Doctors

"THROWING SNOWBALLS INTO HELL"

In June of 1976, a young doctor reluctantly began her shift on call at the Baragwanath Hospital, a huge medical institution on the edge of Soweto, South Africa. Dr Levinson had recently graduated from the University of Witwatersrand (in Johannesburg). "Wits," as it was referred to informally, was one of two English-language universities in South Africa (along with the University of Cape Town) and known for its liberal politics in a country increasingly polarized by the tightening grip of Apartheid. In the immediate postwar period, its medical school had traditionally accepted African, Indian, and Jewish students and a handful of women candidates. But, as the Afrikaans government ramped up measures of racial segregation, nonwhite candidates of the class of approximately 200 medical students were being increasingly squeezed out of its medical school and rerouted to the Durban Medical School in Natal.[1] As part of a sizeable group of Jewish medical trainees, Levinson and her coreligionists occupied an awkward space – part of the "white" ruling class and yet simultaneously, and increasingly, mistrusted by the Afrikaans government.[2]

Baragwanath Hospital was an extraordinary institution. At the time, there were close to two million people – almost all black South Africans – who lived in the Soweto shantytowns bordering Johannesburg, all of who were dependent on this one hospital and a handful of outpatient clinics. At the time of her internship the teaching hospitals in the Johannesburg area were all racially segregated by patient population. Baragwanath was the "black" hospital; Johannesburg General, the white hospital; and Coronation Hospital, was the "coloured" or "East Indian" hospital.[3] As Levinson remembered, the crush of admissions at Baragwanath, even during normal times, was unbearable, with more than one hundred patients admitted each night. "So [each intern was] looking after eighteen to twenty extremely sick people and then having to discharge as many as possible so that you had beds ... later to admit [others]. They were pretty sick when you discharged them."[4] The situation was challenging even in normal times. "They used to talk about it as throwing snowballs into Hell because you let the sick out to let the really sick in."[5]

But these were not normal times. In June of 1976, halfway through her internship, the Soweto riots erupted. There was no avoiding the bloodshed arising from the police repression, which extended to her fellow students who were protesting the attempted closure of some local health clinics. After a nonviolent demonstration against the latest restrictive regulation – that all medical staff had to pass an examination *in Afrikaans* – the government opened fire on the medical students. The surgical wards became overwhelmed with protestors suffering "birdshot" from the police, so they were simply treated in the internal medicine wards by unqualified interns. "I was on the wards," she recalled, "and I had to discharge patients like crazy because of the gunshot wounds and challenges that were happening at that time."[6] As the riots worsened, some of her fellow (white) doctors began arriving armed, working tensely alongside black nurses.[7] "So, there was a huge racial[ly] challenging time where the nurses would challenge the doctors and say 'Who are you going to shoot? Me?' and they'd say 'Well, I've got eight bullets so if I get attacked I'll take eight people down with me.'"[8]

HOP, SKIP, AND JUMP

The medical degrees at Witwatersrand and the University of Cape Town were based loosely on the British medical curriculum, comprising six years of training directly after secondary school. As the capstone experience, all newly graduated doctors were required to complete one year of internship. By the 1970s, it was becoming increasingly common for South African graduates to leave the country during their internship year, a move that was often precipitated (at least for the men) by the call-up for mandatory military service, which many, understandably, were eager to avoid. "The planes were full, going to London, New York, and Canada,"

Levinson recalls. "I'd say of the 200 people in our class, probably 120 left immediately after. Mainly the males left because they were called to the army."[9] Levinson had already travelled to Britain (Scotland and England) and North America (United States and Canada) to assess possibilities, ultimately opting for British Columbia. She decided to go into general practice as a solo practitioner to a community of 500 people in the interior of British Columbia. She was the only doctor for approximately 5,000 square miles, located, in her words, "in the middle of nowhere."[10]

By the mid-1970s, however, landed immigrant status and accreditation in Canada was becoming more difficult for newly arrived medical practitioners, even those willing to service rural and remote areas. Armed with only a temporary one-year work visa, the South African doctor began to hedge her bets, applying and receiving approved immigration status for both New Zealand and Australia. Her anxiety was understandable. She had been working in a salaried position at a 24/7 local community health clinic, paid directly by the provincial government to service small, dispersed communities in the interior and the north. But in 1975, the Social Credit Party returned to power under Bill Bennett; they put the experimental clinics under review, ultimately deciding that they were not cost effective. Levinson moved to a group practice on one of British Columbia's islands for another five years before relocating to a midsize city in Ontario.

Levinson's journey to, and within, Canada highlights several of the emerging themes in Canadian health policy and human resource allocation in the middle of the 1970s. As chapter 7 has pointed out, many provincial ministers of health increasingly concluded over the 1970s that Canada had enough doctors on an aggregate level; rather than a doctor shortage, it was the chronic maldistribution of medical practitioners – both between and within provinces – that was causing headaches. Politicians in Ontario, British Columbia, and to a lesser extent Quebec were feeling that they were awash with doctors (at least those who wanted to practice in urban and suburban areas); other provinces, such as Saskatchewan, Newfoundland, Manitoba, and Nova Scotia lamented that they would not retain many of the doctors they had recruited. Some commentators insinuated that, once foreign-born and -trained doctors had secured Canadian citizenship, they left underserviced regions for other parts of the country. A potential solution to this crisis was to be spearheaded by blunt-spoken Ontario Minister of Health Frank Miller who focussed particularly on foreign-trained doctors. He vowed to stop what he dubbed the "hop, skip, and jump" pattern of medical migration to, and remigration within, Canada.[11]

As Miller well knew, the impact of the previous six years of physician production and immigration had been dramatic. The number of licensed physicians in Ontario, for example, had jumped from 9,862 (in 1968) to 13,365 (in 1972). Moreover, of the 895 *newly* registered medical practitioners in 1973, only 45 per cent were graduates of Ontario medical schools; by contrast, 41 per cent were from non-Canadian schools. Indeed, some specialties in the province boasted a plurality of foreign-trained doctors.[12] What was a good news story for many patients was, of course, a potential headache for ministers of health. The Ontario Provincial Ministry of Health estimated that each new physician who relocated to Ontario from another province, or another country, cost the Ontario taxpayer $250,000 per year (approximately 1 million in current dollars adjusted for inflation). Foreign-trained doctors, in Miller's opinion, were a particular problem because of their inherent mobility once they became Canadian citizens. Some researchers projected a provincial ratio of residents to physicians that would fall below 500:1. "This," opined a frustrated Miller, "was an extravagance that Ontario could not afford."[13]

Given this context of a doctor workforce that had increased 35 per cent in the four years following the launch of Medicare, the province of Ontario established a Requirements Committee on Physician Manpower in April 1973, to explore the possibility of preventing physician oversupply in the near future.[14] A few months later, the possibility of suffering from "too many doctors"[15] was circulating at a 1974 conference of provincial health ministers; a variety of solutions were discussed, including the complete elimination of points attributed to doctors seeking landed immigrant status, though this, of course, required the cooperation of the federal minister of manpower and immigration.[16] With public disquiet over immigration exacerbated by the economic downturn beginning in 1973, this proposal was enshrined in modifications to the immigration regulations the following year when the category "physician or surgeon" was taken off the list earning units for occupations in demand.[17] Halting the interprovincial movement of doctors was a rare moment in Canadian public policy where the interests of have and have-not provinces aligned, at least at the level of provincial ministries of health. The richer provinces wanted to stem the tide of interprovincial medical migration, while the poorer provinces struggled with the problem of offering local incentives and wanted to diminish the ongoing problem of medical attrition.

This new focus on the status and rights of foreign-trained doctors placed the Canadian Medical Association in an awkward position. The leadership was caught between anxieties of physician oversupply (which potentially threatened individual practices of its members) and the continued intrusion of governments into medical decision-making and place of clinical practice, two of the many anxieties that lay behind resistance to Medicare in the 1950s and 1960s. The CMA sponsored a National Committee on Physician Manpower in 1975, which embraced the seemingly defensible goal of national "self-reliance" for future physician needs. In concert with this, federal and provincial ministers of health agreed to restrict the attribution of immigration points that were associated to a letter of offer to individual medical practitioners who had a prearranged job contracts (from a hospital or health authority) that was also *approved by a province* (in contradistinction to those who had job offers from individual hospitals or clinics or even university departments). The combination of these measures would "lift the drawbridge," as Miller vividly put it, on foreign doctors eager to move to richer provinces, while allowing Saskatchewan, Manitoba, Newfoundland, and others to continue to backfill in response to physician attrition. In theory, foreign doctors who received licences in one province would thus find it much more difficult to relocate to more desirable regions of the country after only a few years.

Thus, by the mid-1970s, many provinces were cautiously optimistic that new measures, combined with the new flow of medical graduates arising from the new and expanded Canadian medical schools, would assist them in maintaining adequate health human resources for the next generation. Dalhousie Dean of Medicine Chester Stewart looked back on almost a decade of work toward "self-sufficiency." Using the petroleum metaphor that had come into vogue in 1970s following the OPEC crisis, he declared that "[t]he production pipeline is full and leakproof because the competition for entry is fierce and dropout numbers negligible."[18] Dr Harry Roberts, a member of the admissions committee at the new Memorial University medical school in St John's, likewise expressed optimism about the prospect of retaining more graduates and ultimately of achiev-

ing self-sufficiency for his province. "I think we will gradually be self-sufficient, and we will get the pipeline filled with qualified people graduating
from Memorial ... we could turn off the tap right now and not suffer too
dearly," he pronounced confidently.[19]

TURNING OFF THE TAP

Turning off the tap required cooperation at the federal level as well, particularly in the offices of the Ministry of Manpower and Immigration.
Although Canada had officially embraced "multiculturalism" in 1971, the
public mood towards what was considered to be unrestrained immigration from nontraditional countries began to sour. Inevitably, the oil crisis
of 1973, followed by a decade-long economic stagnation, undermined support for generous immigration measures. Robert Andras, the new Liberal
minister of manpower and immigration, moved quickly to address popular concerns. He wasted little time in asserting his influence; in 1973 he
directed resources at reducing the backlog of applicants for permanent
residence and initiated the Canadian Immigration and Population Study
aimed at outlining policy options for immigration reform. The study
tabled its findings in 1975 as the Green Paper on Immigration. Many credit
his individual determination for the next major consolidation of immigration regulations enshrined in the 1976 Immigration Act.[20]

The 1976 Immigration Act was both progressive in principle and conservative in execution. The act entrenched nondiscrimination on the basis
of race and religion, emphasized humanitarian obligations as a factor influencing the processing of immigration applications, and encouraged
the reunification of families. While many of the precedents for these principles had found their way into immigration policy in the 1960s, their
consolidation in law represented a major new development. The 1976 act
recognized three distinct categories of individuals eligible for landed immigrant status: an "independent class," "family class," and "humanitarian
class." Independent class immigrants were applicants who were evaluated,
as before, on the basis of the points system. The other two categories, however, were more innovative. The humanitarian class included "refugees,"
as defined by UN convention, as well as "persecuted peoples" who did not
qualify for that formal distinction. It marked the first time that refugees

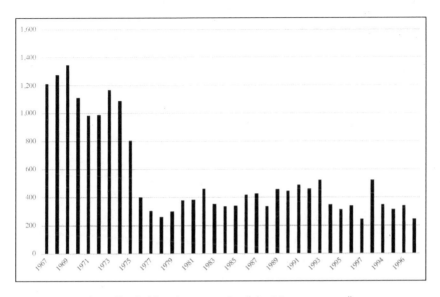

Figure 9.1 Number of landed immigrants stating "physician or surgeon" as intended occupation
Source: E. Ryten, "None Is Too Many – It's Time to Discard This Bankrupt Physician Supply Policy for Canada," ACMC Forum 31; 8–17.

were formally recognized as a distinct status of immigrant in Canada, indicating a greater awareness of the concerns first hinted at in the 1960s. The family class included immediate family members and dependent relatives of Canadians and permanent residents. This class would soon become the largest category, accounting for 45 per cent of all immigrants by the late 1970s.[21]

Perhaps the most influential aspect of the 1976 Immigration Act, however, was its focus on public policy planning. Walter Harris, Liberal minister of what was then called Citizenship and Immigration, observed, shortly after the passing of the 1952 Immigration Act, that "one may say that we do not plan for the distant future ... we merely say that from month to month and at most up to a year in advance, we have certain plans and certain expectations of what can be done by way of migration."[22] Section 7 of the 1976 Immigration Act, by contrast, required the minister to announce annually to Parliament the precise number of immigrants the government intended to admit during the following year. In the context of difficult economic times and increasing public suspicion

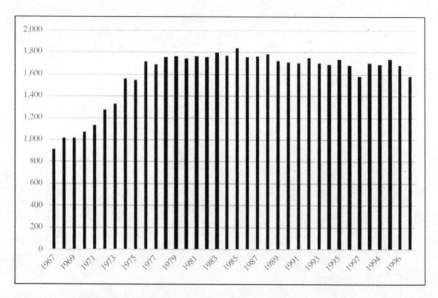

Figure 9.2 Graduates of Canadian medical schools, c. 1967–97
From: E Ryten, "None Is Too Many – It's Time to Discard This Bankrupt Physician
Supply Policy for Canada," ACMC Forum 31; 8–17.

of immigration, this might well result in fewer immigrants being accepted. As a consequence, despite the relatively progressive principles, in
1978 fewer immigrants were accepted into Canada than any year since the
early 1960s.[23]

The confluence of these federal immigration changes, as well as the
provincial restrictions on licensing, resulted in a dramatic drop in the
number of foreign-trained doctors entering Canada, from a peak of more
than 1,200 per annum in the early 1970s to just fewer than 400 in 1976, bot-
toming out at 250 in 1978. For the next twenty years, the number of foreign-trained doctors fluctuated annually but averaged less than 400 per
year, more or less the level that was in place in the pre-1957 era. By contrast,
domestic medical graduates rose to a new plateau of 1,700 in the 1980s (see
figures 9.1 and 9.2). One could argue that this decline in foreign doctors
was an inevitable result of declining (and converging) ratios of residents
per physician across the country. Yet, the improving provincial ratios
masked stark regional differences. While urban and suburban Canada en-

joyed robust communities of doctors, less demographically dense areas of the country struggled with chronic problems of physician retention.

It wasn't just the perception that foreign doctors were allegedly moving from poorer to richer provinces once they were able to do so; it was also that newly graduated doctors from Canadian medical schools were being trained in urban centres and staying in urban (and suburban environments) after graduation. Ministers of health knew there was relatively little they could do with existing medical practices located in urban and suburban areas. However, *new* practitioners (particularly, foreign-trained doctors arriving in the country) offered different opportunities for health policy planners. All ten provinces agreed, in principle at least, to begin to restrict the licensing of foreign-trained doctors to "individuals with pre-arranged job contracts (approved by the province) or those willing to accept a term of indenture to practice in a designated area of need for a specific term" and to explore more aggressive ways of locating doctors in underserviced areas.[24] As discussed in previous chapters, this trend towards issuing "provisional" or "conditional" licenses became an important, if controversial, tool for provincial ministers of health by the late 1970s onwards. By implementing mobility restraints, it could keep immigrant physicians in poorer provinces, and rural and remote areas, without going overboard in the provision of local incentives. The rise of medical indenture also reflected the attempt to continue to fill gaps in health care areas, training positions,[25] or regions while recognizing that the overall (national or even provincial) supply of physicians appeared to be sufficient. The battle over the maldistribution of doctors, and provincial attempts to restrict where doctors could practice, would reach an apex in the 1980s and be constrained, perhaps unexpectedly, by the implementation of the Charter of Rights and Freedoms.

REMUNERECTOMIES

By the time of the 1976 Immigration Act many health economists were concluding that Canada had, in fact, overshot. The country now had too many doctors. For the general public, by contrast, the idea that there could be too *many* medical practitioners seemed odd indeed, both on a practical and cultural level. How could one have too much medical attention? Weren't there still parts of the country that didn't have a family doctor at all? So much newspaper and popular coverage of medical practice in the 1960s and 1970s had been dominated by perceived doctor and nursing shortages that few could fathom that an oversupply suddenly existed. There was also a cultural bias in many journals that reflected a lack of comprehension of the internal logic of how a "market" operated in the new universal health insurance system. A 1974 *Financial Post* editorial outlined a classic model of supply and demand that, it believed, would assist in physician maldistribution – "the aim should be an ample supply of doctors. If this mean a surplus, so much the better. The competition might produce better service in the cities, push more doctors to outlying regions, perhaps even encourage emigration to where medicos [*sic*] are needed instead of draining them from those places."[26]

Some health economists, however, begged to differ and pointed to the fact that universal health insurance systems had created a marketplace that was anything but classical. Traditional concepts of supply and demand and the flexibility of price points for services simply did not apply. The demand for health care – free at the point of delivery – appeared limitless. Moreover, physicians acted as gatekeepers to many other forms of insured and uninsured health services. Through referrals and prescriptions and through deciding among a range of treatment alternatives physicians exercised a significant degree of control over (and demand for) the utilization of services, all of which (if deemed necessary) were paid for by a single payer – the provincial government. Robert G. Evans, among our leading health economists, cautioned Canadians that "suppliers of health care determine customers' perception of need so that consumers believe they need unnecessary care."[27] This view, called "physician generated demand," became sufficiently popular that it was described as orthodoxy by the 1980s.[28]

In a highly influential 1976 article in *Canadian Public Policy*, Evans claimed that a consensus was emerging about physician oversupply and that, in Canada, "nobody loves an immigrant physician" any more.[29] Yet, some did. And one of those to take issue with the claim of consensus was Malcolm C. Brown an expert on the personal financing of health services across Commonwealth nations. In 1977, one year after Evans's article came out, he took on this position directly, debating him in a follow-up special issue of the same journal. Their back-and-forth revealed the ways in which medical liberalism underpinned the physician distribution debates in 1970s Canada, debates that critically influenced policymaking on managing foreign-trained physicians. Restricting physician supply through immigration was simply too risky for researchers like Brown. Indeed, he claimed that it was impossible to predict what would happen to the landscape of service access in Canada when the supply of doctors was restricted in a period when the demand was still expanding (as a result of Medicare but also from new technologies and treatments). "The relation between actual and optimal numbers of practitioners," he argued, was "theoretically indeterminate." Brown was unconvinced by the common premise that more physicians simply meant more billing; instead, he launched a spirited critique of the fee-for-service billing system and how it drove service demand by incentivizing extra visits and procedures, what he called "doctor initiated excess servicing." The overdeployment of routine procedures – dubbed "remunerectomies" in some circles – was the real problem.[30] "Other things being equal," he wrote, "a policy of restricting the number of medical practitioners would probably affect the complete package of medical services."[31] In order to protect physician access in high priority areas – which included rural and remote areas – it would be less risky for the federal government to design programs that facilitated both practitioners' entry into and exit from medical markets in the Canadian provinces, have more salaried positions in health care, and aim for policies that made patients better informed consumers of medical care.

In a rebuttal, Evans, quite surprisingly, agreed. The economist clarified that his policy papers "emphasized the 'second-best' nature of the policy of restricting immigration." One of the reasons his work focused on limiting physician immigration was that it assumed "a more radical restructuring of the health care system" was off the table.[32] Evans, in fact, clearly articulated his own critique of the "paternalistic sovereignty" that underpinned the monopoly power of Canadian physicians. "The most important dimension of [this] monopoly," he explained, "arises from a confusion … between the supply of medical services and that of physicians. One of the most important problems with independent fee-for-service practice is the power and incentive it gives physicians to exclude non-physician personnel (auxiliaries) from supplying services."[33] Evans also agreed that better patient education would make them better able to refuse excessive care. But he added that the health system in Canada needed better pricing mechanisms and the greater deployment of "auxiliary manpower," by which he was referring to mostly female clinicians like nurse practitioners and midwives.[34]

Physicians influencing the level of service utilization may have been a matter of no great significance on its own, but it interacted with the implementation of universal health insurance in specific ways. First, as mentioned earlier, universal health insurance in Canada embraced the fee-for-service system of remuneration, where most physicians were paid for insurable services according to a set fee schedule for "necessary" medical services. Within a particular provincial system, a service was remunerated the same amount regardless of the seniority or location of the practitioner.[35] The 1984 Canada Health Act indirectly outlawed extra billing (see below),[36] and there was no real mechanism for permitting physicians themselves to *discount* fees even if they wished to do so. This meant patients did not respond to fee differentials, since doctors could not reduce or increase their fees in response to competition. As a consequence, in the context of increasing numbers of physicians and thus fewer potential patients per physician, practitioners often responded by prescribing more services for which they would be remunerated. In addition, some doctors gravitated to more expensive and efficient interventions, ones that tended to earn them more. For example, researchers became increasingly aware of an overprovision of surgeries, well beyond the point deemed medically necessary.[37]

Physician oversupply also indirectly affected the fee schedule itself. The schedule was usually determined annually by the provincial governments in consultation with provincial medical associations. When doctors were in oversupply and found themselves with fewer patients, health economists hypothesized that these medical practitioners might well respond by lobbying for higher fees, given that doctors have cultural expectations of earning a certain annual income. This concern was acknowledged in a 1980 federal status report on health care in Canada, in which Justice Emmett Hall wrote, "if an oversupply of doctors in an area persists, pressure will be placed on the provincial government to unnecessarily inflate the payment [fee] schedule to generate the desired income of doctors."[38]

Perhaps unsurprisingly, within a near consensus building around the idea of physician oversupply, the spotlight turned to immigrant doctors.

Although the absolute number of foreign-trained doctors entering the country had declined fourfold from the mid-1970s, they continued to be the focus of sustained attention and not always in predictable ways. As provincial governments witnessed health care costs rising relentlessly at a higher rate than inflation, some health economists saw a cold logic in placing more (not less) emphasis on foreign-trained doctors, since the costs of training them were borne by the countries of origin. Evans himself reasoned that, as immigrant doctors were already trained and immediately available while domestic graduates required public funding and many years to train, the optimal solution might be to close down a few medical schools and rely more heavily on the steady demand of foreign graduates wanting to immigrate to Canada.[39] However, many saw this as a political impossibility due to the strength of the medical lobby and possible backlash from the public to the reduction in medical school placements for young Canadian men and women.[40] As a consequence, provinces further restricted the number and type of medical positions available to graduates of non-Canadian medical schools.

TOO MANY AND TOO FEW

British Columbia, the province in which Levinson originally began practice in Canada, represents an excellent case study in the paradoxical situation of a province having both too many and too few doctors. Despite the province's proliferation of physicians in the late 1960s and early 1970s, 68 per cent of doctors lived in the metropolitan regions of Vancouver and Victoria, a trend towards urban practice that was mirrored nationwide.[41] In response to the concentration of physicians in urban areas, British Columbia began preventing the issuance of billing numbers[42] in areas deemed "overserviced,"[43] apparently a measure that had recently been introduced under the National Health Service in Britain. Although logical from a bureaucratic standpoint, the public policy gambit, first implemented in 1983, was quickly challenged as being a violation of mobility and equality rights under the newly established Canadian Charter of Rights and Freedoms.[44] In the landmark case of *Mia v. Medical Services Commission (British Columbia)* (1985), Justice McEachern granted an administrative law remedy,[45] as the policy was enforced through a policy directive and not enshrined in legislation.[46] He applied sections 6(2) and 7 of the charter, stating, "freedom of movement within the province for the purpose of lawful employment or enterprise, or for the practice of a profession, trade or calling by qualified persons in any community, is indeed a right properly embraced within the rubric of liberty."[47] The policy implications were huge: in effect, the judiciary was overruling the democratically elected provincial legislature in the balance between the right of the province to dictate the geographical location of medical practice versus the right of doctors to practice where they chose. Despite his implicit admonition to elected members of parliament, the government of British Columbia further tested the new constitutional landscape by legislating the provision again as the Medical Service Amendment Act in May 1985.[48] Somewhat surprisingly the new regulations were initially upheld by the BC Supreme Court in *Wilson v. Medical Services Commission (British Columbia)*, in 1987, but struck down by the appeals court the following year.[49] The appeals court decision concluded that "the impugned enactments go beyond mere economic concerns or regulation within the profession. The appellants are all fully qualified and licensed doctors who have been excluded from pursuing the practice of their profession. It matters not whether the exclusion of the opportunity to practice is exclusion from practice everywhere in British Columbia, or exclusion from practice anywhere but specified geographic areas of the province."[50]

Thwarted by the courts, British Columbia tried yet other ways to coerce doctors into rural and remote areas. Instead of restricting (geographically) the ability of physicians to bill for necessary medical services, the government attempted to manipulate the fee schedule itself to provide both inducements and enforce fee penalties. In essence, the Ministry of Health began to restrict, in the early 1990s, what fees physicians could charge. Newly graduated or arrived physicians who qualified to bill the provincial health care system (so-called "new billers") were reimbursed at a rate depending on where they practiced: they received 100 per cent of billings in "underserviced" areas, 75 per cent in "adequately serviced" areas, and 50 per cent in "overserviced" areas. As a way of softening the blow, all doctors were entitled to full compensation after five years of practice and exceptions were made for BC-trained physicians and BC physicians returning to the province after an absence no greater than two years. Supreme court challenges in the 1990s persisted, repeatedly constraining the prerogative of provincial governments to force medical practitioners into underserviced areas. In the wake of the Charter of Rights and Freedoms, some scholars began to question what they termed the "judicialization" of health care policy in the country.[51]

CANADA HEALTH ACT (1984)

The 1970s had been challenging for provincial governments managing the new era of universal health insurance. The great postwar economic boom had come to an end with the oil crisis of 1973 and the following decade of "stagflation" leading to a severe recession in 1981. The federal government struggled with the ongoing economic malaise and the resultant budget deficits; they turned their attention to the hefty annual co-payments for Medicare. In 1977, the Liberal government stepped back from open-ended support of insured services. In its place, it created a system known as Established Program Financing (EPF). In effect, the EPF changed the transfer of health care dollars from the cost sharing enshrined in the 1957 HIDS Act and the 1966 Medical Care Act to block funding through an annual health transfer. The financial constraints, in turn, manifested themselves in near stagnant increases in fee schedules at the provincial level, eroding doctors' real salaries over time. After seeing their salaries augment during the first fifteen years of federally cofunded hospital and medical insurance (1957–72), average take-home salaries began to lose ground compared to other comparable professions.[52]

In response to grumblings from the medical profession, some provinces began to tacitly accept extra billing, the practice of doctors charging patients direct fees above the amount that they were remunerated under their provincial fee schedule.[53] Needless to say, in the era of "free Medicare," extra billing became a major political issue. The general public grew unsupportive of this practice, and the tension between their expectations and that of a significant cohort of high-earning doctors ultimately led to a Royal Commission in 1979, headed (once again) by Justice Emmett Hall. Unsurprisingly, the commission concluded that extra billing contravened a key principle of Medicare – namely that access to medical services ought not to be determined on the basis of individual wealth. Provincial health ministers, however, largely disregarded the commission report, and the

Ottawa Citizen reported one prominent physician as anonymously claiming, unkindly, that "this country does not need to listen to the report of a
man with one foot in the grave."[54] The federal Liberal government took
little action, consumed as it was by the 1980 referendum in Quebec, the
recession of the next year, and the constitutional battles of 1982. Finally,
with the new constitution signed, Liberal Health Minister Monique Bégin
published a position paper stating the government's intention to eliminate extra billing.[55] To that end, the Canada Health Act was introduced into
Parliament 12 December 1983, received royal assent by 1 April 1984, and
came into force 1 July 1984, in the dying days of the Liberal government.

The 1984 Canada Health Act followed many of the protocols outlined
in the 1966 Medical Care Act. It laid out conditions that had to be met by
provincial governments as a prerequisite for receiving federal health
transfers. Sections 8–12 specified five criteria that must be met in order to
receive full federal funding. They included the four from 1966 – public administration, comprehensiveness, universality, portability – and added a
fifth: *accessibility*. Section 12 declared that provinces "must provide for insured health services on uniform terms and conditions and on a basis that
does not impeded or preclude … access to those services by insured persons."[56] Extra billing and medically necessary user charges, though they
could be considered to fall under section 12, were explicitly banned elsewhere in the act. The penalty for allowing them to continue was a reduction in transfers equal to the dollar amount of extra billing taking place
in the province. If provinces eliminated extra billing within three years of
the Canada Health Act coming into force, they would be compensated for
all transfer reductions done as a result of extra billing. Most observers
claim that the Canada Health Act's true purpose was to eliminate those
practices.[57] Bégin describes in her memoir how the only penalty that
existed prior to the Canada Health Act for violating the principles was to
eliminate an entire monthly health transfer to that province. She reasoned
that, faced with this, provinces might close medical services and blame
the federal government for any tragedies that ensued. Seeing this scenario
as unpalatable, the federal government initially took no action on extra
billing. But, to stop the practice, they also decided the country needed a
clear and reasonable synthesis of the five principles and the extra billing
ban, combined with a more "reasonable" punishment mechanism.[58]

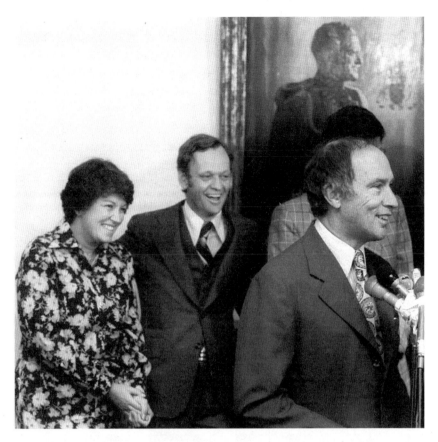

Figure 9.3 Monique Bégin with Jean Chrétien and Pierre Trudeau
From the inauguration of Medicare in 1968 until its revision in the form of the Canada
Health Act (1984), the federal government was controlled by successive Liberal adminis-
trations under the prime ministership of Pierre Trudeau. A key figure in the formula-
tion of the Canada Health Act was one of the few women members of Parliament, the
Québécoise Monique Bégin, who was minister of health at the time of the Canada
Health Act (1984).

Contemporary observers were divided on whether a crisis of access
actually existed as a result of extra billing. In seven of the ten provinces
extra billing was either already banned or virtually nonexistent.[59] Only
Nova Scotia, Alberta, and Ontario exhibited widespread extra billing by
the time of the Canada Health Act, with Ontario taking up forty million
of the estimated 54.6 million of total extra billed dollars in Canada in

1981.[60] Bégin clearly seemed to think that there was a growing problem, claiming that the "government has to take this measure in order to stop the growing erosion of Medicare."[61] Malcolm Brown speculates that, although the rhetoric of an impending crisis was used, the true purpose of the Canada Health Act was to prevent a serious erosion of access further down the road, after an expected Liberal defeat (which, of course, did indeed happen in 1984).[62] He suggests that just as cost sharing was used as a way to incentivize provinces to provide universal access until block grants were introduced in 1977, the Canada Health Act also financially induced provinces towards that end but without exposing the federal government to open-ended financial obligations.[63]

Following the 1984 Canada Health Act, the stage was thus set for a battle over the merits of extra billing and the punitive mechanisms enshrined in the legislation. All ten provinces and every major medical association nationwide lined up against the Canada Health Act, while the bill enjoyed unanimous support from all three federal parties, including the Progressive Conservatives. The reason was clear. A 1984 Gallup poll showed that a staggering 83 per cent of Canadians opposed extra billing. The public debate over the Canada Health Act became conflated with support or opposition of extra billing, which Bégin would later admit was a conscious federal Liberal strategy to polarize the debate.[64] At the end of the battle extra billing had been eliminated in every province, as each province responded to the financial incentive, with the stiffest resistance coming from Ontario.

The debate over extra billing, from the doctors' standpoint, involved both practical and principled issues. The practical issue was simply a desire by a minority of practitioners to continue to bill an amount (government fee + extra charged to the patient) in a manner that was commensurate with their expected income. The principle touched on the longstanding anxiety of the medical profession that a single-payer system would ultimately render doctors little more than modestly paid civil servants rather than the independent professionals that they saw themselves as. They employed strong rhetoric in defending this position. The Canadian Medical Association claimed that the act turned physicians into "a type of state employee," insisting that a system "manned by volunteers" was superior to one "manned by demoralized conscripts."[65] A prominent Ontario surgeon fumed: "I will not be blackmailed into becoming an employee of a government-controlled system."[66] The CMA's president Everett Coffin went so far as to call the new measures "dictatorial legislation."[67] Edwin Urovitz, president of the Scarborough Centenary Medical Association, went a step further, characterising the ban on extra billing "repressive, totalitarian, [and] authoritarian."[68] Dr Ray Holland wrote in a letter to the *Canadian Medical Association Journal* that "there is little doubt that provincial governments will eventually make serfs of doctors."[69] A later CMA president, T.A. McPherson, may have had the most self-righteous response when he borrowed a longstanding historical dictum that, "all that is needed for liberty to be lost is for good men and women to do nothing."[70] Ontario NDP Leader Bob Rae responded to these criticisms by saying "this bill is not Russian. This bill is not fascism … This bill is not terrorism … it is very simply a requirement that the doctors' economic relationship is with the social insurer and not with the individual patient."[71] Rae was not alone in rejecting the hyperbole of some members of the medical profession; the public never became convinced that the loss of physician autonomy was such a terrible thing.[72] As a *Globe and Mail* editorial stated of Bill 94, which sought to ban extra billing in Ontario, "when the doctors speak of being turned into 'civil servants' they are addressing an imagined future scenario which is not justified by Bill 94."[73]

Inflammatory rhetoric aside, many doctors felt that the ban on extra billing was part of a longstanding pattern of government incursion into the realm of physician autonomy that must be resisted in order to prevent a further loss of rights down the road.[74] The overwhelming majority of doctors in Canada did not engage in extra billing, but they feared what would come next – Where they could practice? What patients they had to treat? What treatments they could administer? Some observed with disquiet that the province of Quebec already had quarterly caps on the amount physicians could earn before their rates were heavily discounted and wondered whether or when other provinces would follow suit.[75] These allegations were met with flat denials from politicians. Bégin pronounced, in response, that "no changes are proposed as to government ownership of facilities or imposition of salaried medical practice."[76] In passing Bill 94, Ontario Premier David Peterson concurred that "there is no hidden agenda. This government has no plans beyond this bill."[77]

Extra billing pitted physician autonomy against the newest principle of Medicare – accessibility. Bégin cited the Hall Commission, which observed that "more than one-fourth of those surveyed indicate that it is hard to find a doctor they can afford to see in their home community."[78] In defending the right to extra bill, physicians typically responded that there already existed a tradition of not extra billing "the poor."[79] Bob Rae claimed it would not matter even if the physicians' claim were true, saying that the "institutionalization of charity medicine [is] something this party will never accept."[80] Many criticisms of the Canada Health Act focused not on the merits of extra billing per se but on the methods used to eliminate it. Health care was, of course, a provincial constitutional responsibility, and many pointed out that while using spending power to make it operate a certain way may be technically legal, it was not fair.[81] Provinces claimed that the act forced them to increase medical care funding to compensate for extra billing but that the federal government was not providing the financial support to make this possible. Quebec Health Minister Pierre-Marc Johnson, speaking at a health conference in 1983, piled on, claiming that "declining federal [financial] support is the threat to the Canadian Health care system, not user fees."[82]

It is worth remembering that, even in Ontario, only a minority of practitioners engaged in extra billing, and those practitioners were overwhelmingly specialists.[83] It also allowed for specialists to get paid more when they performed the same services as general practitioners, such as some diagnostic services. However, this justification was clearly less important than that of autonomy, as demonstrated by the OMA's decision to strike in 1986 rather than accept a potential deal that would have offered, somewhat radically, greater fee schedule remuneration for more experienced physicians.[84] Another complaint was that extra billing was the only way to finance some unusual treatments. Doctors claimed that new treatments not yet insured or insured at the wrong level (meaning, in their opinion, below an appropriate amount) would not occur at all if extra billing were banned. Indeed, Ontario had several high-profile cases of doctors closing women's health clinics after the extra billing ban, claiming they couldn't meet costs given the insured remuneration rates for the services they provided.[85] Physicians employed the term "safety valve" in claiming that extra billing provided an "efficient gauge of the satisfaction of doctors and patients"[86] and that the extent of extra billing in the province could be used to demonstrate whether provincial fee schedules were perceived to be fair. Here medical associations often contested the nomenclature of "extra" billing as reinforcing the idea that the provincially negotiated fee schedules were inherently or uniformly "fair" and correctly determined. Nevertheless, neither the provinces nor the medical profession were successful in convincing Canadians that the issue was truly one of autonomy rather than financial self-interest.[87] The public interpreted physician support for extra billing as a straightforward matter of greed. Medical professionals often played into this suspicion. CMA secretary general said on the radio that doctors "traditionally have been leaders in terms of their ability to earn in a community, and they have felt that their traditional position has been undermined,"[88] comments that received wide coverage and reinforced the view that doctors were simply seeking to maximize their incomes. Caricatures in papers across the country, often depicting self-satisfied male doctors returning from the golf course, did little to help the cause of organized medicine.

The perception that doctors were motivated by avarice in opposing extra billing would ultimately undermine the Ontario Medical Association in June 1986 when provincial doctors staged a twenty-six-day strike to protest Bill 94, the provincial legislation enacted pursuant to the Canada Health Act. At the time the Ontario provincial Liberal minority government banned extra billing, with the support of Bob Rae's New Democratic Party. Tellingly, Bill 94 was entitled the "Health Care Accessibility Act," and legislators repeatedly hammered home their only real opposition to extra billing, that it supposedly rendered access to medical services impossible.[89] Ontario was the last province to respond to extra billing, which some speculated was because federal deductions in transfers to that province – which amounted to a total of more than 100 million dollars by the time Bill 94 was passed – cost the province less than it might take to adjust the fee schedule (upward) to compensate for the widespread extra billing. In fact the doctors' claim of being motivated by concerns of autonomy rather than money is supported by the fact that while only 12 per cent of them extra billed by June 1986, somewhere between 50 and 75 per cent of Ontario's doctors participated in the strike, depending on what source one trusts.[90]

The strike, however, proved to be a "public relations disaster"[91] for the Ontario Medical Association. The doctors' association enraged Ontarians by encouraging their members to charge for uninsured services that had previously been "free," such as phone consultations and travel time; these new charges were technically legal but came off as little more than spiteful.[92] Eric Meslin said that Ontarians believed that "by sanctioning a withdrawal of medical services the OMA sought to make a moral issue out of physicians' right to extra-bill, and to elevate that issue to the same moral plane as the Ontario public's right to universal health care."[93] Polling made clear that the vast majority of Ontarians disagreed with this ordering of preferences.[94] Ontarians were further disillusioned by several well-publicized instances of patients being harmed by the strike, weakening the doctors' position even further. In one notable case, a pregnant woman was refused service on the grounds that she was not in an emergency situation, and she miscarried later that day.[95]

Ultimately, most observers thought that the very basis of the strike was misguided and that its failure was predetermined. Jeffrey Simpson called it a "desperate struggle against an irreversible tide of public opinion."[96] A *Globe and Mail* editorial evidently agreed, stating "by calling an indefinite strike, the [OMA] is urging its members to run headlong into a political brick wall."[97] Ann Silversides speculated that the OMA could not possibly believe it could reverse the ban on extra billing and suggested that perhaps they hoped to be legislated back to work, in order to save face, complain of a heavy-handed provincial government, and win future concessions.[98] If this was true they hid it well; nearly three weeks into the strike and after a much-publicized decline in physician participation in strike activities, OMA President Dr Richard Railton encouraged OMA members to vote to continue the strike, claiming that it "is still a win situation for the medical profession,"[99] seeming to justify the claims of those who thought him ill informed. Three years later, the *Globe and Mail* concluded that "it was sheer delusion to think [the extra billing ban] could be rolled back by the 11th-hour demands of a single interest group, but the OMA charged blindly towards the cliff."[100]

In retrospect, the Canada Health Act consolidated the rules governing Medicare into a single piece of legislation but was otherwise unremarkable except for the ban on extra billing. Monique Bégin was correct in calculating that provincial and professional opposition to the banning of extra billing would be overcome by convincing the public that their access to health care depended on it. She later claimed to have received the advice from Pierre Trudeau, based on his experiences with the bitter debates over the patriation of the constitution, that a piece of federal legislation "opposed by the provinces but supported by a majority of Canadians is a sure winner."[101] This prediction proved prescient, as the medical profession was unable to convince Canadians that their professional autonomy should be given preference over the public desire to ensure that no one pay for medical care at the point of delivery. In Manitoba, Nova Scotia, and Saskatchewan the medical profession voluntarily surrendered its right to extra bill after the Canada Health Act was instituted, in exchange for binding arbitration in fee schedule negotiations.[102] However, in Ontario the medical profession drastically overestimated its ability to persuade the provincial government of its views in the face of financial coercion from the federal government and a looming deadline to be compensated for the transfers already deducted. It remains unclear whether the actual level of extra billing was or ever would have been at a point where it meaningfully impeded access for most people and whether physicians were correct that the "poor" were never extra billed as a matter of custom. Nevertheless, the federal Liberals successfully convinced Canadians that the preservation of the system they cherished depended on eliminating extra billing.

SURGEONS DRIVING TAXI CABS

While politicians were fighting medical associations over extra billing, the new reality of the aggregate physician surplus in the country led directly to a new and somewhat peculiar social phenomenon – the un- and under-employment of foreign-trained doctors. From oral interviews and other contemporary documents it is clear that the overwhelming majority of physicians who arrived *before* 1976 found employment as medical practitioners. There was, to be sure, frustration over the requirement to retrain instituted by some provinces, something painful for those who had been practicing already in their country of origin. There was also confusion and a sense of unfairness over the variability of approaches to accreditation adopted by the ten different provinces. The phenomenon of physicians *unable* to get licensed to practice medicine at all, however, was relatively rare. In the latter half of the 1970s, this all changed. Between about 1978 and 1988 a chasm emerged between the number of residency positions (the most common entry point for most foreign-trained doctors) and the number of foreign doctors entering the country and hoping to practice medicine in Canada.

The province of Quebec represents an interesting case study of this phenomenon. The establishment of the medical school at the Université de Sherbrooke at the nadir of the national doctor shortage in the 1960s had provided *la belle province* with a sufficient provincial supply of doctors a decade later. Amidst the recession of the early 80s, Quebec passed a decree (in 1981) limiting the number of new residency (postgraduate) training positions open to foreign graduates to only thirty per year. Over the next few years, foreign-trained doctors kept arriving, apparently unaware of the new restrictions. By 1984 a backlog of 150 foreign-trained doctors were vying for an increasingly miniscule number of dedicated residency positions (only fifteen for the year of the Canada Health Act itself). As frustration mounted and, more importantly, the media began to pick up the story, the Liberal government of Robert Bourassa made repeated one-off attempts to accommodate foreign doctors in the province, only to see the system once again overflow with yet more applicants. Maudlin accounts of underemployed physicians filled the newspapers and medical journals. "They deliver pizzas, wash dishes, drive taxis or work in factories ... The luckier ones find temporary work in hospitals as lab technicians and nurses' aides," one reporter lamented.[103] Many doctors had indeed been waiting years to qualify for a license. As the situation deteriorated over the decade, and frustrations mounted, in March of 1989 seventeen foreign-trained doctors began an unlimited hunger strike for the right to practice.[104]

In retrospect, the provincial government found itself in a no-win situation. The Corporation professionnelle des médecins du Québec (CPMQ), the forerunner to RAMQ[105] (the current provincial health insurance agency), had attempted to warn potential immigrant doctors of the declining availability of residency training positions for non-Canadians. A CPMQ flyer, issued in 1975 and reputedly sent out to immigration consulates around the world in the following years, stated categorically that "due to the increase of Quebec medical graduates and government regulations, there are no posts available for rotating internships in hospitals in the province of Quebec. It is therefore not in your interest to come to

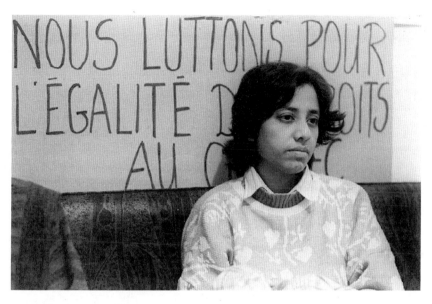

Image 9.4 Hunger Striking Doctors
By the 1980s, many provinces had concluded that they had too many doctors, particularly in urban areas. However, immigrant and refugee doctors continued to arrive from the four corners of the world, only to find that the warm reception afforded to an earlier generation had soured. After years of frustration, one group of Montreal doctors sought to bring light to their situation by engaging in a hunger strike. Eventually, the provincial premier, Robert Bourassa, embroiled in his controversial use of the notwishstanding clause, offered the doctors internships.

the province of Quebec without having obtained an internship appointment and your internship and residency card from the Corporation."[106] It is impossible to determine, however, whether this information reached the intended audience or whether misleading or outdated information continued to circulate internationally about how easy it was to set up a clinical practice in Canada.

By 6 April 1989 outside pressure was mounting with small towns claiming that they would hire the striking doctors and the community health clinics across the province releasing a statement that there was a "physician shortage." On 9 April a Manitoba member of the provincial legislature mischievously released a statement saying that the Manitoba government would be interested in hiring the doctors if the Quebec government was unable to provide placements.[107] On day sixteen of the hunger strike, the

Quebec government sent in a mediator to negotiate with the doctors in order to reach a solution. The next day, the physicians agreed to end their protest after being promised special internship positions by the Quebec health minister.[108] This expedient solution – the Bourassa government was then embroiled in a controversy over the use of the Constitution's not-withstanding clause in December of 1988 and did not want to fight on too many fronts –clearly did not solve the interrelated issues of physician access and the licensing of doctors (and other health care practitioners) from abroad. As health care expenditure would continue to be squeezed by government debt in the coming decade, the theme of doctors driving taxis would become a popular one in the 1990s.

BEYOND DOCTORS?

The Canada Health Act may have enshrined accessibility as the fifth principle of Medicare but the problem of attracting physicians to underserviced areas appeared as unsolvable as ever. Over time, some health policy experts began to question the underlying assumption – Did rural and remote areas of the country really need doctors at all? Was there a preoccupation with physician distribution and too little attention to alternative delivery of medical services? During the same year as the hunger strike in Quebec, Canada's deputy ministers of health commissioned two leading health economists Greg Stoddart and Morris Barer to "provide a framework for a national physician resource policy."[109] In their final report, released in 1991, and in subsequent articles, they delineated a comprehensive plan for addressing the persistent problem of a lack of access to primary care in rural and remote areas (something that had been occasioned by the maldistribution of doctors).[110] As they demonstrated, physician attrition in rural areas was typically 2.5 times the urban rate.[111] Rural physicians were disproportionately foreign-trained, and these physicians tended to express much less satisfaction with rural practice than their Canadian-trained, rural-born counterparts.[112] For Barer and Stoddart, systems that used financial or legal inducements to practice in rural areas too often simply promoted transience among physicians. They were clearly not a long-term solution. The researchers recommended placing more emphasis on "alternatives" to physicians in primary care settings, such as licensed midwives, nurse-practitioners, and physician assistants. A new mix of medical personnel was needed, they concluded, and this should occur concurrent to a restriction of medical school enrolment (by 10 per cent) and a reduction on the reliance of foreign-trained physicians to backfill underserviced areas. Finally, they made sweeping recommendations with regard to what they believed to be the inherent bias in medical school recruitment and training towards urban recruits and urban practice.[113]

The Barer–Stoddart Report was well received by governments, which then proceeded to selectively implement their recommendations, most controversially the restriction of medical school placements in Canada.[114] The more comprehensive primary care reform proposals of the report were not immediately operationalized and some, like the physician assistants proposition, would take almost two decades to gain traction. Other recommendations, such as placing greater emphasis on medical school applicants with an intention to practice in rural areas or the establishment of new medical schools away from the principal cities (such as embodied in the Northern Ontario School of Medicine[115] or the University of Northern British Columbia medical program[116]) would only emerge in the first decade of the twentieth-first century. The asymmetrical implementation of the reforms, combined with the dramatic reduction of health transfers in the debt-ridden mid-1990s, compounded by educational changes in the rotating internship,[117] left many wondering, by the turn of the century, what had happened to the doctor "surplus."[118] By the final years of the twentieth century, Canadian newspapers were once again filled with anxious articles about the doctor and nurse shortage in the country and the "brain drain" to the United States. Remarkably, despite the multiple stresses in the system, no mainstream national party dared countenance the reorganization of universal health insurance in the country to permit a private "tier."

CONCLUSIONS

In the decade following the 1976 Immigration Act, Canada "turned off the taps" and "lifted the drawbridge," convinced that the pipeline of new doctors was sufficient for its needs for the next generation. Census statistics of the period appeared to justify this optimism. It illustrated the absolute and per capita increase in physician supply in 1960s and 1970s that resulted from not only the expansion of domestic medical education but also the influx of approximately 12,000 foreign-trained doctors. Canada now had fifteen medical schools operating at full capacity. By 1981, Canada listed 44,275 physicians, almost exactly double the 21,290 that were practicing in 1961, far outpacing the 31 per cent increase in Canada's population over the same period.[119] During the 1980s, physician immigration did not disappear: following immigration restrictions, immigrant physicians still supplied approximately 20 per cent of new annual licenced doctors or "the output of four medium-sized medical schools."[120]

From 1976 onwards, however, the number of landed immigrants claiming "physician or surgeon" as their intended occupation dropped precipitously from the previous generation. The reason for the fewer number of immigrant doctors must have been multifactorial. Clearly, the changes to the Immigration Act of 1976, with its annual quotas of immigrants and its deprioritization of medicine as an occupation in demand, must have had some significant role to play. The timing of the drop and the implementation of the immigration reforms are simply too close to discount. Other, indirect factors may have contributed. Hospitals and local health authorities must have reduced or eliminated their advertisements in foreign medical journals and word must have got out in the medical community that the job market for physicians in Canada had tightened considerably. Doctors, of course, would continue to arrive in Canada, but their position became increasingly precarious, particularly for those who chose to settle in the more prosperous provinces of Ontario and British Columbia. Indeed, as Shuval and Bernstein have demonstrated in their case study of emigrating physicians following the collapse of the Soviet Union, many of these doctors never found employment as clinicians in their adopted countries.[121]

For those who did arrive in the 1980s, the landscape of medical practice had changed dramatically. The ability to secure a license and the conditions under which one could work, would become considerably more circumscribed for newly arrived practitioners by the time of the Canada Health Act. The preoccupation of ministers of health with controlling costs (in part by capping the absolute numbers of doctors) as well as addressing persistent challenges of accessibility, raised fundamental questions about what restrictions provinces could legally introduce to ensure an equitable distribution of doctors. What would take precedence in the new era of the Medicare – the right of patients to have access to doctors or the right of doctors to practice where they wished? After the immigration of thousands of foreign doctors, and despite the use of provisional licenses by the late 1970s, there was little compelling evidence that there were considerably more foreign-trained doctors practicing in rural areas of Canada than in urban ones by the end of the 1980s. A contemporary study of New Zealand found exactly the same result. The influx of hundreds of foreign-trained doctors had little long-term effect on the internal maldistribution of medical practitioners in that country.[122]

Within the complicated battles over physicians' scope of practice and geographical mobility, the Charter of Rights and Freedoms figured prominently in circumscribing the prerogative of provinces to force doctors to underserviced areas. As the British Columbian situation exemplified, the more coercive approaches adopted by some ministries of health were struck down as running afoul of the new Charter's provisions concerning mobility rights. In this respect, although the medical profession would lament its defeat over extra billing in the 1980s, physicians did safeguard many *geographical* freedoms of practice. Indeed, there is some irony, in retrospect, that the most important dimension to the 1984 Canada Health Act – the addition of *accessibility* as a principle of universal health insurance – would be accompanied by the implementation of a Charter of Rights and Freedoms that would itself constrain governments from better providing increased accessibility to patients. Perhaps a further irony is that, twenty years later, in the early 2000s, the Supreme Court would strike down the "illegality" of private care for medically necessary services *because* of the lack of timely access in the public system.[123]

The period between the 1976 Immigration Act and the 1984 Canada Health Act also provided a fascinating learning experience for health economists into the workings and internal logic of single-payer medical markets. Traditional microeconomic models simply did not hold up to universal health care systems that were structured so that very few individual practitioners opted out of the system and where uniform prices were set centrally. More doctors *might* mean better and more comprehensive care, but they also cost the system more money. As the recession of 1981–82 skewered provincial budgets and the federal debt began to spiral out of control later in the decade, the optimal number of physicians, their geographical distribution, and possible alternatives to them became contested topics of debate amongst health policy experts. Midwifery, nurse-practitioner, and physician assistant programs emerged over two decades, a move to greater interdisciplinarity that was concurrent with and reinforced by the growing proportion of female medical graduates in the country. A new model of primary care and medical education was taking shape, one that was occasioned by the recurrent problem of "doctor shortages"[124] in certain parts of the country. Many believed it was time to look beyond the preoccupation with the supply of doctors in order to solve problems over accessibility to, and equity within, universal health care.

Conclusion

In 2004, a small-budget Quebec comedy delighted film festivals. Entitled *La Grande Séduction*, it portrayed the fictional port village of Sainte-Marie-La-Mauderne and its frantic attempts to persuade a multinational corporation to set up a factory on the outskirts of town. In order to meet the company's insurance requirements, the townsfolk must persuade a physician to set up a local practice. The movie then follows the antics of the local residents who do everything in their power to recruit a doctor – any doctor. In the comic centrepiece scene of the movie, the villagers don cricket whites in order to convince a prospect, Dr Paul Lewis, as to the comeliness of their community. It is a particular Canadian twist on an old movie theme of the doctor "out of place" amongst the unsophisticated, but life loving, locals, and in this case the doctor is an urbane Anglophone Montrealer.[1] However, the predictable plotline proved so popular that an English-language remake of the movie was released a decade later, this time situated in a Newfoundland outport called Tickle Head. In the update, Dr Lewis is an American plastic surgeon based in Los Angeles. The movie retained the same contrived but charming plot, replacing earthy Québécois with salty Newfoundlanders. In both cases, the "seduction" is successful: the doctor stays, the town attracts much-needed industrial jobs, and the medical practitioner realizes greater personal and professional satisfaction in an unfamiliar environment.[2]

Movies such as *La Grande Séduction* resonate with audiences because their plotlines touch upon real-life situations. For, beyond the fictional Sainte-Marie-La-Mauderne and Tickle Head and fifty years after the inauguration of Medicare, many communities across Canada continue to suffer from a significant problem of accessing physician services. One half century after its introduction, millions of Canadians, we are told, still do not have a regular primary care practitioner. Wait lists, not only for family physicians but also elective surgeries and specialist consultations, continue to top popular anxieties. Indeed, one could observe that Canadians have felt their entitlement to free universal medical services has been jeopardized, not by ideologies that espouse two-tiered health care as much as by the fundamental maldistribution of health human resources to staff the existing system. The culmination of these pressures led to a Supreme Court ruling in 2005 – the Chaoulli decision – that concluded that provinces did *not* have a constitutional right to deny parallel private health care if the provinces could not provide timely access to health care in the public system.[3]

This book has shown how the "shortage" of doctors is hardly a recent phenomenon. Indeed, the history of Medicare in Canada has been inextricably linked with the problem of physician access and by recurrent doctor and nurse scarcities erupting across the nation. This vexing problem was identified even before the implementation of universal insurance for medical services, prompting provinces, with the financial assistance of the federal government, to establish four new medical schools. However, in the decade lag between the agreement in principle to establish these new medical schools (in the mid-1960s) and the graduation of new cohorts of doctors (in the mid-1970s) provinces looked abroad to bridge the gap. With the timely assistance of the Immigration (Appeals Board) Act of 1967, provinces dramatically increased their licencing of international medical graduates with the hope that they would eventually solve the problem of access to physicians and respond to the demand unleashed by Medicare. Doctors arrived by the hundreds from all parts of the world. By the end of the 1970s almost one-third of the Canadian medical workforce had been trained abroad. Medical diasporas of Indian, Egyptian, Irish, Taiwanese, and South African doctors dotted the country.

The strategy of relying on foreign-trained doctors to fill the gaping holes in the emerging system of universal health insurance had mixed long-term results. At the most aggregate level there was indeed a surge of licensed physicians and surgeons across the country, as the rate of new practitioners (both Canadian-trained and foreign-trained) dramatically lowered the overall ratio of population to physicians. It also narrowed, over time, the interprovincial differences in the provision of medical services. Newfoundland, for example, would see its number of doctors

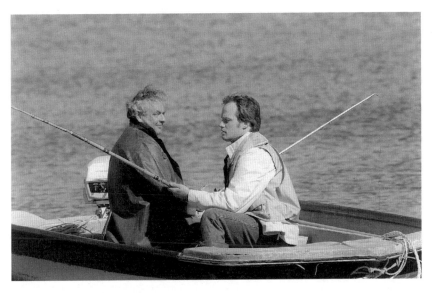

Figure C.1 Seducing Dr Lewis
By the 1990s the unresolved problem of attracting doctors to rural and remote areas
had seeped into popular culture. In the United States this took the form of *Northern
Exposure*, in which a self-centred New York doctor is tricked into relocating to Alaska
to pay off his student debts. In Britain, a popular comedy series entitled *The Indian
Doctor*, involved the adjustment of a South Asian physician amongst the coal miners of
Wales. In Canada, a Québécois film, *La Grande Seduction*, continued this familiar trope,
with the attempts of villages to "seduce" a Montreal Anglophone to relocate to the
Gaspesie. The English remake is set in Newfoundland, where the target of seduction
is an entitled American plastic surgeon.

double in less than a decade, from 345 in 1968 to 605 in 1972, representing
the most dramatic national improvement in resident to physician ratios
for these early years of Medicare. Nova Scotia would place second. Its resident to physician ratio, dropped to below the national average of 618:1.
Although there are many factors that affect physician distribution and retention, the net gain in the first years of Medicare may be attributed
largely to a massive increase in the number of IMGs. As mentioned earlier
in this book, during the first five years of Medicare Canada licensed more
newly arrived doctors than it graduated from domestic medical schools.

The provincial averages and aggregate number of physicians, however,
masked persistent turnover in certain regions. As our oral histories have
demonstrated, some foreign-trained doctors did set up practice and

worked their entire lives in underserviced areas of the country. Some were
recruited to serve group practices, especially in resource towns of Canada's
"new north," while others took up positions in the "Indian hospitals"
and provincial psychiatric facilities across the country. Most foreign-
trained doctors were young, established their families in local communities, and put down roots that would last a lifetime. Others would move
once, maybe multiple times, between practices before settling in more
urban and suburban areas of the country. By the 1990s, a notable few of
this generation of doctors reached significant heights in their respective
specialties, as presidents of medical associations, heads of clinical departments, and deans of medical schools. Taken as a whole, it is likely that
this generation of foreign-trained doctors addressed the *aggregate* problem of physician undersupply in the early era of Medicare, without having
any effect long-term on the maldistribution of doctors *within* provinces
and between regions.

The inability to find a solution to regional doctor shortages lay in the
fact that many of the factors were social, cultural, and demographic and
thus were beyond the control of traditional policy measures. For example,
the twentieth century witnessed a growing trend towards medical specialization, whereby a greater and greater proportion of medical graduates
were not pursuing family practice and where becoming a "generalist" was
looked down upon, a conciliation prize for those not "good enough" for
highly specialized medicine and advanced medical research. Specialization
itself was increasingly dominated by new diagnostic services, which were
invariably located in larger, metropolitan areas of the country. In addition,
the four new medical schools, like the pre-existing dozen, were located in
urban centres. As medical deans knew by observation, and medical researchers began to infer from surveys, medical students from small towns,
for a variety of personal and professional reasons, often did not return
home or to similar small-town locations upon graduation. And urban-
raised young men and women trainees simply did not set up practice in
rural areas of the country. Put simply, young, educated doctors wanted to
live and work on the island of Montreal not the island of Anticosti.

Another means to control the in- and out-flow of doctors was by limiting interprovincial, or even intra-provincial, licensing. However, this
was complicated by the unusual constitutional structure of Canada where

provincial boards regulate licensed practitioners within their jurisdiction but where nationality and mobility arise from a function of being a permanent resident or Canadian citizen. Since specialist qualifications recognized in one Canadian province were almost automatically accepted in another, physicians had a certain national portability of their professional services, particularly after the practitioner received permanent residency.[4] Attempts by provincial governments to restrict the geographical movement of licensed medical practitioners were often struck down by the courts as unconstitutional. With few public policy levers, some provinces continued to suffer from problems of physician transience. Many physicians started out in rural, remote, or otherwise underserviced areas only to relocate to more prosperous regions, to other provinces, or to the United States.

The surge of foreign-trained practitioners entering Canada peaked in the early 1970s and then swiftly returned to pre-1957 levels. This realignment midway through the decade occurred largely as a result of two factors: the coming on line of medical graduates from the new medical schools created in the late 1960s and, secondly, Department of Immigration regulations that ended the priority on assigning generous occupational points to health care practitioners. By 1972 the federal government had implemented a medical service inventory as part of its Health Manpower Directorate organized under the Department of National Health and Welfare. This directorate would analyze the inventory in order to better predict the national need for more physicians. At the time, this included not only select specialties such as internists, neurologists, and obstetricians but also general practitioners. The inventory analysts soon saw signs of oversupply of all kinds of practitioners in British Columbia and Ontario, and as a result, by 1973, the messaging about physician access from the federal government began to shift. Director General of Health Manpower W.S. Hacon began to press for target physician-to-population ratios for Canada. One year later, at a conference of provincial health ministers, the "impending physician surplus" emerged as an official political problem. As a result, the possibility of restricting the immigration of foreign medical graduates was a hot button, and much publicized, concern.

By the mid-1970s, professors in the University of Manitoba's Faculty of Medicine, like Noralou Roos and her colleagues, observed that the public discussion about the doctor shortage had started to "come full circle."[5] With the sudden prospect of too many physicians within Canada's borders, a new debate took shape. One argued that a physician oversupply would be good for underserviced communities, effectively "pushing" doctors to outlying regions and "perhaps even encourage[ing] emigration to where medicos are needed instead of draining them from those places."[6] But government planners worried the glut would merely cause physicians to "overdoctor" some areas and overbill the new Medicare system. By the dawn of the 1980s, provincial ministers of health were looking for ways to curb spiralling health care costs, something made urgent by the recession of 1981–82. Once again, provinces tried to clamp down on the number of new foreign-trained physicians and began to use restricted provincial licences, forcing new foreign-trained licensees into underserviced areas as a form of medical indenture for a particular period of time.[7]

The use of international medical graduates[8] to provide primary care to underserviced communities and institutions, however, was in no way an exclusively Canadian phenomenon. In many respects, what emerged over the last third of the twentieth century was a "regionality" of physician supply that affected many countries in the Western industrialized world. In this way, Manitoba, North Dakota, Wales, and Western Australia bore greater resemblance to each other in terms of their health care challenges than they did to the urban and suburban conglomerations in their own countries.[9] It seems on the surface at least that this disparity and resulting competition for certain kinds of physician services for specific kinds of areas may well have been an example of "functional regionalism" at play in a transnational environment.[10]

Some advocates of Medicare in Canada originally believed that the advent of universal health insurance – with a single fee for specific services regardless of location – would help ameliorate the rural–urban inequalities by raising the remuneration of rural doctors vis-à-vis their urban counterparts. This amelioration did not happen uniformly across Canada, and there was wide variation in accessibility to specialists versus general practitioners across different kinds of rural and remote community life. Medical recruitment to underserved areas became a common concern for many countries, including those characterized by "socialized," "mixed," and "free market" systems. This suggests that the *payment model* of a health care system might be considerably less important in guaranteeing access to health services than the structure of the society and economy. Ultimately, the question of access engages the thorny problem of regional disparities, an issue that underpins the weaker supply of rural doctors no matter which health system was adopted by a given country.[11]

Reading deeply and widely into the contested views about access to medical services we see more debate than consensus around the decision to limit the entry and credentialing of foreign-trained physicians in the years leading up to the Canada Health Act of 1984. Certainly, it is clear that immigration and the implementation of Medicare shifted the medical economics of Canada and influenced the distribution of doctors. Below the surface of public policy discourse, there was little consensus of opinion, mainly because different regions and provinces experienced the immigration of medical professionals in different ways. Examining the postwar history of medical immigration to Canada brings elements of public policy into sharper relief, allowing us to appreciate how service disparities are affected by a range of factors, some of which relate to regional concentration of wealth, local conditions of practice and incentives, while others relate to the larger picture of professional sovereignty and monopoly power.

Additionally, it is important to point out that while governments increasingly put the emphasis on enacting local measures to attract physicians, some received more intervention and incentivization than others. Different provinces saw a range of economic, social, and political relationships emerge between regional "centers" and "peripheries," which can be further complicated by placing it within the legacy of Canadian settler colonialism. The servicing of First Nations reserves and hospitals with foreign-trained physicians, some of whom appeared to be "fast-tracked" through the credentialing system, is a case in point and one that deserves further investigation. This support was to be critical in the pursuit of service access. For, as we have discovered, even the most valiant local efforts can be undermined by macro forces of migration and medical liberalism. These forces have operated since midcentury in an increasingly open, international medical marketplace; local incentives, approaches, and policies work less effectively in environments that have allowed for the easy international flow of highly trained medical personnel.

MEDICAL IMMIGRATION MEETS
GLOBAL HEALTH ETHICS

During the late 1970s and 1980s, the interest in the international migration
of foreign-trained doctors subsided in concert with the dramatic decline
in the licensing of IMGs in most industrialized countries. By the late-
1990s, however, the issue of national doctor and nursing shortages re-
emerged as a major topic of concern and public interest in Canada. By
this time, rural regions of industrialized countries were finding themselves denuded of primary care and looked abroad once again to foreign-
trained doctors as a solution. But, unlike a generation prior, a global
public policy debate had emerged around this phenomenon. In this era
of globalization, politicians and policy makers could no longer claim ig-
norance of the impact of medical migration had on the countries left behind. Within this new global perspective, South Africa played a totemic
role. Devastated by the AIDS pandemic of the 1990s and 2000s, and
struggling with rebuilding a post-Apartheid civil society, the exodus of
(mostly) white doctors, aided and abetted by western countries, touched
raw nerves. And Canada was a principal country recruiting South African
doctors, peaking in the 1990s.[12] The exact number of doctors practicing
abroad is indeterminate, but the South African Medical Association estimated, in 2002, that approximately 50 per cent of its domestically trained
doctors were living abroad.[13] South Africa itself responded by recruiting
African doctors from poorer states, such as Uganda and Tanzania. The
South African Medical Journal described a type of "medical carousel" in
which doctors appeared to be continually moving to countries with a perceived higher standard of living and social stability.[14]

The outstanding question was what could and, for that matter, should
wealthy nations do about it. Critics suggest that Canada embraced, and
continues to embrace, an immigration that is based upon "poaching" the
best and the brightest from less wealthy countries. There can be little denial
that Canada and other countries in the global north made use of the ready
supply of physicians to remedy shortfalls in medical personnel during the
crucial period of the 1960s and 1970s. This pattern has resulted, some argued, in the depletion of health human resources in countries that are not
only poorer but also often plagued by serious public health challenges. Calls
for the prohibition, or at least "ethical regulation," of the transnational mi-

gration of health care practitioners have come and gone.[15] Britain, for
example, pledged in 2001 to tighten the loopholes in its commitment to
stop recruiting from the "developing world,"[16] instead enticing health care
practitioners from poorer countries of the European Union. The World
Health Organization attempted to draw international attention to the issue
by making 2005–15 the decade of global health human resources.[17]

By contrast, some commentators, including some of the doctors we interviewed for this book, suggest that it would be unethical to restrict the
free movement of skilled labour. Physicians, they argued, have as much a
right to optimal working conditions, safe neighbourhoods, or decent pay
as anyone else does.[18] They have a right to personal mobility. While some
argue that the poor public health conditions in Africa are "a result of
factors unrelated to international movement of health professionals,"
others lament that even if a restriction on the emigration of health professionals were desirable it would be largely impossible to enforce.[19] Some
policy experts have suggested that recipient countries could compensate
the countries where the physician trained either in straight monetary
terms or through medical exchange programs.[20] These transfers would
assist in enhanced physician remuneration (in the so-called donor countries) that would reduce one major factor in the decision to emigrate.
Such a global system, however, would necessitate a strong international
organization with the ability to enforce rules and determine levels of compensation. There appears little self-interest in the global north to entertain
formal compensation schemes. Initiatives have thus largely been left to
institutional (hospital and/or university) exchanges and outreach, often
launched my medical émigrés themselves or by large international foundations with particular agendas of their own.

FROM BOMBAY TO GLACE BAY

In 2013, Dr Mohan Virick surprised the communities of Glace Bay and
Sydney, Nova Scotia, when he announced he was giving 140 hectares of
property to the local Mi'kmaq First Nation at Eskasoni. This, Virick insisted, was given as part of their "inheritance." The nearby Eskasoni reserve is the largest in the Atlantic region, comprising a community of
about 4,000 individuals. By 2013, Virick had lived and worked in North

Sydney area for fifty years, and the announcement of this land transfer, which included valuable commercial property in the downtown core, came on the cusp of the physician's retirement. Although he and his wife had four children and nine grandchildren of their own, Virick says he also considered the Eskasoni Mi'kmaq part of his family. Since the community needed support in the here and now, he saw little merit waiting for a posthumous bequest. As he told a reporter from the *Halifax Chronicle-Herald*, "I love them like my kids. When you get older, you pass on things to your children."[21]

Originally of Indian descent but raised in Burma, Virick immigrated to Canada in 1963 after graduating from the Christian Medical College in India. His emigration to Cape Breton fulfilled a long-held dream for the young physician, who had decided in elementary school that he wanted to move to Canada after seeing a documentary on log rolling. He wrote to the Canadian embassy in Burma to get more information, and they advised him to apply after he graduated, which is exactly what he did. As Virick's story goes, he did indeed arrive in Canada several years later, a medical diploma in his hand but only $5 in his pocket. He also possessed little precise knowledge of the geography of Nova Scotia, having arranged no means to get from the airport in the capital city of Halifax to his first Canadian job, in Sydney, which he was not aware was more than 400 kilometres away. It was at this juncture that an Indigenous man, Michael Sappier, helped the newly arrived physician by driving him to Cape Breton so he could be present for his first scheduled day of work. This began a relationship that would last for decades. Sappier became one of Mohan Virick's patients but also his friend. One year later Sappier would loan Virick a suit so the doctor could get married to Mabel Ann, a woman from the area with whom he had also become acquainted soon after his arrival. His connection to Sappier provided Virick with a lifelong friend, as well as entry into the lives of the Eskasoni. This would be the community who, over the years, would comprise the bulk of patients coming through his walk-in family practice clinic in North Sydney.[22] Periodically, he would refer patients to Dr Gupta, the doctor whose life story opened this book.

Virick's emigration to Canada forms part of a larger diaspora of trained health personnel to Canada in the second half of the twentieth century.

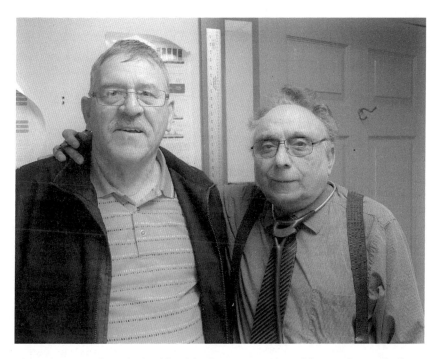

Figure C.2 Dr Mohan Virick with Michael Denny, member of the grand council of the Eskasoni First Nation, Sydney, Nova Scotia, 2012
Fifty years after the Fairclough Directive began the decade-long liberalization of immigration regulations, many foreign-trained doctors were preparing for retirement and looking back on their lives in their adopted countries. Here, Dr Mohan Virick made local news by donating land he had invested in over the previous decades to the Easkasoni First Nation near Sydney, Nova Scotia, situated just next to his family clinic.

His journey in the 1960s was an early ripple in advance of a large-scale migratory wave of tens of thousands of health practitioners relocating across national boundaries. This phenomenon did not go unnoticed and indeed, beginning in this decade, it elicited much concern internationally.[23] Alfonso Mejía, chief medical officer of manpower systems for the World Health Organization, wrote extensively on the phenomenon, observing in 1978 how "anxiety evoked by migration was reach[ing] a peak in both major donor and recipient countries."[24] This "brain drain," according to Mejía, was inextricably linked to economic inequality, and it presaged an uncontrollable loss of medical practitioners from the "developing" world

to the "industrialized" world for the rest of the twentieth century and perhaps beyond. Countries like Britain, the United States, and Canada profited from this mass migration. Physicians were mobile in this era, drawn
to North America at a time of health care service expansion.[25]

This book has traced the history and complexity of the "brain drain"
of doctors and in particular how Canada was situated at the crossroads
of medical migration. Medicare and immigration intersected in powerful
ways in the period 1957–84, dramatically changing the nature of medical
practice in this country. Few communities remained unaware of and un-
affected by the surge of medical immigration. Medical immigration was
diverse, ambiguous, and layered, at once a story of a new era of "racially
blind" immigration to Canada, the early years of a new multicultural nation, and also the first decade of the experiment of Medicare. It also reflected the tumultuous period of decolonization and political upheaval
around the world. Haitian medical professionals leaving the oppression
of the Duvalier regime; Egyptian doctors escaping "Arab socialism"; Czech
medical practitioners taking the brief opportunity of open borders during
the Prague Spring and Warsaw Pact invasion of 1968; American draft doctors who could no longer stomach their role in (medically) approving
young men to serve in Vietnam; Pakistani physicians and surgeons leaving
South Asia during the civil war with East Pakistan (Bangladesh); Jewish
South African doctors who could no longer reconcile themselves to the
growing polarization and oppression of Apartheid South Africa. The early
years of Medicare saw no shortage of good reasons to move oneself and
one's family to the unfamiliar but potentially safe and secure environs of
Canada. And came they did, by the hundreds, leaving a multigenerational
impact on the social and medical history of Canada and the countries
they left behind.

Some arrived, like Dr Virick, with $5 in their pocket and no organized
transportation. Others, however, like Swinson, the ten millionth immigrant to the country, found themselves unexpectedly in the temporary
glare of national media. They constitute, collectively, an important
chapter in the history of contemporary Canada. And, at times, history
would appear to repeat itself. In 2015, at the height of the European and
Middle East refugee crisis, the new Canadian government fast-tracked
the acceptance of 25,000 Syrian refugees. In what was no doubt a signal
event of the new Liberal government, Prime Minister Justin Trudeau

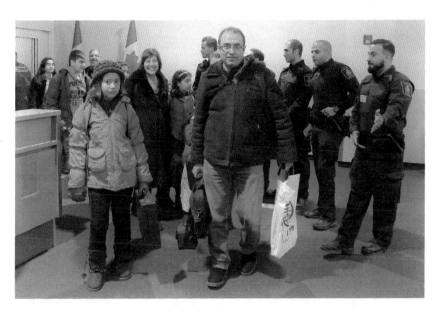

Figure C.3 The Garabedian family arrives at Toronto's Pearson airport, 2015
At the height of the Syrian refugee crisis of 2015, a photo opp of arriving refugees was arranged to reassure Canadians of their nonthreatening nature. One of the first families off the plane were the Garabedians. In multiple interviews that followed, Vanig Garabedian, a gynecologist–obstetrician from Aleppo, spoke movingly of the chaos in Syria and how his clinic had been hit by rockets. Five years later, at the time of this book going to press, Dr Garabedian was still waiting to practice medicine independently in Canada.

waited at Toronto's Pearson airport to personally welcome the first plane-load of refugees to the country. What was less reported is that on the plane the exhausted refugees were asked to wait temporarily before they disembarked, while political attachés shepherded an ideal representative for the inevitable photo-op. Many political leaders in the United States, in the throes of campaigning for the American primaries, had framed the Syrian refugees as potential perpetrators, rather than victims, of terror. As a consequence, the advisors to the new prime minister were eager to provide the most reassuring face to this wave of new Canadians. The selection was Vanig Garabedian, an obstetrician–gynaecologist, his wife Anjilik Jaghlassian, and their three daughters. "Welcome home," Trudeau enthused, as he picked out parkas for the foreign-trained doctor and his tired but photogenic family.[26]

Notes

INTRODUCTION

1 Personal correspondence with Dr Mohini Gupta and Dr Mona Gupta.

2 The precarious status of Indian and Pakistani doctors training under and working for the National Health Service in the 1950s and 1960s has recently been explored in two books: Haynes, *Fit to Practice* and Simpson, *Migrant Architects of the NHS*.

3 "Doctor Returned to Cape Breton to Fulfil Dying Wish," *Cape Breton Post*, 12 September 2011. https://www.pressreader.com/canada/cape-breton-post/20110912/282956741885512.

4 For more on the life of Mohan Virick, see Mullally and Wright, "Connecting to Canada," 230–56.

5 "The Greatest Canadian," Canadian Broadcasting Company, 2004. https://www.cbc.ca/archives/entry/and-the-greatest-canadian-of-all-time-is.

6 We will follow the tradition of capitalizing Medicare, though we recognize that some of the historical literature does not. For a useful summary of the ambiguities of the term, see Marchildon, *Making Medicare*, 5–6.

7 This is not limited to public history but also includes retrospective accounts by well-known medically trained authors. See, for instance, Lam, *Extraordinary Canadians*.

8 Houston, *Steps on the Road to Medicare*.

9 Smith, *Prairie Giant*.

10 Taylor, *Health Insurance and Canadian Public Policy*, 3rd ed.

11 It is instructive that his book was published the same year as the last major doctors' strike in the country. See Naylor, *Private Practice, Public Payment*. See also Naylor, ed., *Canadian Health Care and the State*.

12 Various public prepaid health care schemes came forth in the 1940s and 50s. For Nova Scotia, see McAlister and Twohig, "The Check Off?," 1504–6; and

for British Columbia, see Marchildon and O'Byrne, "From Bennett Care to Medicare," 207–28.

13 New Brunswick had significant difficulty in implementing the system due to competing programs aimed at creating equal opportunity among rural and urban, French and English-speaking populations. See Marchildon and O'Byrne, "Last Province Aboard," 150–67.

14 Marchildon, *Making Medicare*, passim.

15 Maioni, *Parting at the Crossroads*; See also Gray, *Federalism and Health Policy*; Boychuk, *National Health Insurance*; Finkel, "Why Canada has a Universal Medical Insurance Programme."

16 See Jones, "Health and Nation Through a Transnational Lens."

17 Flynn, *Moving Beyond Borders*.

18 Calliste, "Women of Exceptional Merit," 85–102, 87–8. See also previous work by Flynn in "Proletarianization," 57–60.

19 Flynn, "Race, the State, and Caribbean Immigrant Nurses," 247–63. See also Shkimba and Flynn, "'In England We Did Nursing,'" 141–57.

20 Choy, *Empire of Care*.

21 Jones and Snow, *Against the Odds*.

22 Simpson, Esmail, Kalra, and Snow, "Writing Migrants Back into NHS History," 392–6; Simpson, *Migrant Architects of the NHS*.

23 We have preferred to use the term "transnational" in our book, rather than "global." There has been a distinct trend towards so-called "global" histories of various kinds, but the general vagueness of the term has led to a backlash in some historical quarters. Our use of "transnational" simply acknowledges that the migration of doctors and health care providers occurred across and between different national (and regional) domains.

24 Armstrong, "The Common-Health and Beyond."

25 See Mody, "'The Intellectual Boys are the Ones in a Mess,'" 1–20; Mody, "Revisiting Post-war Medical Immigration," 485–509; Mody, "Migrant Medical Women."

26 Greenwood and Topiwala, *Indian Doctors in Kenya*.

27 Jones, "'Strike Out Boldly,'" 55–74.

28 Huish and Kirk, "Cuban Medical Internationalism," 77–92. See also Huish, "Cuba's Latin American School of Medicine," 301–4.

29 Strictly speaking, physicians and surgeons, within the history of medicine and indeed in common nomenclature (Royal College of Physicians and Surgeons), denote the principal two arms of medical practitioners. In practice,

"physicians," as a term, tends to be used ambiguously, particularly in North America, to denote doctors in general.

30   As we emphasize throughout the book, a small proportion of individuals who graduated from foreign medical schools – particularly in Ireland and Britain – were Canadian born.

31   Hoerder, *Cultures in Contact*, 512.

32   Stevens, Goodman, and S.S. Mick, *The Alien Doctors*, 3.

33   For perspectives on the American and international roots of Canadian Medicare, see Duffin, "The Guru and the Godfather," 191–218; and ongoing research by J.T.H. Connor on Dr Frederick Mott and rural health care in the United States and Canada. For a wider international movement, focusing on interwar socialist experimentation with health clinics, see Jones, *Radical Medicine*.

34   This process occurred at different times in different provinces. See Shortt, "Physicians, science, and status," 51–68; See also Naylor, *Private Practice, Public Payment*, chapter 2.

35   The *Canadian Medical Directory* was explicitly based on the British practice, which had existed for more than a century. Prior to 1955 and for several years afterward the medical directories of Canadian provinces were included in the annual editions of the *American Medical Directory*. The 1955 CMD took almost five years to compile and fact check, and resulted in 85 per cent of all doctors confirming the accuracy of their listings. From that point onwards doctors were encouraged to contact the CMD office with updates and/or corrections to their entries. Thousands of copies were distributed to doctors' offices, to medical schools, to hospitals, and to university libraries. The foreword to the 1955 edition (i.e. the first Canadian edition) describes the process of collecting the data and the professional reasons for the publication. See Feasby, *Canadian Medical Directory, first edition*.

36   As discussed in the principal chapters of this book, doctors who were retired, "away"/"abroad" or working for the armed services (for example, stationed in Germany) were not included in the GIS mapping and tables included in this book. In addition, doctors with foreign practicing address were also excluded. Semiretired doctors were included in mapping, based on the principle that they were still providing active medical services, albeit on a reduced basis.

37   The Southam Medical Database has been used for studies of doctors from 1972, including articles (on South African doctors in Canada) by Hugh Grant and contemporary studies of IMGs, such as CIHI's own study of the period

1972–76. See Grant, "From the Transvaal to the Prairies," 681–95; Canadian
Institute for Health Information (CIHI), "International Medical Graduates
in Canada, 1972 to 2007: Analysis in Brief," part of CIHI, *Supply, Distribution
and Migration of Canadian Physicians*.

38 As discussed further in the book, "nationality"" was not a straightforward
concept in terms of the creation of immigration statistics. Indeed, in the
years leading up to 1962, nationality and ethnicity were often conflated, such
as the use of the terms "East Asian," "Chinese," or the collections of statistics
on "Jews."

39 Less well known than the federal Royal Commission on Health Services
(Hall Commission) were provincial commissions of inquiry, such as the
Commission on Health Services (Brain Commission) in Newfoundland,
which reported in January of 1966. See Kealey and Molyneaux, "On the
Road to Medicare."

40 Because the oral interviews were conducted under REB protocols in different
universities (McMaster University, University of Alberta, St Mary's University, the University of New Brunswick, and McGill University) there were different recommendations and requirements as to the anonymity (or not) of
interviewees. As a consequence, some of those interviewed were anonymized
and others were not.

41 Due to the profound practical and financial implications of health care legislation, it was not uncommon for significant laws to be passed in one year
and to take effect later. This occurred in this case (the act took effect in 1947)
but also with HIDS (passed in 1957 and taking effect in 1958) and with the
Medical Care Act (passed in 1966 but taking effect in 1968). See Medical Care
Act [*An Act to authorize the payment of contributions by Canada towards the
cost of insured medical care services incurred by provinces pursuant to provincial medical care insurance plans*], Statutes of Canada 1966, 14–15 Elizabeth II
(Assented to 21 December 1966) chap 64.

42 Maurice Duplessis rejected what he considered a federal intrusion into
provincial jurisdiction. Quebec would have to wait for the new Lesage
government to pass its own Hospitalization Act, in 1961.

43 Fein, *The Doctor Shortage*; Margulies and Bloch, *Foreign Medical Graduates*.

44 Van Hoek, *The Migration of High Level Manpower*; Gish, *Health Manpower*.
See also Gish, *Doctor Migration*.

45 See for example the "Committee on the International Migration of Talent"
(hereafter CIMT).

46 World Health Organization, *Multinational Study* (1973); Mejía, "Migration of Physicians and Nurses."

47 Evans, "Does Canada Have Too Many Doctors?," 155.

48 Interview with Tanya Levinson (pseudonym), June 2013.

CHAPTER ONE

1 Wilbur, "From Family History to Local History," 196.

2 Jones, "'Strike out Boldly,'" 55–74.

3 See Houston and Smyth, *Irish Emigration and Canadian Settlement*; "Obituary: Leatherbarrow, Albert T," *Canadian Medical Association Journal* 132, no. 7 (1 April 1985): 865.

4 "News Items," *Canadian Medical Association Journal* 7, no. 9 (September 1917): 845.

5 "News Items," *Canadian Medical Association Journal* 45, no. 1 (July 1941): 91; "News Items," *Canadian Medical Association Journal* 46, no. 3 (March, 1942): 299.

6 "News Items," *Canadian Medical Association Journal* 63, no. 1 (July 1950): 98. He spent his retirement years active in the provincial Boy Scouts organization. "Provincial News," *Canadian Medical Association Journal* 80, no. 5 (March 1959): 402.

7 Due to the large attendance, universal appeal, and "spirited" discussion that followed, at Leatherbarrow's suggestion, the New Brunswick Medical Society held at least one meeting a year "with an obstetrical viewpoint." See "News Items," *Canadian Medical Association Journal* 26, no. 4 (April 1932): 510–11; "News – New Brunswick," *Canadian Medical Association Journal* 33, no. 5 (November 1935): 584.

8 For the Royal Victoria Hospital and the Scottish influence in Montreal medicine, see Adams, *Medicine by Design*.

9 For the evolution of medicine in Toronto and the central role of the Toronto General Hospital, see Connor, *Doing Good*.

10 Roland, "Ontario Medical Periodicals."

11 For the early medical profession in New France, see Gelfand, "Who Practiced Medicine?" 16–35. For the debate over professional closure in Ontario, see Romano, "Professional Identity," 77–98.

12 Montreal, like Toronto, would witness a handful of short-lived proprietary medical schools before 1880, including the École de Médecine et Chirurgie de Montréal and the St Lawrence School of Medicine. Bishop's University,

then an Anglican English-language university in Lennoxville, also had a short-lived medical school in the 1880s and 1890s, the most famous alumna of which was Maude Abbott who was denied admission to McGill. For a discussion of Quebec medical schools during the Victorian era, see Martin Robert, "La Fabrique du corps médical: dissections humaines et formation médicale dans le Québec du XIXe siècle," unpublished PhD thesis, History Department, Université du Québec à Montréal, 2019, chapter 3.

13 Ostry, *Change and Continuity*, table 9: "Canadian Medical Schools by Year Established and Language of Instruction," 115. See also sources for image 1.
14 Weisz, "Geographical Origins," 93–119.
15 See Haynes, *Fit to Practice*, especially chapters 1–3.
16 The founding year is listed as 1822 or 1829. See McPhedran, *Canadian Medical Schools*, xii; Ostry, *Change and Continuity*, 115: table 9.
17 Hastings, "Territorial Spoils," 459–63. McGill leaders proved reluctant to pressure affiliated Montreal Maternal Hospital to permit black trainees to rotate in OBGYN. Hastings argues that the McGill and Queen's actions made a lasting impression on Caribbean political leaders and undermined nascent proposals of a Canada–West Indies Union at the conclusion of the Great War.
18 Jones, *Radical Medicine*, 195–6.
19 Gidney and Millar, "Medical Students," 39.
20 See Millar, "'We Wanted Our Children Should Have it Better,'" 109–24, 111.
21 Strong-Boag, "Canada's Women Doctors," 207–35.
22 Jacalyn Duffin, "The Quota," 327–50 and figure 1.
23 Gidney and Millar, *Professional Gentlemen*.
24 Mercer, "Edinburgh and Canadian Medicine," 1313.
25 Romano, "Professional Identity," 89–93.
26 Flexner, *Medical Education*.
27 Haynes, *Fit to Practice*, 50–69.
28 See sections 91 and 92 of the British North America Act, 1867. The federal government also retained responsibility for marine hospitals.
29 The federal responsibility gave rise to a network of Indian hospitals throughout the country, which were segregated institutions for Indians often located on or near Indian reserves. Federal jurisdiction in this area, under the authority of the Indian Health Services, continued until the 1950s, when, during the negotiations over cofunded hospitalization insurance, the federal government forced the province to take responsibility for status Indians. See Marchildon, "Three Dimensions of Universal Medicare," 367.

30 Marble, *Surgeons, Smallpox, and the Poor.*

31 Ostry, *Change and Continuity*, 118.

32 Penfield, "Health Insurance and Medical Education," 528.

33 Kelley and Trebilcock, *The Making of the Mosaic*, chapter 8 (311–45).

34 Palmer, "Anglo-Canadian Views of Multiculturalism," 314.

35 Kelley and Trebilcock, *The Making of the Mosaic*, 312, 529n3.

36 Knowles, *Strangers at Our Gates*, 168–9.

37 Green, *Immigration and the Postwar Canadian Economy*, 24.

38 At the time, South Asian immigration continued to be limited formally by treaties and quotas. Kelley and Trebilcock, *The Making of the Mosaic*, 329. See also Knowles, *Strangers at Our Gates*, 169–70.

39 Roy, *The Triumph of Citizenship*, 263.

40 The reasons for exclusion were many and included 1. nationality, citizenship, ethnic group, occupation, class of geographical area of origin; 2. peculiar customs, habits, modes of life, or methods of holding property; 3. unsuitability having regard to the climate, economic, social, industrial, educational, labour, health, or other conditions or requirements existing ... in Canada; or, 4. probable inability to become readily assimilated or to assume the duties and responsibilities of Canadian citizenship. Kelley and Trebilcock, *The Making of the Mosaic*, 325.

41 Knowles, *Strangers at Our Gates*, 163; for the reference to Indian relatives, see 187.

42 Miller, "Public Health and Medical Care in Newfoundland," 53.

43 Ibid.

44 "Special Article: The Refugee Doctor," *Canadian Medical Association Journal* 57, no. 6 (December 1947): 591–3.

45 "Medical Societies: The N.B. Medical Society Annual Meeting," *Canadian Medical Association Journal* 69, no. 5 (November 1953): 538.

46 "Voice of the Public Press," *Canadian Medical Association Journal* 75, no. 9 (1 November 1956): 770.

47 Ibid.

48 Ibid.

49 A series of eight rural municipalities created community clinics with the combined support of the Rockefeller Foundation and the provincial government in 1928, for instance. See "Editorial Comments: Establishment of Rural Health Units in Saskatchewan," *Canadian Medical Association Journal*, 18, no. 4 (April 1928): 436.

50 Houston, *Steps on the Road to Medicare*, chapter 5.

51 Duffin and Falk, "Sigerist in Saskatchewan," 658–83; see also Duffin, "The Guru and the Godfather," 191–218.

52 Connor, "One Simply Doesn't Arbitrate Authorship of Thoughts," 245–71.

53 For a similar example of the Beveridge report and the National Health Service as the emblem of state-run medical care, see Digby, "'Vision and Vested Interests,'" 486 and passim. For the NHS as a comparator used to measure other national public systems, see Freeman, "A National Health Service, by Comparison," 503–20.

54 Jones, *Radical Medicine*.

55 Taylor, *Health Insurance and Canadian Public Policy* (1978), 87.

56 Houston and Massie, *36 Steps on the Road to Medicare*, 97–8.

57 The plan covered "an almost complete range of hospital services as benefits at the standard ward level with no limitation on entitlement days as long as in-patient care was medically necessary." Taylor, *Health Insurance and Canadian Public Policy* (1978), 102.

58 Johnson, *Dream No Little Dreams*, as quoted in Houston and Massie, *36 Steps on the Road to Medicare*, 100.

59 Mott, "A Pattern of Local Services," 216–20.

60 See Sigerist, *Report of the Saskatchewan Health Services Survey Commission*.

61 Houston and Massie, *36 Steps on the Road to Medicare*, 177.

62 Mott, "A Pattern of Local Services," 216.

63 Ibid.

64 Kelly observed that this "ha[d] been a troublesome and expensive feature of certain other plans." Kelly, "Medical Economics," 508.

65 Ibid., 506.

66 Ibid., 508.

67 Kelly was unhappy with the lack of medical representation on the health region board, a body that was "made up entirely of laymen." Moreover, the provincial Health Service Planning Commission had only "medical men who are civil servants" as opposed to those in active private practice in the province. Kelly, "Medical Economics," 509.

68 Ibid., 511.

69 Mott, "A Pattern of Local Services," 219–20.

70 Kelly, "Swift Current, Twelve Years Later," 812. Naylor sees as a key measure of the success of the Swift Current Health Region the quick rise in the number

of general practitioners: in 1946 there were about twenty active general practitioners in Swift Current; by 1948 the number had risen to thirty-six. Naylor,
Private Practice, Public Payment, 141–2.

71 Kelly, "Swift Current, Twelve Years Later," 812.

72 Mott, "A Pattern of Local Services," 219.

73 J. Lloyd Brown, "Problems Arising," 750.

74 Twohig, "'Everything Possible Is Being Done.'"

75 Midwifery became marginalized in urban and suburban Canada for much of
the twentieth century. However, in rural and remote regions of the country,
it continued to play an important role. See Mitchinson, *Giving Birth in
Canada.*

76 Lawson and Noseworthy, "Newfoundland's Cottage Hospital System," in
Gregory P. Marchildon (ed.), *Making Medicare,* 477–98.

77 For a study of nurses arriving in midcentury, see Walsh and Beaton, *Come
from Away.*

78 Lawson and Noseworthy, "Newfoundland's Cottage Hospital System,
1920–1970," 229.

79 Connor, "Twillingate," 13.

80 Johnson, "Health Insurance," 68.

81 The Canadian Medical Association, "A Submission Respecting Health
Insurance," 386.

CHAPTER TWO

1 "The Memoirs of Stanley H. Kryszek," Pier 21. The lengthy personal memoir
can be retrieved at the Pier 21 website https://pier21.ca/content/the-memoirs
-of-stanley-h-kryszek-polish-immigrant. See also the biography published
by his daughter Jean Kryzsek Chard, *Reminiscences of Stanley H. Kryszek* (2007).

2 Ibid.

3 Ibid. *Canadian Medical Directory,* 1961.

4 For an overview of development of the National Insurance Act of 1911,
see E.P. Hennock, *The Origins of the Social Welfare State in England and
Germany.*

5 See Webster, *The National Health Service,* 28–44 and passim. For a general
survey of postwar health care in Britain, see Berridge, *Health and Medicine
in Britain since 1939.*

6   For an examination of the interplay of race, employment, and immigration in postwar Britain, see Paul, *Whitewashing Britain*.

7   By 1971, more than 31,000 Irish and 5,000 Jamaican nurses worked in the NHS. See Simpson, *Migrant Architects of the NHS*, 72.

8   Haynes, *Fit to Practice*, chapter 5.

9   For an excellent analysis of the tradition of Indian doctors immigrating to Britain for medical training, see Simpson, *Migrant Architects of the NHS*.

10 Gelfand, "Who Practiced Medicine in New France?"

11 See, inter alia, Marble, *Surgeons, Smallpox, and the Poor*; Romano, "Professional Identity."

12 Mukharji, *Doctoring Traditions*.

13 For an analysis of the diverse origins and startling dispersion of Scottish medical graduates, see Crowther and Dupree, *Medical Lives*.

14 Armstrong, "A System of Exclusion."

15 For a case study of this in the British Caribbean, see De Barros, "Imperial Connections."

16 Wright, Flis, and Gupta, "The 'Brain Drain' of Physicians."

17 As cited in Simpson et al, "Writing Migrants back into NHS history," 392. For an examination of refugee European doctors and scientists in Britain during and immediately after WWII, see Weindling, "Medical Refugees."

18 Ministry of Health [Great Britain] and Department of Health for Scotland, *Report of the Committee*.

19 Abel-Smith and Gales, *British Doctors at Home and Abroad*, 9.

20 Royal Commission on Doctors' and Dentists' Remuneration. Dental coverage was, in the early years of the National Health Service, comprehensive. However, for financial reasons as well as a competing, parallel private system (with higher remuneration), the array of dental services offered under the NHS began to erode over the decades.

21 Abel-Smith and Gales, *British Doctors at Home and Abroad*, 9–10.

22 Wright, Mullally, and Cordukes, "'Worse than Being Married.'"

23 Judek, *Medical Manpower in Canada*, 38–44.

24 Seale, "Medical Emigration," figures derived from figure 1, 1173.

25 Slight deviations were made from the original outline in the Spens report. The position of senior hospital medical officer (SHMO) was added as a junior specialist grade just slightly below a consultant post and that of junior hospital medical officer (JHMO) as a permanent post approximately equal to

that of junior registrar. Thereafter, there were seven different grades. Finally, it needs to be remembered that general practice was not seen as a specialty at the time, and so general practitioners were not required to do any postgraduate training. While some performed voluntary work in hospital for a few years after graduation, many did not. It was not until the early 1960s that specific postgraduate training for general practitioners began to emerge. Hannay, "Undergraduate Medical Education and General Practice," 182.

26 We are grateful to one anonymous reviewer of the manuscript for making this additional analytical point.

27 Stevens, *Medical Practice in Modern England*, 144, 139–45.

28 Ibid., 145.

29 Ibid., 145–50.

30 Cutler, "Dangerous Yardstick?," 217–38; and Cutler, "A Double Irony," 201–20.

31 Simpson, *Migrant Architects*, 38–40.

32 John Bowman [pseudonym], interview, May 2008.

33 Charles Crowther [pseudonym], interview, May 2009.

34 Ronald Zaretsky [pseudonym], interview, May 2008.

35 Donald Holt [pseudonym], interview, May 2008.

36 Ibid.

37 John Bowman [pseudonym], interview, May 2008.

38 Jeremy Davidson [pseudonym], interview, April 2009.

39 Although she was not British and fleeing the National Health Service, one female Irish physician remembered following a friend to Canada, intending to stay only a year, "do Paediatrics, see the world and go home." But she met her future husband at Dalhousie University in Halifax and stayed. Melissa Mahoney [pseudonym], interview, April 2009.

40 David Charlton [pseudonym], interview, April 2009.

41 One physician started at a salary that seemed a "fantastic amount of money" at the time: Can$19,000. It was his plan to work and save for a year and then travel the world with his wife before returning to England. Charles Crowther [pseudonym], interview, May 2009.

42 Richard Gartner [pseudonym], interview, June 2008; Melissa Mahoney [pseudonym], interview, April 2009.

43 See, for instance, interview with Melissa Mahoney [pseudonym], April 2009.

44 Hampshire, *Citizenship and Belonging*, 19.

45 Hansen, *Citizenship and Immigration*, 180.

46 Hampshire, *Citizenship and Belonging*, 29.

47 Ibid., 30.

48 Spencer, *British Immigration Policy since 1939*, 139.

49 Paul, *Whitewashing Britain*, 171–2.

50 Spencer, *British Immigration Policy since 1939*, 137. The General Medical Council of Medical Education and Registration of the United Kingdom (hereafter General Medical Council or GMC), was responsible for the registration of all licensed doctors in Britain, from the Medical Registration Act of 1858 to 1978. For an institutional history of the GMC, See Haynes, *Fit to Practice*.

51 Haynes, *Fit to Practice*, 142.

52 "Doctors: 1600 in UK," *Journal of the Indian Medical Association* 39, no. 9 (1 November 1962): 487.

53 Haynes, *Fit to Practice*, 106.

54 Hampshire, *Citizenship and Belonging*, 31.

55 Kelley and Trebilcock, *The Making of the Mosaic*, 332n124.

56 "Manitoba Doctors Suggest Program to Ease Shortage," *Financial Post*, 18 July 1964.

57 Abel-Smith and Gales, *British Doctors at Home and Abroad*, passim.

58 Powell criticized Republican American representatives and senators who were using the figures over emigrant British doctors to undermine attempts, at that time, to introduce state-run health insurance in the United States. Ironically, Powell, whose 1968 "Rivers of Blood" speech would later excite racial tensions in the country, had, as minister of health, purposefully downplayed the extent to which immigration of Commonwealth doctors to Britain had been facilitated to fill the gaps in NHS hospital positions. Ibid., 14–15.

59 Abel-Smith and Gales, *British Doctors at Home and Abroad*, 10.

60 See Flynn, *Moving Beyond Borders*, especially chapter 4, 94–126; and Flynn, "Race, the State, and Caribbean Immigrant Nurses, 1950–1962." For the treatment of visible minority nurses in Anglo-America during this period see Calliste, "Women of Exceptional Merit," 85–102.

61 For the United States, see Brush, "'Exchangees' or Employees?"

62 "Correspondence: British Health Service," *Canadian Medical Association Journal* 73 (December 1955): 991.

63 Ibid.

64 Armstrong, "Correspondence."

CHAPTER THREE

1 The names of some individuals and towns have been changed in accordance with specific Research Ethics Board protocols. In these cases, ethnicity and gender (of the interviewee) and the locations have been maintained.

2 Robert MacDonald [pseudonym], interview, April 2009.

3 Ibid.

4 Ibid.

5 Ibid.

6 Ibid.

7 Jean, "Family Allowances and Family Autonomy."

8 The health grants program consolidated all existing and conditional grants to provinces for tuberculosis, venereal disease, mental health, children's programs, and cancer treatment. Ostry, *Change and Continuity*, 37–8.

9 Martin, "An Address," 140.

10 Ibid.

11 Hospital Insurance and Diagnostic Services Act [*An Act to Authorize Contributions by Canada in respect of Programmes Administered by the Provinces, Providing Hospital Insurance and Laboratory and Other Services in Aid of Diagnosis*]. Statutes of Canada 1957, 5-6 Elizabeth II (Assented to 12 April 1957) Chap. 28 (155).

12 The contribution, paid by Ottawa, would be the total of several costs. First, it would pay 25 per cent of the per capita cost of inpatient services; 25 per cent of the per capita cost of inpatient services in the province less the per capita amount of authorized charges, multiplied by the average for the year of the number of persons in the province who were eligible for and entitled to insured services at the end of each month in that year. Secondly, Ottawa was to pay an amount that was in the same proportion to the cost of outpatient services in the province, less the amount of authorized charges, similarly to the case of inpatient services. However, the cost did not include the following: any amount expended on the capital cost of land, buildings, or physical plant; any amount expended for the payment of any capital debt or interest; any amount expended for the payment of any debt incurred prior to the coming into force of an agreement or interest. The contributions were to be paid by the minister of finance from the Consolidated Revenue Fund upon the certificate of the minister of national health and welfare, with all payments subjected to the conditions of the act.

13 Except for a general charge through a general provincial health care pre-
    mium or other amount not related to a specific service.

14 Hospital Insurance and Diagnostic Services Act.

15 He believed, as did many, that more work would be done under hospitaliza-
    tion, especially childbirth, more of a physician's work would be redefined
    and under review under a hospital setting, and how a physician is paid
    would change, with more income flowing through the institution than
    previously in a private practice. See Young, "The Impact of Hospital Insu-
    rance," 756–7.

16 MacMillan, "The Impact of Hospital Insurance," 767.

17 Royal Commission on Health Services, *Report of the Royal Commission on
    Health Services*, vol. 1, 727.

18 Morgan, "The Impact of Hospital Insurance," 747.

19 Taylor, "The Canadian Health System in Transition," 180.

20 Royal Commission on Health Services, *Report of the Royal Commission on
    Health Services*, vol. 1, xix.

21 James and Blishen, "Review of Royal Commission on Health Services," 44, 94.

22 Royal Commission on Health Services, *Report of the Royal Commission*,
    Appendix B.

23 Judek, *Medical Manpower in Canada*, 4.

24 "Newfoundland's Doctor Shortage Acute: Many Outports without Medical
    Care," *The Globe and Mail*, 10 December 1960, 3.

25 "Manitoba Doctors Suggest Program to Ease Shortage," *Financial Post*, 18
    July 1964.

26 For an illuminating contemporary study, see Fish, Farmer, and Nelson-Jones,
    "Some Social Characteristics of Students," 950–4.

27 Ibid, 128–33.

28 Judek, *Medical Manpower in Canada*, 26–31.

29 Ibid, 23–31.

30 Ibid, 108–12.

31 The Saskatchewan College of Physicians and Surgeons should not be con-
    fused with other provincial colleges with a similar title. For example, the
    Ontario College of Physicians and Surgeons is the government organization
    designed to protect the interests of patients and, if necessary, discipline
    doctors. This is also the case in most other provinces. The Saskatchewan
    College of Physicians and Surgeons, by contrast, was the name of the doc-

tors' organization, roughly the equivalent at the time of the Ontario Medical Association.

32 Taylor, *Health Insurance and Canadian Public Policy*, 245, 247.

33 Johnson, *Dream No Little Dreams*, 269–70.

34 Naylor, *Private Practice, Public Payment*, 198–9.

35 Johnson, *Dream No Little Dreams*, 276, quotation 259.

36 Marchildon and Schrijvers, "Physician Resistance," 212.

37 Naylor, *Private Practice, Public Payment*, 198–9.

38 Johnson, *Dream No Little Dreams*, 277–8.

39 Naylor, *Private Practice, Public Payment*, 205.

40 Marchildon and Schrijvers, "Physician Resistance," 212.

41 Johnson, *Dream No Little Dreams*, 287.

42 Spasoff and Wolfe, "Trends in the Supply and Distribution," 526.

43 Daniell, "4 Doctors Fly to Saskatchewan," 10.

44 Johnson, *Dream No Little Dreams*, 285; Naylor, *Private Practice, Public Payment*, 203; Taylor, *Health Insurance and Canadian Public Policy*, 315.

45 Saskatchewan Federation of Labour, *The First Fight for Medicare*, 10.

46 See, inter alia, Daniell, "4 Doctors Fly to Saskatchewan," 10; "Saskatchewan Sends Circulars to UK Doctors," *The Globe and Mail*, 4 July 1962, 8; "Service Dwindling, Battle of Medicare Reaches a New Pitch," *The Globe and Mail*, 7 July 1962, 9; Merry, "More British Medics Fly to Help Canada," A4; Griffin, "British Medics Irk Canada," 1.

47 Naylor, *Private Practice, Public Payment*, 203.

48 "Canadian Appeal for 200 Doctors," *The Times* (London) 11 July 1962, 8.

49 Badgley and Wolfe, *Doctors' Strike*, 51–2.

50 "Saskatchewan Sends Circulars," 8.

51 "Service Dwindling," 9. Physicians were offered $1,925 per month; interns, residents, and assistants $1,200, with transportation and expenses covered. "U.K. MDs Get Leave for Prairie Service," *The Globe and Mail*, 5 July 1962, 8.

52 Merry, "Doctors Sign in Britain to Aid Canadians," 2.

53 As well, the government "was prepared to invoke the Emergency Measures Act, permitting foreign graduates to practice [without a formal provincial license]." Badgley and Wolfe, *Doctors' Strike*, 67.

54 Marcus, "Think Before Moving," 11.

55 Marchildon and Schrijvers, "Physician Resistance," 217.

56 "U.K. MDs Get Leave For Prairie Service," 8.

57　MPU statement, quoted in "London Advice to Volunteers," *The Times* [London, England], 5 July 1962, 10.

58　"British Doctors Shy Off Canada," *Los Angeles Times*, 20 July 1962, 8.

59　Naylor, *Private Practice, Public Payment*, 208–9.

60　Taylor, "Saskatchewan Adventure," 725.

61　Taylor, *Health Insurance and Canadian Public Policy*, 323.

62　Badgley and Wolfe, *Doctors' Strike*, 62.

63　Marchildon and Schrijvers, "Physician Resistance," 216.

64　Taylor, *Health Insurance and Canadian Public Policy*, 315; Johnson, *Dream No Little Dreams*, 283; Tollefson, *Bitter Medicine*, 110.

65　Johnson, *Dream No Little Dreams*, 289.

66　Marchildon and Schrijvers, "Physician Resistance," 217.

67　Johnson, *Dream No Little Dreams*, 292.

68　Taylor, *Health Insurance and Canadian Public Policy*, 299.

69　Saskatchewan Federation of Labour, *The First Fight for Medicare*, 8.

70　Marchildon and Schrijvers "Physician Resistance," 218.

71　Badgley and Wolfe, *Doctors' Strike*, 87. See also "Across the Land," *The Globe and Mail*, 14 July 1962, 9; Merry, "More British Medics," A4.

72　Badgley and Wolfe, *Doctors' Strike*, 83–4.

73　Ibid.

74　"British Doctors Given Assurance," *The Times* [London, England], 14 July 1962, 7.

75　Taylor, *Health Insurance and Canadian Public Policy*, 325.

76　"Our Correspondent, 'Doctors Begin Return to Surgeries,'" *The Times* [London, England] 25 July 1962, 8.

77　Spasoff and Wolfe, "Trends in Supply and Distribution," 524.

78　Mullally and Wright, "La Grande Séduction?," 41, 73.

79　Royal Commission on Health Services, *Report of the Royal Commission*, 69–73.

80　Ibid.

81　The second school would have likely been attached to York University. Indeed, oral interviewees recall that colleagues were already being sounded out, in 1967 and 1968, as potential service chiefs and department heads.

82　Royal Commission on Health Services, *Report of the Royal Commission*, 69–73.

83　Calliste, "Women of Exceptional Merit," 6, 85.

84　Royal Commission on Health Services, *Report of the Royal Commission*, 62–9.

85   Ibid., 241–2.

86   Ibid., 521–48.

87   Ibid., 521–8.

88   Maioni, *Parting at the Crossroads*, chapter 7.

89   Inequality of billing practice would not exist at the level of gender or seniority but rather in the different fees set by different provinces.

CHAPTER FOUR

1   "Immigration: An Ideal Family," *Time Magazine* (Canada), 12 July 1972, column two.

2   Ibid. See also "Ten Millionth Immigrant Lands," *Toronto Sun*, 30 May 1972, 94.

3   For the expansion of higher education in Canada during this period, see, inter alia, Panayotidis and Stortz, *Historical Identities*; Cormier, *The Canadianization Movement*.

4   Russell, "Enlarge Immigration Staff," 8.

5   Knowles, *Strangers at Our Gates*, 137–8.

6   Hawkins, *Canada and Immigration*, chapter 6.

7   Ibid., 143.

8   Knowles, *Strangers at Our Gates*, 139.

9   Raska, "Welcoming the Sick and Afflicted," 173, 171–92.

10   Order in Council PC 1962-86 (1 February 1962).

11   For a particularly illuminating documentary of the subjectivity and scope of immigration officers in the mid-1960s, view the interviews by Judith Jasmin, for Radio Canada, entitled "Des Immigrants à leur arivée." We are grateful to Sean Mills for this reference.

12   Raska, "Welcoming the Sick and Afflicted," 189. Other examples of the asymmetry include the reaction to different types of refugees. For example, Canada responded to the Hungarian refugee crisis of 1956–57 as well as the calls by UNHCR to help close its displaced persons camps in Europe and accepted Czech "refuges" during the Prague Spring of 1968, but Canada was more circumspect in the welcoming of Chinese refugees at the same time. See Madokoro, *Elusive Refuge*.

13   "Selective Immigration," editorial, *The Globe and Mail*, 13 March 1962, 6.

14   *House of Commons Debates* (29 May 1966), 5435.

15   Italics added. Ibid. (30 May 1966), 5731.

16   As one immigration agent recalled, "The form … was the IMM1067 or Immigration Assessment Record which comprised 3 transaction sheets (T1,

T2, and T3). The T1 was the initial assessment (preselection) and the T2 recorded the points at interview, officer's comments, as well as medical, security/criminality and other requirements. The sheets were sent off to Ottawa each Friday. A similar form, the IMM1054, was used inland." Gerry Maffre, email correspondence, forwarded to David Wright.

17 P.C. 1967-1616, 434–5. Needless to say, the implementation in practice was somewhat more complicated. These units were maximum amounts, and immigration agents were given formulas for those, for example, whose age did not fall between eighteen and thirty-five or whose understanding of English and/or French was not fluent. Other exceptions include the discretion to deny approval to those who achieved 50+ units but whose occupational demand was "0." A former immigration agent referred to this as the "safety valve" for years of exceptional demand. [Name/anonymized], personal correspondence with David Wright.

18 Kent, *A Public Purpose*, 408.

19 Joe Bissett and Gerry Maffre, email correspondence shared with David Wright, 11 July 2019.

20 Ibid.

21 Ibid.

22 Michael John McCormick, Immigration, Refugees and Citizenship Canada, email correspondence with David Wright, 11 July 2019.

23 Knowles, *Strangers at the Gates*, 139–41.

24 Hawkins, *Canada and Immigration*, 402.

25 Richmond and Rao, "Recent Developments in Immigration," 188.

26 Troper, "Canada's Immigration Policy Since 1945," 267.

27 Figures derived from Van Hoek, *The Migration of High Level Manpower*, 73, table I. 21.

28 Marchildon and O'Byrne, "Last Province Aboard," 156.

29 Clause 2 stated that insured persons were those "lawfully entitled to be or to remain in Canada" and made it their home, excluding tourists, visitors, prisoners, and members of the armed forces and RCMP (Clause 2). The health care for prisoners (in federal penitentiaries), members of the armed forces, and the RCMP was technically provided directly by the federal government.

30 Marchildon, *Making Medicare*, 8–9 and table 2.

31 Naylor, *Private Practice, Public Payment*.

32 There were also individuals who worked in hybrid situations – that is, those

who were guaranteed a "base" salary but were also permitted to bill the provincial health insurance system for clinical services. This hybrid was common, at least until the 1990s, in academic–clinician settings. It should be noted that those medical graduates who were still in postgraduate training (called residents) were almost always on a salary until they graduated and became fully independent practitioners.

33 Maioni, *Parting at the Crossroads*, 133.
34 Langley and Langley, "A Tense and Courageous Performance," 19–20.
35 Shillington, *The Road to Medicare in Canada*, 157.
36 Quiñonez, "Why Was Dental Care Excluded?," 2.
37 "With approval of the bill, Parliament had committed the federal government to paying half the average cost, nationally, of provincially organized and operated medical care plans which embraced the conditions set out in the prime minister's statement of July 1965," Shillington, *The Road to Medicare in Canada*, 157.
38 Maioni, *Health Care in Canada*, 27.
39 Tudiver, *Universities for Sale*, 24–5.
40 Hacon "Improving Canada's Health Manpower Resources," 1104–8. See also "An Act to provide a Health Resources Fund," Revised Statutes of Canada (1970), chap. H-4, 3739–43; and the Department of National Health and Welfare, *Annual Report of the Minister of National Health and Welfare*, 1.
41 Hacon "Improving Canada's Health Manpower Resources," 1104–8.
42 Hastings, "Toward a National Health Program," 73.
43 Westell, "$500 Million Is Allocated," 1; see also Hacon "Improving Canada's Health Manpower Resources," 1104–8.
44 "Provinces Give Approval to Health Resources Fund," *The Globe and Mail*, 24 September 1965, 1; "Group Reports on Division of Health Fund," *The Globe and Mail*, 23 December 1965, 2.
45 Westell, "Ontario to Get $100,000,000," 1; "Crash Plan Pressed to Boost MD Ranks," *The Globe and Mail*, 22 June 1966, 4; Bain, "Money for Hospitals," 7.
46 Hacon "Improving Canada's Health Manpower Resources," 1104–8; "House Approves Bill Providing $500 Million for Medical Facilities," *The Globe and Mail*, 28 June 1966, 2.
47 Hacon, "Letter to the Editor," 25.
48 Waring, "Report from Ottawa," 36.
49 For a case study, see Wright, *SickKids*, chapter 11.
50 McPhedran, *Canadian Medical Schools*, 29–30.

51 Ibid., 232.

52 Lampard, *Alberta's Medical History*, 416; "History of the Cumming School of Medicine," University of Calgary Cumming School of Medicine. See also "Medical Education: The Revolution Has Already Begun," *Canadian Doctor* 34, no. 6 (June 1968): 44–7.

53 "The Med School Dilemma: Part Two – Lack of Research Money Real Villain in Education Crisis," *Canadian Doctor* 33 no. 1 (January 1967): 48.

54 "$500 Million Health Fund is Termed Pittance," *The Globe and Mail*, 6 June 1967, 12; "MacEachen Criticizes CMA Chief for Calling Health Fund 'Pittance,'" *The Globe and Mail*, 7 June 1967, 10.

55 "The Med School Dilemma, " 46–8.

56 These concerns were voiced, on their behalf, in the Parliamentary debates. "What is the use of putting $500 million in new buildings if we have not the personnel to open them? It comes back to the point that we are not providing the [research] funds to do it." Mr Rynard, House of Commons, Debates 27th Parliament, 2nd Session vol 2 (12 June 1967), 1408.

57 The Honorable Mr Lang, Senate Debates, 27th parliament, 1st Session, vol 1 (29 June 1966), 831.

58 University of Sherbrooke, *Université de Sherbrooke Annuaire General 1970–71*, 11.

59 Evans, "Future Manpower Needs," 1592–6, quotation 1595–6.

60 Bowers and Purcell, *New Medical Schools at Home and Abroad*, 232. Forty new schools of medicine were opened between 1960 and 1980 in the United States. Schofield, *New and Expanded Medical Schools*, 46.

61 Spaulding and Cochran, *Revitalizing Medical Education*, 26, quotation 35–6, 180.

62 "Top MD Leaves UK for McMaster Post," *The Globe and Mail*, 16 September 1968, 17. "By 1968 he was the most chair-worthy clinical academic in the United Kingdom without a chair, probably because his academic brilliance was offset by his ability to be outrageously frank. However, this frankness did not deter the selection committee of the innovative new medical school at McMaster University." Howell, Dickinson, and Hamilton, "Edward James Moran Campbell," 1105.

63 Campbell, "Medical Community, Family Say Farewell to Dr Campbell," 12.

64 Campbell, *Not Always on the Level*, 189.

65 Spaulding and Cochran, *Revitalizing Medical Education*, 182.

66 Ibid., 54–5, 184.

67 Spinks, *Decade of Change*, 77–8.
68 The University of Western Ontario, uwo *Composite Calendar 1970–71*, D-4. See also "Ontario Grants $30 Million for Province's First On-Campus Teaching Hospital," *The Globe and Mail*, 25 January 1967, 3.
69 Rusted, "Faculty of Medicine Memorial University," 232.
70 MacLeod, "Crossroads Campus," 136.
71 Rusted, "Faculty of Medicine Memorial University," 235.
72 "New Brunswick Medical School Plans Discussed," *Canadian Doctor* 35, no. 2 (February 1969): 9; "Want Med School for NB," *Canadian Doctor* 35, no. 6 (June 1969): 18; "Three New Brunswick Cities Bidding to Be Chosen As New Med School Site," *Canadian Doctor* 32, no. 10 (October 1966): 7.
73 "No Need for New Brunswick Med School Says Report," *Canadian Doctor* 33, no. 8 (August 1967): 7.
74 McPhedran, *Canadian Medical Schools*, 220.
75 Horn, *York University*, 128–9.
76 See Tesson, Hudson, Strasser, and Hunt, *Making of the Northern Ontario School of Medicine*.
77 "Dr Walter Campbell Mackenzie, 1909–78," Alberta Medical Association. Last modified 21 May 2014. https://web.archive.org/web/20190504190457/ https://www.albertadoctors.org/about/medical-history/patients-1st-for-over-100-years/mackenzie [Archived 4 May 2019]. See also Lampard, *Deans, Dreams and a President*, xvi–ii, 129.
78 McPhedran, *Canadian Medical Schools*, 171.
79 Ibid., 171–2.
80 "$1.5 Million in Grants Made to Four Cities," *The Globe and Mail*, 12 April 1969, 15.
81 Ibid., 99.
82 "Medical Research in Canada – An Analysis of Immediate and Future Needs (The Gundy Report)," *Canadian Medical Association Journal* 94, no. 15 (9 April 1966): 806–8. See also "A Penny-Wise Approach to Medicine," *The Globe and Mail*, 24 September 1966, 6; and "Medical Faculty Shortages Feared as Universities in Ontario Expand," *The Globe and Mail*, 18 January 1967, 1.
83 Hollobon, "Freeze on Research Funds Blamed," 37.
84 Mustard, "The Choice," 43–53.
85 Collishaw and Grainger, "Enrolment in Canada's Medical Schools, 1970–71," 167.

86 Lamarche and Hébert, "Enrolment in Canadian Medical Schools, 1974–75," 737.

87 Barr, *A Century of Medicine at Western*, 602.

88 Corbet, *Frontiers of Medicine*, 134 and table 10.

89 "Expansion of Medical Education in Canada and the US," *Forum/The Association of Canadian Medical Colleges* 7, no. 3 (May–June 1974): 12; Nelson-Jones and Fish, "Projections of Graduates From Canadian Medical Schools, 1970–81," 853.

90 Lamarche and Hébert, "Enrolment in Canadian Medical Schools, 1974–75," 737. Other such reports include Nelson-Jones and Fish, "Medical Student Enrolment in Canada: Report of Statistics, 1968–69," 647; Nelson-Jones and Fish, "Canadian and Landed Immigrant Applicants to Canadian Medical Schools for 1968–69," 186; Collishaw and Grainger, "Medical Student Enrolment in Canada, 1969–70: Report of Statistics," 916.

91 Korcok, "Restriction of Physician Immigration," 509–13.

CHAPTER FIVE

1 Ďurčanský and Dhondt, "Great Anniversaries," 40.

2 Slovak universities would continue, under German surveillance.

3 "An agreement between the Czechoslovak Government in Exile and the University Vice Chancellor [of Oxford] allowed 44 Czech and Slovak students to receive medical degrees of the three Czechoslovak Universities from Oxford University on the basis of studies completed in Britain." Svobodny, "The Medical Faculty," 221–2.

4 Zarecor, *Manufacturing a Socialist Modernity*, 9–11.

5 Chatham-Kent physician tribute, "Mirko 'Mike' Vaclav Havlas," https://web.archive.org/web/20180913214806/http://ckphysiciantribute.ca/doctors/mirko-mike-vaclav-havlas/; Chatham-Kent physician tribute, "Vlasta 'Vivian' Bozena Havlas" [Archived 13 September 2018]. https://web.archive.org/web/20180914153251/http://ckphysiciantribute.ca/doctors/vlasta-vivian-bozena-havlas/.

6 Heimann, *Czechoslovakia*, 150.

7 Ibid., 207–8.

8 Connelly, *Captive University*, 249–51; quotation 270.

9 Alfred Breslau, interview, 24 July 2019.

10 Raska, "Freedom Voices," 3–4.

11 Vaněk and Mücke, *Velvet Revolutions*, 30; see also Weinerman and Weinerman, *Social Medicine in Eastern Europe*, 44.

12 Bren, *The Greengrocer and His TV*, 178.

13 Ibid., 18–19.

14 Bolton, *Worlds of Dissent*, 6.

15 Leff, *The Czech and Slovak Republics*, 59.

16 Raska, "Freedom Voices," 4.

17 Chatham-Kent physician tribute, "Vlasta 'Vivian' Bozena Havlas."

18 Madokoro, "Good Material," 167.

19 Ibid., 161–2; 165.

20 Chatham-Kent physician tribute, "Vlasta 'Vivian' Bozena Havlas."

21 A further 457 (1.3 per cent) doctors submitted insufficient information to make a determination as to whether they were Canadian- or foreign-trained.

22 The "counting" of doctors in the country was (and is) an imprecise science. However, the figures listed above are corroborated by contemporary reports. For example, according to a 1977 government report, 31 per cent of all active physicians in Canada were immigrants as of 1972. Roemer and Roemer, *Health Manpower Policy*, 27.

23 Goldschmidt, *Modern Egypt*, 109, 111, 133.

24 Pearson and the role of Canada as "Middle Power" peacemaker would become a dominant motif of Canada in the 1960s and 1970s. See Chapnick, "The Canadian Middle Power Myth," 188–206. Along with Medicare, there were few more potent symbols of Canadian identity, and pride, as the blue helmets and Canadians self-gratulatory conception of themselves as world peacekeepers.

25 Tignor, *Egypt*, 14.

26 Roussillon, "Republican Egypt Interpreted," 353; Sayyid Marsot, *A History of Egypt*, 137.

27 Goldschmidt, *Modern Egypt*, 109, 131, 133.

28 Tignor, *Egypt*, 10.

29 Amin, *Whatever Happened to Egyptians*, 154.

30 Ayubi, "The Egyptian 'Brain Drain,'" 432–4, quotation 434.

31 Amin, *Whatever Happened to Egyptians*, 68–73, 72–3.

32 Goldschmidt, *Modern Egypt*, 162.

33 Laskier, *The Jews of Egypt*, 264; Kramer, *The Jews in Modern Egypt*, 233.

34 Laskier, *The Jews of Egypt*, 264.

35 Philipp, "Copts and Other Minorities," 143; Dalachanis, *The Greek Exodus from Egypt*, 227. See also Talani, *From Egypt to Europe*, 68.

36 Dessouki, "The Shift in Egypt's Migration Policy," 55–61. See also Roman, "Emigration Policy in Egypt," 5.

37 Talani, *From Egypt to Europe*, 64.

38 Dessouki, "The Shift in Egypt's Migration Policy," 57.

39 Zohry, "Migration and Development in Egypt," 75.

40 Previously known as Farouk University until the revolution of 1952.

41 The Cairo-based medical school was originally called the "el-Demerdash School of Medicine" and was funded by several large bequests and donations. It became a faculty of medicine within the university, when the latter was founded, in 1950. It was written most often as "Ein Shams" in the CMD.

42 At the time this was usually after one year of satisfactory internship. See annual reports of the CPSO; some physicians were referred back for further training based on the reports submitted by hospitals to the CPSO. *Report of the College of Physicians and Surgeons of Ontario* (1962), 13; *Report of the College of Physicians and Surgeons of Ontario* (1963), 13.

43 *Report of the College of Physicians and Surgeons of Ontario* (1964).

44 *Report of the College of Physicians and Surgeons of Ontario* (1965), 27.

45 Ibid.

46 "Indians, Pakistanis Barred: 150 Foreign MDs to Write Exam," *The Globe and Mail*, 23 August 1965," 5.

47 "Thompson Issues Challenge: Charges Doctors Run Closed Shop," *The Globe and Mail*, 13 July 1965," 5.

48 "Foreign-trained Doctors Appeal on Human Rights," *Toronto Daily Star*, 23 August 1965, 5; "4 Asians 100 Foreign Doctors Barred," *Toronto Daily Star*, 26 August 1965, 4.

49 "Foreign Doctors Who 'Aren't Good Enough,'" *Maclean's Reports* 78, no. 18 (18 September 1965): 1.

50 "Help Settle MD Row," *The Globe and Mail*, 5 July 1965, 5.

51 "Fall in India's Education Level Blamed for Ban on MDs Here," *The Globe and Mail*, 31 August 1965," 5.

52 "Help Settle MD Row," 5.

53 "Dymond's 3 to Probe Asian Doctors' Case," *Toronto Daily Star*, 26 January 1966, C5.

54 "Lift that Scalpel! Claim that Vein!" *Toronto Daily Star*, 28 June 1965, 6.

55 *Report of the College of Physicians and Surgeons of Ontario* (1966), 8.

56 "Fall in India's Education Level Blamed," 5; "Rule Standards Inferior: College Upholds Refusal to License Doctors From Asia," *The Globe and Mail*, 27 November 1965," 4.

57 *Report of the College of Physicians and Surgeons of Ontario* (1966), 7.

58 "Help Settle MD Row," 5; "Foreign Doctors Appeal Ont. Ban," *The Leader-Post* (Regina), 23 August 1965, 5.

59 "Licensing Rules Same, Doctors' Spokesman Says," *The Globe and Mail*, 25 August 1965," 5.

60 "Indian Doctors' Plea," *The Times of India*, 3 July 1965, 9; "Licence Review for MDs," *The Leader-Post* (Regina), 2 July 1965, 11.

61 "Indians, Pakistanis Barred," 5.

62 "Fall in India's Education Level Blamed," 5.

63 "Rule Standards Inferior," 4.

64 "Doctors, Health Workers Favor Medical Review," *The Globe and Mail*, 27 January 1966, 4.

65 "No Discrimination Against Colored MDs: Dymond," *The Globe and Mail*, 1 July 1966," 10.

66 *Report of the College of Physicians and Surgeons of Ontario* (1966), 9.

67 Roy, *Taiwan*, 56.

68 Brown, *Is Taiwan Chinese?*, 60.

69 Davison, *Short History of Taiwan*, 83.

70 Wang, "From Elitism," 209.

71 Copper, *Taiwan*, 86, 88.

72 As a result, the percentage of students continuing into junior high school jumped from 51 to 80 per cent in 1971. Davison, *Short History of Taiwan*, 94.

73 Wang, "From Elitism," 262. See also Wu, Chen, and Wu, "The Development of Higher Education in Taiwan," 126.

74 Hsu, *Nianqing Yishi de banghuang yu jueze* [Confusion and Dilemma] 11.

75 Lily Cheung [pseudonym], interview, 24 March 2019.

76 Arrigo, "Fifty Years After '2-2-8,'" 47.

77 Ibid., 48.

78 Copper, *Taiwan*, 95.

79 Xierali, "The Characteristics and Distribution," 141.

80 Talbot, *Pakistan*, 80.

81 Qadeer, *Pakistan – Social and Cultural Transformations*, 26–50.

82 Ibid., 24, 70.

83 Talbot, *Pakistan*, 9.

84   Chatterji, Alexander, and Jalais, *The Bengal Diaspora*, 52.
85   Lewis, *Bangladesh*, 59, 61.
86   Van Schendel, *A History of Bangladesh*, 118.
87   Qadeer, *Pakistan – Social and Cultural Transformations*, 242.
88   Lewis, *Bangladesh*, 63–4, 66.
89   Van Schendel, "The Pakistan Experiment," 181. See also Talbot, *Pakistan*, 70.
90   Lewis, *Bangladesh*, 62–3.
91   Talbot, *Pakistan*, 81.
92   Schendel, *A History of Bangladesh*, 120.
93   Raghavan, *1971: A Global History*, 7.
94   Van Schendel, *A History of Bangladesh*, 135.
95   Lewis, *Bangladesh*, 68.
96   Van Schendel, *A History of Bangladesh*, 156–7.
97   Talbot, *Pakistan*, 85–6.
98   See Qadeer, *Pakistan – Social and Cultural Transformations*, 229.
99   Lewis, *Bangladesh*, 71.
100 This figure is almost certainly an underestimate due to those practitioners, like Dr Gupta in the opening vignette of the book, who began medical studies in pre-Partition Punjab.
101 Newfoundland had only one Pakistani-trained doctor by 1976; PEI had none.
102 "Senate Passes Nixon Draft Lottery Scheme," *The Harvard Crimson*, 20 November 1969. https://www.thecrimson.com/article/1969/11/20/senate-passes-nixon-draft-lottery-scheme/.
103 Kusch, *All American Boys*.
104 "Draft Lottery Concerns Army," *Lodi News-Sentinel*, 26 November 1969, 5.
105 Public Law 779 of the 81st Congress. The 1950 law had amended the Selective Service Act of 1948. This law had authorized a separate draft for physicians for the first time in US history. United States Congress, Senate Committee on Armed Services, *Doctor Draft Substitute*. For responses in the early 1950s, see Myers, "Doctor-Draft Law," 743; Gamble et al. "Comments on the Doctor Draft," 705–6; Swope, "Doctor Draft Regulations," 232–4.
106 Unlike the general draft, doctors were eligible to serve until they reached thirty-five years of age (rather than twenty-six for regular draftees). *Nelson v. Peckham*, 210 F.2d 574, 577 (1954).
107 If the health care professional was under age twenty-six at time of appointment, there was a further requirement of forty-eight months of inactive reserve service comprised of thirty-six months ready reserve and twelve

months of standby reserve, which could be satisfied before or after active duty service – a combined total obligation of six years. United States Congress, Senate Committee on Armed Services, *Armed Services Security Cases*.
108 Khot, Park, and Longstreth, "The Vietnam War and Medical Research," 502.
109 Alexander Nemec [pseudonym], interview, 22 May 2008.
110 Emphasis added. Rousselot, "Doctor Draft," 87.
111 Ibid., 88.
112 Alfred Breslau, interview, 24 July 2019.
113 Hall, "Brain Drain and the Draft," 764.
114 Andrew Taylor [pseudonym], interview, 10 July 2008,
115 Ibid.
116 Jonas Molnar [pseudonym], interview, 22 August 2008.
117 Ontario Medical Association, *The Submission*, 112.
118 53.3 per cent in Saskatchewan and 62.5 per cent in Newfoundland. Roemer and Roemer, *Health Manpower Policy*, 27–8.
119 In 1972, for example, 42.8 per cent of foreign medical graduates were located in smaller towns while 45.5 per cent of Canadian med school graduates were also in smaller towns. Ibid.

CHAPTER SIX
1 Jonathan Murphy [pseudonym], interview, September 2008. The name has been changed pursuant to REB agreements.
2 Ibid.
3 Ibid.
4 Ibid.
5 Goldsmith-Kasinsky, *Refugees from Militarism*; Kusch, *All American Boys*; Hagan, *Northern Passage*.
6 Hess, "A UN Report on Brain Drain: The Rich Get Richer and the Poor Get Poorer," 9.
7 "The Cruel Doctor Drain," *The Globe and Mail*, 15 September 1967, 6.
8 World Health Organization, *Multinational Study of the International Migration of Physicians and Nurses* (1973).
9 Canada had adopted official bilingualism by 1968, but it is fair to say that its medical establishment was dominated by an English-speaking majority and anglophone medical elite. Indeed, part of the reforms (and indeed attraction) of the separatist movement in Quebec in the 1970s was to address the dominance of the English in areas of business, politics, and the professions.

10 Dublin, "Migration of Physicians," 870.
11 Stevens, Goodman, and Mick, *The Alien Doctors*.
12 Fein, *The Doctor Shortage*.
13 Ibid.
14 Margulies and Bloch, *Foreign Medical Graduates*.
15 "Discrimination Charges Denied: Foreign MDs in Canada Face Tangle of Regulations," *The Globe and Mail*, 18 January 1966, 3.
16 Bowden, "The Brain Drain," 7. See also "The Brain Drain Grows: Can Scientists Resist US Temptation?," *Toronto Daily Star*, 17 March 1967, B6.
17 MacFarlane, "Brain Gain from Immigrants," 29.
18 "The Cruel Doctor Drain," *The Globe and Mail*, 15 September 1967, 6.
19 Van Hoek, *The Migration of High Level Manpower*.
20 Margulies and Bloch, *Foreign Medical Graduates*.
21 The Committee on the International Migration of Talent (CIMT), *The International Migration of High-Level Manpower*.
22 Ibid.
23 Gish, *Doctor Migration and World Health*.
24 Ibid.
25 Ibid.
26 World Health Organization, *Multinational Study of the International Migration of Physicians and Nurses*, 1973; World Health Organization, *Multinational Study of the International Migration of Physicians and Nurses: An Analytical Review of the Literature*, 1976; Mejía, "Migration of Physicians and Nurses," 207–15; Mejía, Pizurki, Royston, *Physician and Nurse Migration*.
27 Mejía, "Migration of Physicians and Nurses," 207–15.
28 "Doctors: 1600 in UK," *Journal of the Indian Medical Association* 39, no. 9 (1 November 1962): 487.
29 Mullally and Wright, "Connecting to Canada."
30 "Current Topics," *The Times of India*, 20 October 1967, 8.
31 Stevens and Vermeulan, *Foreign Trained Physicians*.
32 Bhalla, "'We Wanted to End Disparities At Work,'" 40–78.
33 Commonwealth Consultative Committee on South and South-east Asia, "The Colombo Plan."
34 Ferguson, "The Indian Medical Graduate in America, 1965," 291–8.
35 Sackley, "Foundation in the Field," 247–8.
36 "Activities of the Institute of Applied Manpower Research in India," *International Labour Review* 90, no. 2 (August 1964): 184–5.

37 See IAMR, "Preface," *Indian Scientists in the United States*, n.p.

38 IAMR, "Manpower 1968," 186. The study is based on data compiled by the American Medical Association. See IAMR, *Indian Physicians in the United States*, 33.

39 IAMR, *The Brain Drain Study, Phase I*, 41.

40 Ibid., table 1, "Index of Annual Increase in Passports Issued," 6; table 2, "Distribution of Passport-holders by Educational Category and Year of Passport Issue," 8; chart 1, "Distribution of Passport-holders by Educational Category and Year of Passport Issue," 9; table 3, "Distribution of Passport-holders by Educational Category and Regional Passport Office," 10; table 17, "Percentage Distribution of Passport-holders to Annual Outturn by Educational Category and Year of Passport Issue," 42–3.

41 See also ibid., table 18, "Gross Addition to the Total Stock of Indian Personnel Abroad by Educational Categories (1960–67)," 46.

42 Ibid., 48.

43 Bannerjee, "Immigration of Doctors," 194.

44 Ibid.

45 Ministry of External Affairs Annual Report 1965–1966, quoted in IAMR, *The Brain Drain Study*, 22.

46 "Indian Doctors Bid to Beat 'Brain Drain' Laws," *Journal of the Indian Medical Association* 55 (16 December 1970): 427.

47 "Indian Doctors take ECFMG Examination at Kuala Lumpur," *Journal of the Indian Medical Association* 57 (16 November 1971): 393.

48 For an insight into the complicated reciprocal understandings of Canadian provinces and Britain's General Medical Council qualification, see "Foreign MDs in Canada Face Tangle of Regulations," *The Globe and Mail*, 18 January 1966, 3.

49 Licensing of doctors in the United States, in parallel to Canada, differed between individual states. Some states were known as being relatively "liberal" in the recognition of foreign credentials. Others were more conservative. This resulted in clustering patterns in the United States, such as the prominence of Indian-trained doctors in three states in particular: Michigan, New Jersey, and New York. Canadian-trained doctors appear to have had a comparatively easy time having their credentials recognized south of the border.

50 Abraham, "Stopping The Brain Drain," 10.

51 "Doctors Serving Abroad Offered Jobs in India," *Journal of the Indian Medical Association* 56 (16 January 1971): 57.

52 32.7 per cent of the 2,370 individuals in this scheme were designated as doctors. Abraham, "Stopping the Brain Drain," 10.

53 Davis, *The Serpent and the Rainbow*, 256.

54 Girard, *Haiti: The Tumultuous History*, 111.

55 Pegram, *Choosing Their Own Style*, 36–7.

56 Polyné, *From Douglass to Duvalier*, 181.

57 Mooney, *Faith Makes Us Live*, 250.

58 Mills, *A Place in the Sun*.

59 Ibid., chapter 1.

60 Contemporary reports suggested as many as 150 at one point in time.

61 Minn, *Where They Need Me*.

62 A controversial racial term in North America and Europe, it generally denoted "mixed" (ie black/white) individuals until recent decades. In the Haitian context, the appellation *mulatto* was widely used by Duvalier and his supporters as a way of identifying (and critiquing) the elite and/or American sympathizers. This racial division between "true blacks" and mixed-race Haitians was central to Duvalier's ideology of *noirisme*.

63 Makere University has a complicated history, being part of the University of East Africa system and offering degrees that were granted in conjunction with the University of London.

64 Susser and Cherry, "Health and Health Care," 455–75.

65 Digby, "'The Bandwagon'?," 829, 827–51.

66 Marks and Andersson, "Diseases of Apartheid," 192.

67 Coovadia et al., "Health in South Africa 1," 826.

68 Digby, "Black Doctors and Discrimination," 273.

69 Digby, *Diversity and Division*, 421. See also Coovadia et al., "Health in South Africa 1," 820: "Early 1970s: in the Bantustans, the doctor to population ratio was estimated at 1:15 000 compared with 1:1700 in the rest of the country."

70 Digby, *Diversity and Division*, 426.

71 By the late 1970s two other "black" medical schools were created: MEDUNSA (1977) and the University of Transkei (1985). Digby, "Black Doctors and Discrimination," 270.

72 Digby, *Diversity and Division*, 198, 205–6, quotation 208.

73 Digby, "Black Doctors and Discrimination," 277–8.

74 Digby, *Diversity and Division*, 213–14.

75 Ibid.

76 See Armstrong, "A System of Exclusion," passim. The South African medical degree bore similarities to many Western European countries. Students were

admitted directly from secondary school and embarked on basic sciences courses before entering clinical training. The undergraduate medical sciences degree (MBChB) thus took approximately six years. Most programs then required one year of internship, in which students were required to choose surgery, medicine, or OBGYN. It was these internships that often witnessed students going abroad.

77 Ronald Eichenberg [pseudonym], interview, June 2013.

78 Grant, "From the Transvaal to the Prairies," 681–95.

79 Ronald Eichenberg [pseudonym], interview, June 2013.

80 Interview with David Dowitsky [pseudonym], May 2013.

81 Gish, *Health Manpower & the Medical Auxiliary*.

82 McKenzie, "Canada Found Stopover Point," B21.

83 See, inter alia, "The Brain Shortage," *The Globe and Mail*, 15 April 1966, 6, in which the editors lamented the loss of "thousands of skilled Canadians" to the United States on an annual basis. Arguably, with the various national research projects in the United States, the drain of research scientists was even greater than clinicians. Citing an OECD report, the same article claimed that Canada lost 50 per cent of its graduates in engineering in 1959.

84 Kirk and Erisman, *Cuban Medical Internationalism*. See also Huish and Kirk, "Cuban Medical Internationalism," 77–92.

85 Jones, "A Mysterious Discrimination," 139–56.

86 Choy, *Empire of Care*.

87 Mejía, "Migration of Physicians and Nurses," 207.

88 Gish, "Doctor Migration and World Health."

89 Brown, Cueto, and Fee, "The World Health Organization," 87–9.

90 Richard Eidelman [pseudonym], interview, June 2013.

91 David Dowitsky [pseudonym], interview, May 2013.

92 Rehka Gupta, interview, June 2008.

93 Arvin Akas, interview, March 2014.

94 Ruchika Akash, interview, March 2014.

95 "The Brain Shortage," *The Globe and Mail*, 15 April 1966, 6.

96 "The Cruel Doctor Drain," 6.

CHAPTER SEVEN

1 For details on both the history and mythology surrounding Wilfred Grenfell and the International Grenfell International, see Rompkey, *Grenfell of Labrador*.

2 Kealey and Molyneaux, "On the Road to Medicare," 90–111.

3 Paul Minc, correspondence to Sasha Mullally, 31 August 2013.

4 Evans, "Does Canada Have Too Many Doctors?," 147–60.

5 Saskatchewan Farmer's Union, *Submission of the Saskatchewan Farmer's Union*, table D, 7. These data were drawn from Saskatchewan Advisory Planning Committee on Medical Care, *Interim Report of the Advisory Planning Committee on Medical Care.*

6 Medical Society of Prince Edward Island, "Exhibit No. 28," Appendix A: "Physician Distribution in Prince Edward Island. Number of physicians in private practice and type of work done," 1791.

7 The brief was formally submitted by the provincial CMA representatives in conjunction with the local medical society.

8 Medical Society of Prince Edward Island, "Exhibit No. 28," 1752.

9 Ibid., 1755.

10 Medical Society of Prince Edward Island and Canadian Medical Association Prince Edward Island Division, *The Submission*, 1.

11 Which they attributed in part to the lack of administrative, research, and teaching posts. Medical Society of Prince Edward Island, "Exhibit No. 28," 1779.

12 Ibid., 1845–6.

13 Dewar, *Life at Leighwood.*

14 Ibid., 1759.

15 Ibid., 1843–5.

16 Ibid., 1759.

17 Ibid., 1780, see also 1845–6.

18 Medical Society of Prince Edward Island and Canadian Medical Association Prince Edward Island Division, *The Submission of the Medical Society of Prince Edward Island and CMA PEI Division*, 7–8.

19 Ibid., 5, 6.

20 Ontario Public Health Association, "Exhibit No. 344," 11902.

21 They recommended that the government of Ontario through a program of subsidization encourage students from rural areas to seek admission to a faculty of dentistry and subsequent to graduation return to a rural area to practise. $30,000 per year would provide subsidization for ten students in each of the first three years in dental school. Royal College of Dental Surgeons of Ontario and Ontario Dental Association, "Exhibit No. 325," 11491–2, 11498–9.

22 Ibid., 11499.

23 Ontario Medical Association, "Exhibit No. 238," 8834.

24 Ibid., 8862.

25 Ontario Medical Association, *The Submission*, 18, para. 64.

26 Ibid., para. 169.

27 Ibid., 8843 and para. 73.

28 Ibid., 20–1.

29 Mair and Hatcher, "The Pattern of Health Organization," 542, 543.

30 Ontario Medical Association, *The Submission*, Appendix #7: Survey of First-Year Medical Students, 126.

31 Ibid., 127.

32 Ontario Medical Association, *The Submission*, Appendix #15 Results of Questionnaire sent to Branch Societies, 254. The OMA reported there were hospital waiting lists in the Sudbury area – 775 for 725 beds – as more cases were being referred there "that would otherwise (or previously) go to Toronto; these are drawn from Manitoulin, Blind River, Elliot Lake, Timmins, Sturgeon Falls, etc." Ibid., 243.

33 Ibid., 112.

34 Ibid., Appendix 4, 111, 113, 269–70.

35 Ibid., Appendix 7.

36 Corbett, "Immigration and Canadian Politics," 212–13.

37 There are many sources that discuss the landscape of reciprocal licensing, but this is confirmed in Kelly, "Medical Practice in Canada," 35–6.

38 Mullally, "Policing Practitioners on the Periphery," 153–68.

39 Kealey, "Delivering Health Care," 183–98.

40 Historically, the province relied heavily on medical graduates from American medical colleges, although by midcentury one can discern a "Canadianization" of medical education in physician registries. See Mullally and MacDonald, "Call the Doctor?" 41–68.

41 The margin of error is estimated at approximately 3 per cent. Eleven physicians have no place of training listed and could not be identified from subsequent CMDs (fourteen not listed in 1961 but subsequently identified in 1966 edition). Of those identified elsewhere, one physician was identified as Estonian, one as trained in Ottawa, and another at Dalhousie from the 1966 CMD. Of those left, half were listed as interns or residents at hospitals and have surnames that suggest Chinese, Yugoslavian, Italian, and Polish ethnic backgrounds. While it is not possible to be certain, it is somewhat likely that these seven physicians were licensed in New Brunswick with foreign medical training, which would bring the proportion up to about 16 per cent.

42 Using the same methodology, the margin of error for this sample is 1.2 per cent, with nine physicians listed without medical education. All but one have Asian or South Asian surnames, and all are affiliated with hospitals as interns and residents. Were they included in our calculations, the proportion of foreign-trained physicians in New Brunswick would exceed 33 per cent.

43 Kelly, "Medical Practice in Canada," 35.

44 Ibid., 36.

45 Ibid., 35.

46 Mair and Hatcher, "The Pattern of Health Organization," 542.

47 Ibid., 543.

48 Ibid.

49 Davidson, "Medical Immigration," 786.

50 Ibid., 787.

51 Chamberlain, "Where Shall John Go? Canada," 693.

52 Ibid.

53 Ibid., 694.

54 Ibid.

55 Roos, Gaumont, and Horne, "The Impact of the Physician Surplus," 169.

56 "Better Facts Needed on MDs," The Financial Post, 2 March 1974, 5, quoted in Roos, Gaumont, and Horne, "The Impact of the Physician Surplus," 169.

57 Hawkins, "Canadian Immigration Policy," 149.

58 Ibid., 148.

59 See Evans, Price Formation.

60 Roos, Gaumont and Horne, "The Impact of the Physician Surplus," 198.

61 Ibid., 197.

62 Spaulding and Spitzer, "Implications of Medical Manpower Trends," 527–33.

63 Copeman, "177 of 203 Doctors Stay," 774–6.

64 Roos, Gaumont, and Horne, "The Impact of the Physician Surplus," 169.

65 Copeman, "177 of 203 Doctors Stay," 774–6.

66 Hacon, "Health Manpower Development," 10.

67 Ibid., 7.

68 Ibid.

69 Barer and Stoddart, "Toward Integrated Medical Resource Policies," 620.

70 The provinces were Newfoundland, Nova Scotia, New Brunswick, Ontario, and Manitoba.

71 Wright, "Factors Influencing," 44.

72 Hacon, "Health Manpower Development," 11.

73 Ibid., 78.
74 Hurley, "Simulated Effects of Income-based Policies," 221.
75 Evans, "Does Canada Have Too Many Doctors?," 155.

CHAPTER EIGHT

1 See Webster, *The National Health Service*, 28–45. For a survey of postwar health care in Britain, see Berridge, *Health and Medicine in Britain since 1939* and a special issue of *Social History of Medicine* 21, no. 3 (2008).
2 John Carter (pseudonym), interview, 3 May 2009.
3 Ibid.
4 Ibid.
5 The physician arrived at the high point of medical immigration from Britain. Wright, Mullally, and Cordukes, "Worse Than Being Married," 45–51.
6 Carter, interview.
7 Ibid.
8 Madison, "Preserving Individualism," 442–83. See also Madison, "Notes on the History," 52–4, 56–60, 86–93.
9 Newell and Mahon, "Medical Group Income Distribution Accounting," 224–5. How-to articles became more common by the 1960s and 1970s. See Lyon, "Aspects of Group Medical Practice," 799–803.
10 Several obituaries credit Rorem's Depression-era policy work with laying the foundation for both programs. See, for instance, Fowler, "C. Rufus Rorem, 93, Economist."
11 He was part of a group of economists committed to resisting the push toward socialized medicine. The historiography on medical economics at midcentury is underdeveloped, but for context to the debates on socialized medicine in the United States, see Numbers, *Almost Persuaded*.
12 Rorem, "Economics of Private Group Practice," 462–6.
13 Ibid.
14 Vayda, "Prepaid Group Practice," 72–3, 75, 77.
15 Some of these pre-Medicare plans are described in Marchildon's edited collection of essays on Medicare. See the collection of articles that review early health insurance schemes on the lines of the universal system in British Columbia, Quebec, Saskatchewan, Newfoundland, and Alberta. "Part Two: Individual Provincial Histories of Medicare," in Marchildon, ed., *Making Medicare*, 137–276.
16 Acheson, "Public Interest Cited," 929.

17 Korcok, "Group Medicine a Growing Force," 135–7.

18 Paulick and Roos, "The Young Physician," 276–8.

19 Carter (pseudonym), interview.

20 Between 1950 and 1960 alone, Canadian provinces licensed approximately 5,000 new international medical graduates (IMGs), and of these, 2,000 had British training credentials. See, for instance, Judek, *Medical Manpower in Canada*, 38–44.

21 According to historian Jacalyn Duffin, since 1958 physicians in Canada have been the highest paid professional group in Canada. When the British physician cited above came to Canada in 1968, the average physician would have reported an income of about $17,500, which translates to $115,000–$120,000 in today's Canadian dollars. By contrast, his reported annual salary of $19,000 yields an income of $130,000 in 2013 Canadian dollars. For trends in the historical census reported and taxation reported physician incomes in Canada, see Duffin, "The Impact of Single-Payer Health Care," 1198–208.

22 The Canadian Medical Association circulated a survey/questionnaire to their membership on the desirability of salaried positions. According to J.B. MacMillan, CMA president at the time, 84 per cent of all doctors answering said they would refuse to work for salary. See MacMillan, "Letter to the Editor," 800.

23 Wright, Mullally, and Cordukes, "Worse Than Being Married," 574–5.

24 See Lucas, *Minetown, Milltown, Railtown*; Randall and Ironside, "Communities on the Edge," 17–35; Bowles, "Single-Industry Resource Communities," 63–83; Bowles, *Little Communities and Big Industries*.

25 This precarity precipitated a late-century decline that is explored through oral history in High, *Industrial Sunset*.

26 Freudenburg and Frickel, "Digging Deeper," 266–88.

27 For a history of Cobalt, see Angus and Griffin, *We Lived a Life and Then Some*.

28 For a historical overview of municipal expansion, see Halseth and Sutherland, "From Kitimat to Tumbler Ridge," 134–60.

29 In 1951, a pulp mill was built on nearby Watson Island, which became the major employer in the region. See Bowman, *Muskeg, Rocks and Rain* and Large, *Prince Rupert*.

30 See, for instance, McAlister and Twohig, "The Check Off?," 1504–6.

31 Turnover at the community health centre was very high by the late 1960s,

while patient demand for specialty services prompted an expansion of physician staff at the community health centre from forty-seven in 1968 to 145 in 1977. Lomas, *First and Foremost*, 80–3, 94.

32 David McNair, interview, 11 September 2013.

33 Lomas, *First and Foremost*, 63.

34 McNair, interview.

35 Ibid.

36 Ibid.

37 Ibid.

38 Lomas, *First and Foremost*, 94–6. See, also, Korcok, "The Sault Experience," 879; Hastings, Mott, Barclay, and Hewitt, "Prepaid Group Practice," 91–103.

39 Lomas, *First and Foremost*, 66.

40 Leah, "A Most Extraordinary Mining Town."

41 This was part of approximately 8.5 million dollars the company invested in building the community, administered by officials occupying a local government district board. Henderson, "Community Planning of the Town Site," 1193, 1197. Quoted in Robson, "Manitoba's Resource Towns."

42 But the development of the resource frontier had become a publicly controlled endeavour. Ibid.

43 Brodie, *The Political Economy of Canadian Regionalism*, 135–80. See also Fowke, "The National Policy."

44 This meant the influence of local business interests lessened [while large foreign/multinationals increased], technical [planning] expertise was emphasized, and a broad mandate for enticing and supporting large-scale capital projects made provincial funds available to promote resource development. This, with the general continentalist orientation in Canadian economic affairs during the era of the Second National Policy, created, in the words of Jim Kenney, "an underlying logic to the growth strategy in this era which promised material and political benefits to ... utilit[ies], business[es] and government; and each of these interests was actively involved in the [promotion] process." See Kenny and Secord, "Public Power for Industry," 87.

45 Kenney and Secord, "Public Power for Industry," 101. According to Kenney and Secord, "Some Canadian political economists have suggested that the American stockpiling effort, and the Paley Report [Resources for Freedom, 1952] in particular, can be seen as a factor in the increasing ownership of Canadian resources by American multinationals during the decade following

the Second World War. The unusually high demand created by American stockpiling efforts combined with lowered duties drew many American-based corporations to Canada."

46 Innis, "The Canadian Mining Industry," 309–20.

47 President's Materials Policy Commission, *The Outlook for Key Commodities*, 118.

48 Richards and Pratt, *Prairie Capitalism*, chapters 4–8. Saskatchewan had mixed results trying to do this with potash in the 1970s. See Taylor, "The Pursuit of Industrial Development," chapter 3.

49 This term describes the Canadian economic growth regime of the period. See Clark-Jones, *A Staple State*. See also Aronson, *American National Security*.

50 This would include a large indoor mall – the largest of its kind in Canada. "It is a one-industry town, but it won't be a company town," Nesbitt was quick to point out. "[INCO] will be the main employer of the 8,000 people who will live there eventually. But we want as much private ownership as possible in the town itself." Desbarats, "Thompson's 'Nickel Curtain,'" 3.

51 Desbarats, "Thompson's 'Nickel Curtain,'" 3.

52 The first reference to the needs of this reserve is in 1962 when a community development officer was hired by the town and assessing the employment needs of this population became part of his mandate. "Development Officer Named for Thompson," *Winnipeg Tribune*, 4 December 1962, 17.

53 "First Permanent Elementary School for Nickel Town," *Winnipeg Tribune*, 11 September 1959, 4. It was constructed by the company but deeded to the local government authorities during an opening ceremony that September.

54 Louttit, "Thompson: Mining Town," n.p.

55 Town authorities were crying for more housing in 1961, as production ramped up and overcrowding started to become a problem. The town was planned to house 8,000 workers but in reality mine operations required double that population to produce the seventy-five million tons of nickel a year. "Planner's Dream Realized at Thompson," *The Winnipeg Evening Tribune*, 24 March 1961, 19. Consultants projected that Thompson would service up to 17,500 people by the mid-1960s. "17,500 by 1966," *Winnipeg Tribune*, 2 November 1961, 25.

56 "Planner's Dream Realized at Thompson," 19.

57 Ibid.

58   Ibid.
59   Canadian Medical Association, *Canadian Medical Directory* (1960, 1964, 1968, 1972).
60   Ibid.
61   Surajit Ghosh, interview, 26 September 2013.
62   Ibid.
63   Lachlan McIntosh, interview, 5 September 2013.
64   Ghosh, interview.
65   McIntosh, interview.
66   Ghosh, interview.
67   McIntosh, interview.
68   Ghosh, interview.
69   McIntosh, interview.
70   Ibid.
71   Ibid.
72   Ghosh, interview.
73   Ibid.
74   McIntosh, interview.
75   Ibid.
76   Ghosh, interview.
77   McIntosh, interview.
78   Ghosh, interview.

CHAPTER NINE

1   For a history of the Durban Medical School, see Noble, *A School of Struggle*.
2   Tanya Levinson [pseudonym], interview, June 2013.
3   Horwitz, *Baragwanath Hospital, Soweto*.
4   Tanya Levinson [pseudonym], interview, June 2013.
5   Ibid.
6   Ibid.
7   Marks, *Divided Sisterhood*.
8   Tanya Levinson [pseudonym], interview, June 2013.
9   Ibid.
10   Ibid.
11   Korcok, "Restriction of Physician Immigration," 509–13.
12   Ibid., 512.

13 Ibid., 509.

14 This committee was "to work with a Task Force of Health and Welfare Canada and the specialists' associations to develop recommendations on the overall requirements for physicians of all kinds." Roos et al., "The Impact of the Physician Surplus," 171.

15 Evans, "Does Canada Have Too Many Doctors?" 147–60.

16 See Roos et al, "The Impact of the Physician Surplus," 171, for details on these events.

17 Ibid.

18 Chester Stuart, *Canadian Medical Association Journal*, 1975, 517; Hacon and Aziz, "The Supply of Physicians in Canada," 517.

19 Korcak, "Restriction of Physician Immigration," 513.

20 Green, *Immigration and the Post-War Canadian Economy*, 25.

21 Knowles, *Strangers at Our Gates*, 211.

22 House of Commons Debates (24 April 1953), 4383.

23 86,313 immigrants were accepted that year, down from 218,465 in 1974. Ibid.

24 Korcok, "The Restriction of Physician Immigration," 509.

25 One gap was, paradoxically, mismatches in the annual allocation of residency (postgraduate) positions affiliated to academic units in the country. Under the "match" system, graduating doctors (from their MD programs) would choose their postgraduate specialty and then rank their training programs. Medical schools' postgraduate directors would concurrently rank their choice of applicant doctors. Inevitably, unfilled positions would emerge, some of which would become available to graduates of foreign medical schools. The anomalies of the "match" system continue to this day. I am grateful to Greg Stoddart for alerting me to this persistent problem that dates back to this period.

26 Quoted in Roos et al, "The Impact of the Physician Surplus," 169; see also Noether, "The Growing Supply of Physicians," 503–37.

27 Evans, "Health Services in Nova Scotia," 357.

28 Manga, "Arbitration and the Medical Profession," 675.

29 Evans, "Does Canada Have Too Many Doctors?," 147–60.

30 Brown and Evans, "Does Canada Have Too Many Doctors," 369.

31 Ibid., 367.

32 Ibid., 369.

33 Ibid., 371–2.

34 Ibid., 372.

35 Though remuneration for the same service might vary *between* provincial plans.

36 The Canada Health Act of 1984 insisted on accessibility and prohibited matching federal funds to provincial health insurance systems that permitted extra billing. The financial coercion led inevitably the abolition of extra fees, though not without considerable battles at the provincial level and a doctors' strike in Ontario (in 1986). See Canada Health Act, [*An Act relating to cash contributions by Canada and relating to criteria and conditions in respect of insured health services and extended health care services*] R.S.C., 1985, c. C-6.

37 Evans extensively reviews the evidence that fee-for-service payment structures lead to excessive provision of surgeries. See Evans, "Does Canada Have Too Many Doctors?" 151.

38 Hall, *Canada's National–Provincial Health Program for the 1980s*, 33.

39 Evans, "Does Canada Have Too Many Doctors?" 154.

40 Manga, "Arbitration and the Medical Profession," 675. Sam Freedman, dean of medicine at McGill University, even mused in 1983 that "it might be agreed to close completely at least two of the less viable [medical] schools," though presumably he did not mean his own. Woods, "The Alleged MD Surplus," 1171.

41 This figure is for 1974. Wright, *Factors Influencing the Location*, 24.

42 Once a doctor was approved to practice in a province, the respective minister of health would issue a unique billing number to that doctor. This number would be used on all relevant forms requesting reimbursement for insurable services.

43 Administratively this was relatively straightforward to introduce. Bureaucrats could simply discount or prohibit billing by doctors whose place of practice was in an area code deemed to be overserviced, which almost always corresponded to urban and suburban areas.

44 Ibid, 38.

45 Administrative law is the branch of law that deals with appropriate actions of the government.

46 Grey, "Does Section 7 of the Charter Protect," 935.

47 *Re Mia and Medical Services Commission of British Columbia*, [1985] 17 D. L.R. (4th) 414.

48 Wright, *Factors Influencing the Location of Practice*, 39.

49 *Wilson v. Medical Services Commission of B.C.* [1987] 3 W.W.R. 48 and *Wilson v. Medical Services Commission of B.C.*, 30 B.C.L.R. (2d) 97, 53 D.L.R. (4th) 171.

50 *Wilson v. Medical Services Commission of B.C.*, 30 B.C.L.R. (2d) 97, 53 D.L.R. (4th), 193.

51 Manfredi and Maioni, "Courts and Health Policy," 224.

52 Duffin, "The Impact of Single-Payer Health Care," figure 1. According to Duffin's calculations based on taxation data, the average income of Canadian doctors, adjusted for inflation, peaked around 1971–72 when their pay eclipsed even that of American doctors. It then fell in both real and comparative terms during the rest of the 1970s.

53 Stevenson, Williams, and Vayda, "Medical Politics and Canadian Medicare," 68.

54 Bégin, *Medicare*, 76.

55 "1983: The Year in Review. The National View: Canada Health Act Looms Large," *Canadian Medical Association Journal* 130 (1 January 1984): 63.

56 Brown, "Health Care Financing," 111.

57 Stevenson, Williams, and Vayda, "Medical Politics and Canadian Medicare," 68.

58 Bégin, *Medicare*, 87.

59 Stevenson, Williams, and Vayda, "Medical Politics and Canadian Medicare," 70.

60 Heiber and Deber, "Banning Extra-Billing in Canada," 63.

61 "Federal Health Minister Tables Canada Health Act," *Canadian Medical Association Journal* 130, no. 1 (1 January 1984): 1C.

62 Brown, "Health Care Financing," 127.

63 Ibid, 111.

64 Bégin, *Medicare*, 108.

65 Stevenson, Williams, and Vayda, "Medical Politics and Canadian Medicare," 70.

66 French, "Exodus of One in the Works," A7.

67 Coffin, "CMA President Responds to the Act," 1D.

68 Fine, "Child, 3, Waits Two Hours for Treatment," A19.

69 Holland, "The Ontario Doctors' Strike," 728.

70 McPherson, "The Canada Health Act 'illegal'?," 78.1.

71 Peterson, "Doctors Strike Day 10," A16.

72 Silversides, "Money Is Still Central Issue," A17.

73 "Physicians' Folly," *The Globe and Mail*, 11 June 1986, A6.

74 Stevenson and Williams, "Physicians and Medicare," 507.

75 Meslin, "The Moral Costs of the Ontario Physicians' Strike," 12.

76 Bégin, "Health Minister Bégin Comments," 731.

77 Peterson, "Doctors Strike Day 10," A16.

78 Bégin, "Health Minister Bégin Comments," 731.

79 Kravitz et al., "Risk Factors Associated," 1229.

80 Peterson, "Doctors Strike Day 10," A16.

81 For example, Manning, "Canada Health Act," 1166–7.

82 Bégin, *Medicare*, 149.

83 Silversides, Douglas, and Todd, "Doctors Wrestle with Call to Strike," A1.

84 McLaren, "OMA Rejects Compromise," A1.

85 "Doctor's Strike Could Affect Earnings," *Toronto Star*, 1 July 1986, C6.

86 Brownridge, "MDS and Extra-billing," A7.

87 Silversides, "Money is Still Central Issue"; Stevenson and Williams, "Physicians and Medicare," 518.

88 Bégin, *Medicare*, 81.

89 Meslin, "The Moral Costs," 11.

90 Stevenson, Williams, and Vayda, "Medical Politics and Canadian Medicare," 70, suggest 65–70 per cent of doctors went out on strike. Later (91) they report the OMA's claim of 75 per cent and a *Globe and Mail* newspaper poll claiming 60 per cent. Meslin, by contrast, estimated 50 per cent. Meslin, "The Moral Costs," 12. Kravitz and Shapiro demonstrate that part of the confusion in the numbers stems from differing duration and intensity of strike activities among Ontario's physicians. They show that Ontario Health Insurance Plan (OHIP) billings actually declined only 9 per cent in June 1986 from June of the previous year, which may also indicate that the strike was not as widespread as the media's reporting implied. Kravitz and Shapiro, "Duration and Intensity," 742.

91 Kravitz and Shapiro "Duration and Intensity," 742.

92 Meslin, "The Moral Costs," 12.

93 Ibid, 13.

94 Hancock, "A Need to Erase the Doctor's Empire," A7.

95 Todd, "Patient Having Miscarriage Turned Away," A22.

96 Simpson, "A Losing Battle," A6.

97 "Physicians' Folly," A6.

98 Silversides, "Non-participation by Many MDS," A1.

99   Silversides, "OMA Votes to Continue Strike Action," A1.

100   Micay, "The Strike That Backfired," A7.

101   Bégin, *Medicare*, 119.

102   Stevenson, Williams, and Vayda, "Medical Politics and Canadian Medicare," 70.

103   Lowry, "Quebec's Hunger-Striking MDs," 1342.

104   "17 Physicians Stage Hunger Strike in Montreal," *The Globe and Mail*, 29 March 1989, A9; Alexander, "Foreign Trained MDs," A3.

105   *Régie de l'assurance maladie du Québec* (the government department, in Quebec, responsible for administering health insurance in the province).

106   As cited in Lowry, "Quebec's Hunger-Striking MDs," 1345.

107   Buchignani, "Manitoba MLA Wants Doctors," A3.

108   "Quebec Doctors Halt Hunger Strike After Govt. Concessions," *Ottawa Citizen*, 13 April 1989, A5.

109   Barer and Stoddart, *Toward Integrated Medical Resource Policies*, v.

110   The report was more than 300 pages long. In response to the deputy ministers, the authors reduced the full report into a shorter, abbreviated one. Many of the themes were also parceled into articles published in the *Canadian Medical Association Journal* in the subsequent years. Greg Stoddart, personal correspondence with the authors.

111   Lepnurm and Trowell, "Satisfaction of Country Doctors," 14–20.

112   Ibid., 18.

113   Barer and Stoddart, *Towards Integrated Medical Resource Policies*, passim.

114   For two perspectives on the legacy of the Barer–Stoddart report, see Beck and Thompson, "The Health Care Philosophy," 65; and Evans and McGrail, "Richard III, Barer-Stoddart, *et la fille de temps*," 18–28.

115   The Northern Ontario Medical School is shared by Lakehead University (in Thunder Bay) and Laurentian University (in Sudbury) and accepted its first medical school students in 2005. It has an explicit mandate to train medical practitioners for underserviced areas including, but not limited to, First Nations reserves in northern Ontario. Laurentian is also noteworthy as the only other university in Ontario (in addition to Ottawa) to be nominally bilingual.

116   The Northern Medical Program (of British Columbia) is not a self-standing UGMD but rather coordinates undergraduate and postgraduate training of the medical school of the University of British Columbia.

117   We are grateful to Greg Stoddart for this point.

118 Chan, *From Perceived Surplus to Perceived Shortage*, 1. Stoddart also attributes the renewed doctor shortage in the mid- to late-1990s to the termination of the rotating internship, something which he argues eliminated, in effect, a whole cohort of practitioners. Greg Stoddart, personal correspondence with the authors, May 2012.

119 Aizenman, "The Oncoming Hordes," 1177. This augmentation of national physician supply was consistent with general trends in the "industrialized" world, which witnessed a growth in the physician *ratios*, between 1950 and 1979, of 96 per cent (from 10.2 per 10,000 to 19.6 per 10,000). Canada's figure for 1981 was approximately 18 per 10,000. See Kindig and Taylor, "Growth in the International Physician Supply," 3130, table 1 and passim. Canadian figure derived from Statistics Canada census of population, 1851–2006.

120 Figures for 1977–78. ACMC Position Paper, "Physician Manpower," 38.

121 Shuval and Bernstein, *Immigrant Physicians*.

122 See Barnett, "Foreign Medical Graduates in New Zealand," 1049–60.

123 Now known as *Chaoulli v Quebec*, the Supreme Court in a split decision (four to three) ruled that the Quebec Health Insurance Act and the (Quebec) Hospital Insurance Act violated the rights of Jacques Chaoulli by infringing upon his right to "life, liberty, and security of the person." See *Chaoulli v. Quebec* (2005) 1 SCR 791, 2005 SCC 35.

124 See Chan, *From Perceived Surplus to Perceived Shortage*.

CONCLUSION

1 *La Grande Séduction*. The movie won the Audience Award at the 2004 Sundance Movie Festival. The remake – *The Grand Seduction* (2013) – was directed by Don McKellar and distributed by Entertainment One.

2 The cosmopolitan, arrogant city doctor living unexpectedly amongst country bumpkins is an enduring comedic trope. One thinks of Michael J. Fox as the status-obsessed plastic surgeon whose car breaks down in hillbilly Appalachia in the 1991 movie *Doc Holiday*. There was also the long-running, if somewhat quirky, 1990 CBS series *Northern Exposure*, where a New York medical graduate agrees to work in Alaska only to find out that he failed to read the fine print. Like *La Grande Séduction*, the physicians in both of these examples are, at first, appalled by the lack of technological interventions in rural practice but are eventually won over by the kindness of the people and, of course, a local love interest. For a rare medical migration variation, there was also the British comedy *The Indian Doctor*, depicting an erudite South

Asian physician and his long-suffering wife working in rural Wales amongst suspicious working-class coal miners.

3   *Chaoulli v. Quebec* (2005) 1 SCR 791, 2005 SCC 35.

4   Near the end of our period under study, Quebec would impose French-language requirements for practitioners wishing to relocate to the province from the rest of Canada or from abroad.

5   Roos, Gaumont, and Horne, "The Impact of the Physician Surplus," 169.

6   "Better Facts Needed on MDS," *The Financial Post*, 2 March 1974, 5 quoted in Roos, Gaumont, and Horne, "The Impact of the Physician Surplus," 169.

7   Audas, Ross, and Vardy, "Provisionally Licensed," 1315–16.

8   This term clarified the essential licensing distinction between those trained outside of Canada and those who graduated from Canadian medical schools. The older term of foreign doctor, or foreign-trained doctor, was ambiguous, due to the minority of foreign-trained doctors who were, in fact, Canadian students who graduated from medical schools abroad. This last phenomenon became pronounced with the popularity of Caribbean-based medical schools in the 1990s.

9   A geographical analysis of IMGs in rural America, outside of our time period of study, has also suggested that the regional physician disparity in Canada is part of a broader transnational phenomenon. Baer, *Doctors in a Strange Land*.

10 Friesen, "The Evolving Meaning of Region in Canada," 529–45; Conrad, "Past Imaginings," 6–9.

11 See Mullally and Wright, "La Grande Séduction?," 69–89.

12 For a comprehensive examination of South African physician emigration to Canada from 1975–2000 including a discussion of what compensation might look like, see Grant, "From the Transvaal to the Prairies."

13 Hagopian et al., "The Migration of Physicians," 17.

14 As cited in Bundred and Levitt, "Medical Migration," 245–6.

15 Itano, "Condition Critical"; Mullan, "Doctors and Soccer Players," 6.

16 Department of Health, Great Britain, *Code of Practice for NHS Employers*.

17 World Health Organization, "World Health Assembly Concludes."

18 Alkire and Chen, "Medical Exceptionalism."

19 Clemens, "Do Visas Kill?"; Clemens and Petterson, "New Data," 1.

20 See, inter alia, Mullan, "The Metrics," 1810–8; Benatar, "An Examination of Ethical Aspects," 2–7.

21 "MD's Gift to Eskasoni: 140 Hectares," *Halifax Chronicle Herald*, 24 April 2014, 2.

22 Ibid.

23 This literature is voluminous but in addition to the work produced by Alfonso Mejía and colleagues cited below influential titles that drew attention to the problem include Committee on the International Migration of Talent, *The International Migration of High-level Manpower* and Van Hoek, *The Migration of High Level Manpower*.

24 Mejía, "Migration of Physicians and Nurses," 207. Mejía himself helped raise these concerns in the early 1970s with the publication of an earlier study of this brain drain phenomenon: *World Health Organization: Multinational Study of the International Migration of Physicians and Nurses* (1973). For additional works published on this theme, see also Mejía, Pizurki, and Royston, *Physician and Nurse Migration*; Mejía, "Health Manpower Migration in the Americas"; and Mejía, Pizurki, and Royston, *World Health Organization Multinational Study* (1981).

25 Health insurance became tied to employment in the United States, but Canada adopted a universal health care system. For background information, consider Numbers, *Almost Persuaded*.

26 "Canada Welcomes in First Group of 25,000 Syrian Refugees," *The National* [Associated Press], 11 December 2015. https://web.archive.org/web/2015121819 1600/http://www.thenational.ae/world/americas/canada-welcomes-in-first-group-of-planned-25000-syrian-refugees [Archived 18 December 2015].

Bibliography

Abel-Smith, Brian, and Kathleen Gales. *British Doctors at Home and Abroad*. Published for the Social Administration Research Trust. Welwyn, Hertfordshire: Codicote Press, 1964.

Abraham, P.M. "Stopping The Brain Drain: No Easy Solution." *The Times of India*, 10 December 1968.

Acheson, C.B. "Public Interest Cited as Restrictive Covenant Fails Court Case in Ontario." *Canadian Medical Association Journal* 106, no. 8 (22 April 1972): 929–30.

ACMC. Position Paper: "Physician Manpower." ACMC *Forum* 11 (December 1978): 38.

Adams, Annmarie. *Medicine by Design: The Architect and the Modern Hospital, 1893–1943*. Minneapolis: University of Minnesota Press, 2008.

Aizenman, A.I. "The Oncoming Hordes: Physicians in Canada." *Canadian Medical Association Journal* 127, no. 12 (1982): 1177–9.

Alexander, Peter. "Foreign Trained MDs Threaten Hunger Strike." *Montreal Gazette*, 28 February 1989, A3.

Alkire, S., and L. Chen. "'Medical Exceptionalism' in International Migration: Should Doctors and Nurses Be Treated Differently?" Draft paper prepared for the workshop Global Migration Regimes, Stockholm, 2004. http://www.fas.harvard.edu/~acgei/Publications/Akire/ Migration%2010-25.pdf.

Amin, Galal. *Whatever Happened to the Egyptians? Changes in Egyptian Society from 1950 to the Present*. Cairo and New York: American University in Cairo Press, 2000.

Angus, Charlie, and Brit Griffin. *We Lived a Life and Then Some: The Life, Death, and Life of a Mining Town*. Toronto: Between the Lines, 1996.

Armstrong, J.G. "Correspondence: British National Health Service." *Canadian Medical Association Journal* 74 (1 April 1956): 582.

Armstrong, John. "The Common-Health and Beyond: New Zealand Trainee Specialists in International Medical Networks, 1945–1975." PhD diss., University of Waikato, 2013.

– "A System of Exclusion: New Zealand Women Medical Specialists in International Medical Networks, 1945–75." In *Doctors Beyond Borders: The Transnational Migration of Physicians in the Twentieth Century*, edited by Laurence
Monnais and David Wright, 118–41. Toronto: University of Toronto Press, 2016.

Arnold, Peter. *A Unique Migration: South African Doctors Fleeing to Australia.*
Edgecliff, NSW: Createspace, 2011.

Aronson, Lawrence Robert. *American National Security and Economic Relations
with Canada, 1945–1954*. Westport and London: Praeger, 1997.

Arrigo, Linda Gail. "Fifty years after '2-2-8': the Lingering Legacy of State Terror in
the Consolidation of Bourgeois Democracy in Taiwan." *Humboldt Journal of
Social Relations* 23, no. 1–2 (1997): 47–69, https://www.jstor.org/stable/23263489.

Audas, Rick, Amanda Ross, and David Vardy. "The Use of Provisionally Licensed
International Medical Graduates in Canada." *Canadian Medical Association
Journal* 173, no. 11 (2005): 1315–16, https://doi.org/10.1503/cmaj.050675.

Ayubi, Nazih. "The Egyptian 'Brain Drain': A Multidimensional Problem." *International Journal of Middle East Studies* 15 (November 1983): 432–4.

Badgley, Robin F., and Samuel Wolfe. *Doctors' Strike: Medical Care and Conflict
in Saskatchewan*. New York: Atherton Press, 1967.

Baer, L.D. *Doctors in a Strange Land: The Place of International Medical Graduates
in Rural America*. Lanham, MD: Lexington Books, 2002.

Bain, George. "Money for Hospitals: Deciding How Much to Whom." *The Globe
and Mail*, 3 February 1966.

Bannerjee, R.N. "Immigration of Doctors." *Indian Medical Journal* 59 (August
1965): 194.

Barer, Morris L., and Greg L. Stoddart. *Toward Integrated Medical Resource Policies
for Canada*. Vancouver: Health Policy Research Unit, Centre for Health Services
and Policy Research, University of British Columbia, 1991.

– "Toward Integrated Medical Resource Policies for Canada: 8. Geographic Distribution of Physicians." *Canadian Medical Association Journal* 147, no. 5 (1 September 1992): 617–23.

Barnett, J.R. "Foreign Medical Graduates in New Zealand 1973–79: A Test of the
'Exacerbation Hypothesis.'" *Social Science and Medicine* 26 (1988): 1049–60.

Barr, Murray L. *A Century of Medicine at Western: A Centennial History of the Faculty of Medicine, University of Western Ontario*. London, ON: University of Western Ontario, 1977.

Beaton, Marilyn, and Jeanette Walsh. *From the Voices of Nurses: An Oral History of
Newfoundland Nurses Who Graduated Prior to 1950*. St John's, NL: Jesperson, 2004.

Beck, Ivan T., and Matthew Thompson. "The Health Care Philosophy That Nearly Destroyed Medicare in Canada in a Single Decade." *Clinical and Investigative Medicine* 29, no. 2 (2006): 65–76.

Bégin, Monique. "Health Minister Bégin Comments on Proposed Canada Health Act." *Canadian Medical Association Journal* 128, no. 6 (15 March 1983): 731.

– *Medicare: Canada's Right to Health.* Montreal: Optimum Publishing International, 1988.

Benatar, S.R. "An Examination of Ethical Aspects of Migration and Recruitment of Health Care Professionals from Developing Countries." *Clinical Ethics* 2, no. 2 (2007), 2–7.

Berridge, Virginia. *Health and Medicine in Britain Since 1939.* Cambridge: Cambridge University Press, 1999.

Bhalla, Vibha. "'We Wanted to End Disparities at Work': Physician Migration, Racialization, and a Struggle for Equality." *Journal of American Ethnic History* 29, no. 3 (Spring 2010): 40–78.

Bolton, Jonathan. *Worlds of Dissent: Charter 77, the Plastic People of the Universe, and Czech Culture Under Communism.* Boston: Harvard University Press, 2012.

Bowden, Lord. "The Brain Drain Felt Around the World." *The Globe and Mail*, 16 March 1967.

Bowers, John Z., and Elizabeth F. Purcell, eds. *New Medical Schools at Home and Abroad: Report of a Macy Conference.* New York: Josiah Macy, Jr Foundation, 1978.

Bowles, R.T. *Little Communities and Big Industries: Studies in the Social Impact of Canadian Resource Extraction.* Toronto: Butterworth Press, 1982.

– "Single-Industry Resource Communities in Canada's North." In *Rural Sociology in Canada*, edited by D.A. Hay and G.S. Basran, 63–83. Toronto: Oxford University Press, 1992.

Bowman, Phylis. *Muskeg, Rocks and Rain: Prince Rupert.* Prince Rupert: n.p., 1973.

Boychuk, Gerard. *National Health Insurance in the United States and Canada: Race, Territory, and the Roots of Difference.* Washington: Georgetown University Press, 2008.

Brand, Joshua, and John Falsey. *Northern Exposure.* Six seasons, 110 episodes. Aired 1990–95 on CBS.

Bren, Paulina. *The Greengrocer and His TV: The Culture of Communism after the 1968 Prague Spring.* Ithaca, NY: Cornell University Press, 2010.

Brodie, Janine. *The Political Economy of Canadian Regionalism.* Toronto: Harcourt Brace Jovanovich Canada, 1990.

Brown, J. Lloyd. "Problems Arising Through Operation of the Saskatchewan Hospital Services Plan." *Canadian Medical Association Journal* 78, no. 10 (15 May, 1958): 749–51.

Brown, M.C. "Health Care Financing and the Canada Health Act." *Journal of Canadian Studies* 21, no. 2 (1986): 111–32.

Brown, Malcolm C., and R.G. Evans. "Does Canada Have Too Many Doctors: Two Views." *Canadian Public Policy* 11, no. 3 (Summer 1977): 365–72.

Brown, Melissa J. *Is Taiwan Chinese? The Impact of Culture, Power and Migration on Changing Identities.* Berkeley: University of California Press, 2004.

Brown, Theodore, Marcos Cueto, and Elizabeth Fee. "The World Health Organization and the Transition from 'International' to 'Global' Health." In *Medicine at the Border: Disease, Globalization and Security, 1850 to the Present*, edited by Alison Bashford, 76–94. London: Palgrave MacMillan, 2006.

Brownridge, Ronald. "MDs and Extra-billing: A Question of Rights." *The Globe and Mail*, 12 June 1986.

Brush, B.L. "'Exchangees' or Employees? The Exchange Visitor Program and Foreign Nurse Immigration to the United States, 1945–1990." *Nursing History Review* 1 (1993): 171–80.

Buchignani, Walter. "Manitoba MLA Wants Doctors on Hunger Strike to Work There." *The Montreal Gazette*, 9 April 1989.

Bundred, P.E., and C. Levitt. "Medical Migration: Who are the Real Losers?" *The Lancet* 356, no. 9225 (15 July 2000): 245–6.

Calliste, Agnes. "Women of Exceptional Merit: Immigration of Caribbean Nurses to Canada." *Canadian Journal of Women and the Law* 6 (1993): 85–102.

Campbell, Craig. "Medical Community, Family Say Farewell to Dr. Campbell." *Ancaster News* [Ancaster, ON], 16 April 2004.

Campbell, E.J. Moran. *Not Always on the Level.* London: British Medical Journal Press, 1988.

Canada, Research and Statistics Division, Department of National Health and Welfare. *Recommendations in Health Survey Report of Manitoba.* Ottawa: August 1952.

Canadian Institute for Health Information (CIHI). *Supply, Distribution and Migration of Canadian Physicians.* Ottawa: CIHI, 2007.

Canadian Medical Association. *Canadian Medical Directory.* Don Mills, ON: Seccombe House, 1956–76.

Canadian Society of Radiological Technicians. "Exhibit No. 64: Submission of the Canadian Society of Radiological Technicians." In *Hearings of the Royal Commission on Health Services 1961-1962*, vol. 14, *Hearings Held at Winnipeg, Manitoba*, 3575–3888. Handbound at the University of Toronto Press [1964].

Caton-Jones, Michael, dir. *Doc Hollywood*. Burbank, CA: Warner Bros, 1991.

Chamberlain, M.J. "Where Shall John Go? Canada." *British Medical Journal* 1, no. 6062 (12 March 1977): 693–6.

Chan, Benjamin T.B. *From Perceived Surplus to Perceived Shortage: What Happened to Canada's Physician Workforce in the 1990's?* Ottawa: Canadian Institute for Health Information, 2002.

Chapnick, Adam. "The Canadian Middle Power Myth." *International Journal* 55, no. 2 (2000): 188–206.

Chard, Jean Kryszek. *Reminiscences of Stanley H. Kryszek*. Xlibris, 2007.

Chatterji, Joya, Claire Alexander, and Annu Jalais. *The Bengal Diaspora: Rethinking Muslim Migration*. London: Routledge, 2015.

Chaudhuri, B. Ray. "Unemployment among Doctors." *Journal of the Indian Medical Association* 69, no. 3 (1 August 1977): 64–6.

Chiang, Lan-hung Nora. "Different Voices: Identity Formation of Early Taiwanese Migrants in Canada." In *Immigrant Adaptation in Multi-Ethnic Societies: Canada, Taiwan, and the United States*, edited by Eric Fong, Lan-Hung Nora Chiang, and Nancy Denton, 255–84. New York: Routledge, 2013.

Chilton, Lisa. *Receiving Canada's Immigrants: The Work of the State before 1930*. Ottawa: Canadian Historical Association, 2016.

Choy, Catherine. *Empire of Care: Nursing and Migration in Filipino American History*. Durham, NC: Duke University Press, 2003.

Clark-Jones, Melissa. *A Staple State: Canadian Industrial Resources in Cold War*. Toronto: University of Toronto Press, 1987.

Clemens, Michael Andrew. "Do Visas Kill? Health Effects of African Health Professional Emigration." Center for Global Development Working Paper No. 114; iHEA 2007 6th World Congress: Explorations in Health Economics Paper. March 2007. http://dx.doi.org/10.2139/ssrn.980332.

Clemens, Michael Andrew and G. Petterson, "New data on African Health Professionals Abroad." *Human Resources for Health* 6, no. 1 (2008): 1–11, https://doi.org/10.1186/1478-4491-6-1.

Coffin, Everett. "CMA President Responds to the Act." *Canadian Medical Association Journal* 130, no. 1 (1 January 1984): 1D.

College of Physicians and Surgeons of Ontario. *Report of the College of Physicians and Surgeons of Ontario*. Toronto: College of Physicians and Surgeons of Ontario, 26 April 1962.

– *Report of the College of Physicians and Surgeons of Ontario*. Toronto: College of Physicians and Surgeons of Ontario, 26 April 1963.

– *Report of the College of Physicians and Surgeons of Ontario.* Toronto: College of Physicians and Surgeons of Ontario, 26 April 1964.
– *Report of the College of Physicians and Surgeons of Ontario.* Toronto: College of Physicians and Surgeons of Ontario, July 1965.
– *Report of the College of Physicians and Surgeons of Ontario.* Toronto: College of Physicians and Surgeons of Ontario, January 1966.
Collishaw, N.E., and R. M. Grainger. "Enrolment in Canada's Medical Schools, 1970–71." *Canadian Medical Association Journal* 106, no. 2 (1972): 163–8.
– "Medical Student Enrolment in Canada, 1969–70: Report of Statistics." *Canadian Medical Association Journal* 104, no. 10 (1971): 916–22.
Committee on the International Migration of Talent (CIMT). *The International Migration of High-Level Manpower: Its Impact on the Development Process.* New York: Praeger Publishers, 1970.
Commonwealth Consultative Committee on South and South-east Asia. *The Colombo Plan for Co-Operative Economic Development in South and South-east Asia: Annual Report of the Consultative Committee.* [13th Annual Report of the Consultative Committee] London: HMSO, 1964.
Connelly, John. *Captive University: The Sovietization of East German, Czech, and Polish Higher Education, 1945–1956.* Chapel Hill: University of North Carolina Press, 2000.
Connor, J.T.H. *Doing Good: The Life of Toronto's General Hospital.* Toronto: University of Toronto Press, 2000.
– "'One Simply Doesn't Arbitrate Authorship of Thoughts': Socialized Medicine, Medical McCarthyism, and the Publishing of *Rural Health and Medical Care* (1948)." *Journal of the History of Medicine and Allied Sciences* 72, no. 3 (2017): 245–71.
– "Thinking the Unthinkable? Dr. Frederick D. Mott, Socialized Medicine, and Contemplating Canadian Medicare as a Yankee Invention." Paper presented at the Canadian Society for the History of Medicine Annual Conference, Calgary, AB, May 2016.
– "Twillingate," *Newfoundland Quarterly* 100, no. 1 (2007): 13–15, 30–4.
Conrad, Margaret. "Past Imaginings: Reflections on Nation, Region and Culture in Canada." Paper presented at the Canadian American Research Symposium [CARS], 2004. The Atlantic Canada Portal E-Print Repository, University of New Brunswick, http://atlanticportal.hil.unb.ca:8000/archive/00000041/01/past imaginings.pdf.
Coovadia, Hoosen, Rachel Jewkes, Peter Barron, David Sanders, and Diane McIntyre. "The Health and Health System of South Africa: Historical Roots of

Current Public Health Challenges." *The Lancet* 374, no. 9692 (5 September 2009): 817–34.

Copeman, W.J. "177 of 203 Doctors Stay in Underserviced Areas." *Ontario Medical Review* 40, no. 12 (December 1973): 774–6.

Copper, John F. *Taiwan: Nation-state or province?* 6th ed. Boulder, CO: Westview Press, 2013.

Corbet, Elise. *Frontiers of Medicine: A History of Medical Education and Research at the University of Alberta.* Edmonton: University of Alberta Press, 1990.

Corbett, David. "Immigration and Canadian Politics." *International Journal* 6, no. 3 (1951): 207–16.

Cormier, Jeffrey. *The Canadianization Movement: Emergence, Survival, and Success.* Toronto: University of Toronto Press, 2004.

Crawford, P. Ralph. *The Canadian Dental Association: A Century of Service, 1902–2002.* Ottawa: Canadian Dental Association, 2002.

Crellin, John K. *The Life of a Cottage Hospital: The Bonne Bay Experience.* St John's, NL: Flanker Press, 2007.

Crowther, M. Anne, and Marguerite W. Dupree. *Medical Lives in the Age of Surgical Revolution.* Cambridge: Cambridge University Press, 2007.

Culter, Tony. "Dangerous Yardstick? Early Cost Estimates and the Politics of Financial Management in the First Decade of the National Health Service." *Medical History* 47, no. 2 (2003): 217–38.

– "A Double Irony: The Politics of National Health Service Expenditure in the 1950s." In *Financing Medicine: The British Experience Since 1750* edited by Martin Gorsky and Sally Sheard, 200–20. London: Routledge, 2006.

Dalachanis, Angelos. *The Greek Exodus from Egypt: Diaspora Politics and Emigration, 1937–1962.* New York: Berghahn Books, 2017.

Daniell, Raymond. "4 Doctors Fly to Saskatchewan as Province Seeks Aid in Strike." *New York Times*, 3 July 1962, 10.

Davidson, R.H. "Medical Immigration to North America." *British Medical Journal* 1, no. 5280 (17 March 1962): 786–7.

Davis, Wade. *The Serpent and the Rainbow.* New York: Simon & Schuster, 1997.

Davison, Gary Marvin. *A Short History of Taiwan: The Case for Independence.* Westport, CT: Praeger, 2003.

De Barros, Juanita. "Imperial Connections and Caribbean Medicine, 1900–1938." In *Doctors Beyond Borders: The Transnational Migration of Physicians in the Twentieth Century,* edited by Laurence Monnais and David Wright, 20–41. Toronto: University of Toronto Press, 2016.

Department of Health, Great Britain. *Code of Practice for NHS Employers Involved in the International Recruitment of Healthcare Professionals*. London: Department of Health, 2001.

Department of National Health and Welfare. *Annual Report of the Minister of National Health and Welfare Respecting Operations Under the Health Resources Fund Act for the Fiscal Year Ended March 31, 1981*. Ottawa: Queen's Printer, 1981.

"Des immigrants à leur arrivée." Les Archives de Radio-Canada. Société Radio-Canada. Last updated 28 October 2009. http://archives.radio-canada.ca/societe/immigration/clips/17176/.

Desbarats, Peter. "Thompson's 'Nickel Curtain' Protects Planner's Dream." *Winnipeg Tribune*, 16 August 1958, 3.

Dessouki, Ali E. Hillal. "The Shift in Egypt's Migration Policy: 1952–1978." *Middle Eastern Studies* 18, no. 1 (1982): 55–68.

Dewar, L. George. *Life at Leighwood: the Doctor's Home*. Summerside, PEI: Williams and Crue, 1983.

Digby, Anne. "'The Bandwagon of Golden Opportunities'? Healthcare in South Africa's Bantustan Periphery." *South African Historical Journal* 64, no. 4 (2012): 827–51.

– "Black Doctors and Discrimination Under South Africa's Apartheid Regime." *Medical History* 57, no. 2 (2013): 269–90.

– *Diversity and Division in Medicine: Health Care in South Africa from the 1800s*. New York: Lang, 2006.

– "'A Medical El Dorado?': Colonial Medical Incomes and Practice at the Cape." *Social History of Medicine* 88 (1995): 463–79.

– "'Vision and Vested Interests': National Health Service Reform in South Africa and Britain during the 1940s and Beyond." *Social History Medicine* 21, no. 3 (2008): 485–502.

Dublin, Thomas D. "Migration of Physicians to the United States." *New England Journal of Medicine*, 286 (1972): 870–7.

Duffin, Jacalyn. *History of Medicine: A Scandalously Short Introduction*. Toronto: University of Toronto Press, 2010.

– "The Impact of Single-Payer Health Care on Physician Income in Canada, 1850–2005." *American Journal of Public Health* 101, no. 7 (2011): 1198–208.

– "The Guru and the Godfather: Henry Sigerist, Hugh MacLean, and the Politics of Health Care Reform in 1940s Canada." *Canadian Bulletin of Medical History* 9 (1992): 191–218.

– "The Quota: 'An Equally Serious Problem' for Us All," *Canadian Bulletin of Medical History* 19, no. 2 (2002): 327–49.

Duffin, Jacalyn, and Leslie A. Falk. "Sigerist in Saskatchewan: the Quest for Balance in Social and Technical Medicine." *Bulletin of the History of Medicine* 70, no. 4 (1996): 658–83.

Ďurčanský, Marek and Pieter Dhondt. "Two Great Anniversaries, Two Lost Opportunities: Charles University in Prague, 1848 and 1948." In *University Jubilees and University History Writing: A Challenging Relationship*, edited by Pieter Dhondt, 21–56. Leiden: Brill, 2014.

Evans, John R. "Future Manpower Needs in Teaching and Research." *Canadian Medical Association Journal* 97, no. 26 (1967): 1592–6.

Evans, R.G. "Does Canada Have Too Many Doctors? Why Nobody Loves an Immigrant Physician." *Canadian Public Policy* 2, no. 2 (1976): 147–60.

– "Health Services in Nova Scotia: The View From the Graham Report." *Canadian Public Policy* 1, no. 3 (Summer 1975): 355–66.

– *Price Formation in the Market for Physician Services*. Ottawa: Queen's Printer, 1973.

Evans, R.G., and Kimberlyn M. McGrail. "Richard III, Barer–Stoddart and the Daughter of Time." *Healthcare Policy* 3, no. 3 (2008): 18–28.

Faculty of Dentistry of the University of Manitoba. "Exhibit No. 59: Submission of the Faculty of Dentistry of the University of Manitoba." In *Hearings of the Royal Commission on Health Services, 1961–1962*. Vol. 14: Hearings Held at Winnipeg, Manitoba. 3450–3483. Handbound at the University of Toronto Press [1964].

Faculty of Medicine, University of Manitoba. "Exhibit No. 50: Submission of the Faculty of Medicine, University of Manitoba. In *Hearings of the Royal Commission on Health Services, 1961–1962*. Vol. 12: Hearings Held at Winnipeg, Manitoba. 3156–3174. Handbound at the University of Toronto Press [1964].

Feasby, W.R., ed. *Canadian Medical Directory, First Edition*. Toronto: Current Publications, Ltd., 1955.

Fedunkiw, Marianne. *Rockefeller Foundation Funding and Medical Education in Toronto, Montreal, and Halifax*. Montreal and Kingston: McGill-Queen's University Press, 2005.

Fein, Rashi. *The Doctor Shortage: An Economic Diagnosis*. Washington, DC: The Brookings Institution, 1967.

Feldstein, Paul J., and Irene Butter. "The Foreign Medical Graduate and Public Policy: A Discussion of the Issues and Options." *International Journal of Health Services* 8, no. 3 (1978): 541–58.

Ferguson, Donald C. "The Indian Medical Graduate in America, 1965: A Survey of Selected Characteristics." *Journal of the Indian Medical Association* 48 no. 6 (March 1967): 291–8.

Fine, Sean. "Child, 3, Waits Two Hours for Treatment." *The Globe and Mail*, 17 June 1986, A19.

Finkel, Alvin. "Why Canada has a Universal Medical Insurance Programme and the United States Does Not: Accounting for Historical Differences in American and Canadian Social Policies." In *Locating Health: Historical and Anthropological Investigations of Place and Health*, edited by Erika Dyck and Christopher Fletcher, 71–88. London: Pickering and Chatto, 2010.

Fish, D.G., C. Farmer, and R. Nelson-Jones. "Some Social Characteristics of Students in Canadian Medical Schools, 1965–66." *Canadian Medical Association Journal* 99, no. 19 (1966): 950–4.

Flexner, Abraham. *Medical Education in the United States and Canada: A Report to the Carnegie Foundation for the Advancement of Teaching*. Boston: Merrymount Press, 1960. First published 1910 by the Carnegie Foundation for the Advancement of Teaching.

Flynn, Karen. *Moving Beyond Borders: A History of Black Canadian and Caribbean Women in the Diaspora*. Toronto: University of Toronto Press, 2011.

– "Proletarianization, Professionalization, and Caribbean Immigrant Nurses." *Canadian Women's Studies* 18, no. 1 (1998): 57–60.

– "Race, the State, and Caribbean Immigrant Nurses, 1950–1962." In *Women, Health, and Nation: Canada and the United States Since 1945*, edited by Georgina Feldberg, Molly Ladd-Taylor, Alison Li, and Kathryn McPherson, 247–63. Montreal and Kingston: McGill-Queen's University Press, 2003.

Fowke, Vernon C. "The National Policy – Old and New." *Canadian Journal of Economics and Political Science/Revue canadienne de economiques et science politique* 18, no. 3 (1952): 271–86.

Fowler, Glenn. "C. Rufus Rorem, 93, Economist; His Ideas Led to Blue Cross Plan." *New York Times*, 21 September 1988.

Freeman, Richard. "A National Health Service, by Comparison." *Social History of Medicine* 21, no. 3 (2008): 503–20.

French, Orland. "Exodus of One in the Works." *The Globe and Mail*, 1 May 1986, A7.

Freudenburg, William R., and Scott Frickel. "Digging Deeper: Mining-Dependent Regions in Historical Perspective 1." *Rural Sociology* 59, no. 2 (1994): 266–88.

Friesen, Gerald. "The Evolving Meanings of Region in Canada." *Canadian Historical Review* 82, no. 3 (2001): 529–45.

Gamble, James L., Charles D. Cook, William C. Wigglesworth, and George E. LaCroix. "Comments on the Doctor Draft." Letters to the Editor. *New England Journal of Medicine* 248, no. 16 (1953): 705–6.

Gelfand, Toby. "Who Practiced Medicine in New France? A Collective Portrait."
In *Health, Disease, and Medicine: Essays in Canadian History*, edited by Charles
Roland, 16–35. Toronto: Clark Irwin/Hannah Institute for the History of Medi-
cine, 1984.

Gidney, R.D., and W.P.J. Millar. "Medical Students at the University of Toronto,
1910–40: A Profile." *Canadian Bulletin of Medical History* 13, no. 1 (1996): 29–52.

– *Professional Gentlemen: The Professions in Nineteenth-Century Ontario*. Toronto:
University of Toronto Press, 1984.

Girard, Philippe R. *Haiti: The Tumultuous History – From Pearl of the Caribbean
to Broken Nation*. London: Palgrave Macmillan, 2010.

Gish, Oscar. *Doctor Migration and World Health: The Impact of the International
Demand for Doctors on Health Services in Developing Countries.* London: G. Bell
& Sons, 1971.

– ed. *Health Manpower & the Medical Auxiliary*. London: Intermediate Technology
Development Group, 1971.

Goldschmidt, Arthur, Jr. *Modern Egypt: The Formation of a Nation-State*. London:
Hachette, 2004.

Goldsmith-Kasinsky, Renee. *Refugees from Militarism: Draft-age Americans in
Canada*. New Brunswick, NJ: Transaction Books, 1976.

Gorsky, Martin. "The British Health Service 1948–2008: A Review of the Historiography." *Social History of Medicine* 21 (2008): 437–60.

Grant, Hugh. "From the Transvaal to the Prairies: the Migration of South African
Physicians to Canada." *Journal of Ethnic and Migration Studies* 32, no. 4 (2006):
681–95.

Gray, Gwendolyn. *Federalism and Health Policy: The Development of Health Systems
in Canada and Australia*. Toronto: University of Toronto Press, 1991.

Green, Alan G. *Immigration and the Postwar Canadian Economy*. Toronto: Macmillan of Canada, 1976

Greenwood, Anna, and Harshad Topiwala. *Indian Doctors in Kenya, 1895–1940: The
Forgotten History*. Basingstoke: Palgrave Macmillan, 2015.

Grey, Julius H. "Does Section 7 of the Charter Protect the Right to be a Professional?" *Les Cahiers de Droit* 31, no. 3 (1990): 933–43.

Griffin, Eugene. "British Medics Irk Canada." *Chicago Daily Tribune*, 17 July 1962, 1.

Gullet, D.W. *A History of Dentistry in Canada*. Published for the Canadian Dental
Association. Toronto: University of Toronto Press, 1971.

Hacon, W.S. "Health Manpower Development in Canada." *Canadian Journal of
Public Health/Revue Canadienne de Sante Publique* 64, no. 1 (January/February
1973): 5–12.

– "Improving Canada's Health Manpower Resources." *Canadian Medical Association Journal* 97 (28 October 1967): 1104–8.

– Letter to the Editor. *Canadian Doctor* 33, no. 11 (November 1967): 25.

Hacon, W.S., and Jawed Aziz. "The Supply of Physicians in Canada." *Canadian Medical Association Journal* 112, no. 4 (1975): 514–20.

Hagan, John. *Northern Passage: American Vietnam War Resisters in Canada.* Cambridge, MA: Harvard University Press, 2001.

Hagopian, Amy, Matthew J. Thompson, Meredith Fordyce, Karin E. Johnson, and L. Gary Hart. "The Migration of Physicians From Sub-Saharan Africa to the United States of America: Measures of the African Brain Drain." *Human Resources for Health* 2, no. 17 (2004): n.p. [10pp].

Hall, Anthony. "Brain Drain and the Draft." *British Medical Journal* 1, no. 5542 (1967): 764.

Hall, Emmett M. *Canada's National-Provincial Health Program for the 1980s – A Commitment for Renewal.* Ottawa: National Health and Welfare, 1980.

Halseth, Greg and Lana Sullivan. "From Kitimat to Tumbler Ridge: A Crucial Lesson Not Learned in Resource-Town Planning." *Western Geography* (*Western Division, Canadian Association of Geographers*) 13–14 (2003/2004): 132–60.

Hampshire, J. *Citizenship and Belonging: Immigration and the Politics of Demographic Governance in Postwar Britain.* London: Palgrave Macmillan, 2005.

Hancock, Trevor. "A Need to Erase the Doctor's Empire." *The Toronto Star*, 21 April 1986.

Hannay, David. "Undergraduate Medical Education and General Practice." In *General Practice Under the National Health Service 1948–1997*, edited by Irvine Loudon, John Horder, and Charles Webster, 165–81. London: Clarendon Press, 1998.

Hansen, Randall. *Citizenship and Immigration in Postwar Britain: the Institutional Origins of a Multicultural Nation.* Oxford: Oxford University Press, 2000.

Hastings, J.E. "Toward a National Health Program: Canadian Experience." *Bulletin of the New York Academy of Medicine* 48, no. 1 (January 1972): 66–82.

Hastings, J.E., F.D. Mott, A. Barclay, and D. Hewitt. "Prepaid Group Practice in Sault Ste Marie, Ontario. Analysis of Utilization Records." *Medical Care* 11, no. 2 (1973): 91–103.

Hastings, Paula. "Territorial Spoils, Transnational Black Resistance, and Canada's Evolving Autonomy during the First World War." *Histoire sociale/Social History* 47, no. 94 (2014): 443–70.

Hawkins, Freda. *Canada and Immigration: Public Policy and Public Concern.* Montreal and Kingston: McGill-Queen's University Press, 1972.

– "Canadian Immigration Policy and Management." *The International Migration Review* 8, no. 2 (1974): 141–53.

Haynes, Douglas M. *Fit to Practice: Empire, Race, Gender, and the Making of British Medicine, 1850–1980*. Rochester: University of Rochester Press, 2017.

Heiber, S. and R. Deber. "Banning Extra-Billing in Canada: Just What the Doctor Didn't Order." *Canadian Public Policy* 13, no. 1 (March 1987): 62–74.

Heimann, Mary. *Czechoslovakia: The State That Failed*. New Haven, CT: Yale University Press, 2011.

Henderson, D.G. "Community Planning of the Townsite of Thompson." *The Canadian Mining and Metallurgical Bulletin* 57, no. 631 (November 1964): 1192–200.

Hennock, E.P. *The Origins of the Welfare State in England and Germany, 1850–1914: Social Policies Compared*. Cambridge: Cambridge University Press, 2007.

Hess, John. "A UN Report on Brain Drain: The Rich Get Richer and the Poor Get Poorer." *The Globe and Mail*, 11 April 1966, 9.

High, Steven. *Industrial Sunset: The Making of North America's Rust Belt, 1969–1974*. Toronto: University of Toronto Press, 2003.

"History of the Cumming School of Medicine." University of Calgary Cumming School of Medicine. https://web.archive.org/web/20150503090634/http://cumming.ucalgary.ca/about/history.

Hoerder, Dirk. *Cultures in Contact: World Migrations in the Second Millennium*. Durham, NC: Duke University Press, 2002.

Holland, Ray. "The Ontario Doctors' Strike." Letter to the editor, *Canadian Medical Association Journal* 135, no. 7 (October 1, 1986): 728.

Hollobon, Joan. "Freeze on Research Funds Blamed: Report Warns of Limit on Medical School Expansion." *The Globe and Mail*, 14 November 1968, 37.

Horn, Michiel. *York University: The Way Must Be Tried*. Montreal and Kingston: McGill-Queen's University Press, 2009.

Horwitz, Simonne. *Baragwanath Hospital, Soweto: A History of Medical Care, 1941–1990*. Johannesburgh: Wits University Press, 2013.

Houston, C. Stuart. *Steps on the Road to Medicare: Why Saskatchewan Led the Way*. Montreal and Kingston: McGill-Queen's University Press, 2003.

Houston, C. Stuart, and Merle Massie. *36 Steps on the Road to Medicare: How Saskatchewan Led the Way*. Montreal and Kingston: McGill-Queen's University Press, 2013.

Houston, Cecil J., and William J. Smyth. *Irish Emigration and Canadian Settlement: Patterns, Links and Letters*. Toronto: University of Toronto Press, 1990.

Howell, Jack, John Dickinson, and John Hamilton. "Edward James Moran Campbell." *British Medical Journal* 329, no. 7474 (November 2004): 1105.

Hsu, H. B 許宏彬. *Nianqing Yishi de banghuang yu jueze: Cong "Qing xing" kan
   1950–1960 niandai Taiwan yixue jiaoyu, yishi chulu ji wailiu wenti* 年輕醫師的徬徨
   與抉擇：從《青杏》看 1950 1960 年代臺灣醫學教育、醫師出路及外流問題. [Con-
   fusion and Dilemma: An observation of the Education, Career Path, and Exodus of Medical Graduates in 1950 and '60s Taiwan], *Xing da lishi xuebao*
   (December 2013): 11.

Huish, Robert. "How Cuba's Latin American School of Medicine Challenges the
   Ethics of Physician Migration." *Social Science & Medicine* 69, no. 3 (2009): 301–4.

Huish, Robert and John Kirk. "Cuban Medical Internationalism and the Development of the Latin American School of Medicine." *Latin American Perspectives*
   34, no. 6 (2007): 77–92.

Hurley, Jeremiah. "Simulated Effects of Income-based Policies on the Distribution
   of Physicians." *Medical Care* 28, no. 3 (1990): 221–38.

Innes, Abby. *Czechoslovakia: The Short Goodbye*. New Haven: Yale University Press,
   2001.

Innis, Harold. "The Canadian Mining Industry." In *Essays in Canadian Economic
   History*, edited by Mary Q. Innis, 309–20. Toronto: University of Toronto Press,
   1956.

Institute of Applied Manpower Research. *The Brain Drain Study, Prepared for the
   Inter Ministerial Group on the Brain Drain*. New Delhi: Institute of Applied
   Manpower Research, 1970.

– *Indian Physicians in the United States, A Stock Study*. New Delhi: Institute of
   Applied Manpower Research, 1969.

– *Indian Scientists in the United States, A Stock Study*. Report No. 1. New Delhi:
   Institute of Applied Manpower Research, 1969.

– *Manpower 1968*. New Delhi: Institute of Applied Manpower Research, 1968.

Itano, Nicole. "Condition Critical as African Doctors Head Overseas." *Christian
   Science Monitor*, 1 October 2002. https://web.archive.org/web/20150925033315/
   https://www.csmonitor.com/2002/1001/p07s02-woaf.html. [Archived 25
   September 2015].

Jackman, Martha. "The Implications of Section 7 of the Charter for Health Care
   Spending in Canada." Commission on the Future of Health Care in Canada,
   Discussion Paper No. 31 Saskatoon, SK: Privy Council, 2002. http://publications
   .gc.ca/pub?id=9.558259&sl=0.

James, George, and Bernard R. Blishen. "Review of Royal Commission on Health Services." *Milbank Memorial Fund Quarterly* 44, no. 1 (1966): 92–117.

Jean, Dominique. "Family Allowances and Family Autonomy: Quebec Families Encounter the Welfare State, 1945–1955." In *Canadian Family History: Selected Readings*, edited by Bettina Bradbury, 401–37. Toronto: Irwin, 2000.

Johnson, A.W. (With the assistance of Rosemary Proctor.) *Dream No Little Dreams: A Biography of the Douglas Government of Saskatchewan, 1944–1961.* Toronto: University of Toronto Press, 2004.

Johnson, William Victor. "Health Insurance from the Viewpoint of the General Practitioner." *Canadian Medical Association Journal* 51, no. 1 (July 1944): 68–70.

Jones, E.L., and S.J. Snow. *Against the Odds: Black and Minority Ethnic Clinicians and Manchester, 1948 to 2009.* Manchester: Manchester NHS Primacy Care Trust, 2010.

Jones, Esyllt. "Health and Nation Through a Transnational Lens: Radical Doctors and the History of Medicare in Saskatchewan." In *Within and Without the Nation: Canadian History as Transnational History*, edited by Karen Dubinsky, Adele Perry, and Henry Yu, 293–310. Toronto: University of Toronto Press, 2015.

– *Radical Medicine: the International Origins of Socialized Health Care in Canada.* Manitoba: ARP Books, 2019.

Jones, Greta. "A Mysterious Discrimination: Irish Medical Emigration to the United States in the 1950s." *Social History of Medicine* 25, no. 1 (2011): 139–56.

– "'Strike Out Boldly for the Prizes That Are Available to You': Medical Emigration from Ireland 1860–1905." *Medical History* 54, no. 1 (2010): 55–74.

Judek, Stanislaw. *Medical Manpower in Canada.* Ottawa: Queen's Printer/Royal Commission on Health Services, 1964.

Kealey, Linda. "Delivering Health Care in Rural New Brunswick: Outpost Nursing in the 20th Century." In *Medicine in the Remote and Rural North, 1800–2000*, edited by J.T.H. Connor and Stephan Curtis, 183–98. London: Chatto and Pickering Press, 2011.

Kealey, Linda, and Heather Molyneaux. "On the Road to Medicare: Newfoundland in the 1960s." *Journal of Canadian Studies* 41, no. 3 (2007): 90–111.

Kelley, Ninette, and Michael J. Trebilcock. *The Making of the Mosaic: A History of Canadian Immigration Policy.* Toronto: University of Toronto Press, 1998.

Kelly, A.D. "Medical Economics: The Swift Current Experiment." *Canadian Medical Association Journal* 58, no. 5 (May 1948): 506–11.

– "Medical Practice in Canada." *Supplement to The British Medical Journal* 1, no. 5012 (26 January 1957): 35–7.

- "Swift Current, Twelve Years Later." *Canadian Medical Association Journal* 83, no. 15 (8 October 1960): 812–13.

Kenney, James L. and Andrew Secord. "Public Power for Industry: A Re-examination of the New Brunswick Case, 1940–1960." *Acadiensis* 30, no. 2 (Winter/Spring, 2001): 84–108.

Kent, Tom. *A Public Purpose: An Experience of Liberal Opposition and Canadian Government.* Montreal and Kingston: McGill-Queen's University Press, 1988.

Khot, Sandeep, Buhm Soon Park, and W.T. Longstreth Jr. "The Vietnam War and Medical Research: Untold Legacy of the US Doctor Draft and the NIH 'Yellow Berets.'" *Academic Medicine* 86, no. 4 (2011): 502–8.

Kindig, David A., and Charles M. Taylor. "Growth in the International Physician Supply, 1950 through 1979." *Journal of the American Medical Association* 253, no. 21 (7 June 1985): 3129–32.

Kirk, John, and Michael Erisman. *Cuban Medical Internationalism: Origins, Evolution, and Goals.* London: Palgrave MacMillan, 2009.

Knowles, Valerie. *Strangers at Our Gates: Canadian Immigration and Immigration Policy, 1540–2006.* Toronto: Dundurn Press, 1992.

Korcok, Milan. "Group Medicine a Growing Force Worldwide." *Canadian Medical Association Journal* 133, no. 2 (1985): 134–7.

- "Restriction of Physician Immigration seen as Method of Curtailing Health Costs." *Canadian Medical Association Journal* 112, no. 4 (1975): 509–13.

- "The Sault Experience: After Ten Years a Pioneer Health Centre Feels the Pinch." *Canadian Medical Association Journal* 107, no. 9 (1972): 897–902.

Kramer, Gudrun. *The Jews in Modern Egypt 1914–1952.* Seattle: University of Washington Press, 1989.

Kravitz, Richard L., and Martin F. Shapiro. "Duration and Intensity of Striking among Participants in the Ontario, Canada Doctors' Strike." *Medical Care* 30, no. 8 (1992): 737–43.

Kravitz, Richard L., Martin F. Shapiro, Lawrence S. Linn, and Erika S. Sivarajan Froelicher. "Risk Factors Associated with Participation in the Ontario, Canada Doctors' Strike." *American Journal of Public Health* 79, no. 9 (1989): 1227–33.

Kusch, Frank. *All American Boys: Draft Dodgers in Canada from the Vietnam War.* Westport, CT: Praeger, 2001.

Lam, Vincent. *Extraordinary Canadians: Tommy Douglas.* Toronto: Penguin, 2011.

Lamarche, G., and G. Hébert. "Enrolment in Canadian Medical Schools, 1974–75." *Canadian Medical Association Journal* 112, no. 6 (1975): 734–7.

Lampard, Robert. *Alberta's Medical History: "Young and Lusty, and Full of Life."* Red Deer County, AB: Robert Lampard, 2008.

— *Deans, Dreams and a President: The Deans of Medicine at the University of Alberta's Faculty of Medicine & Dentistry 1913–2009 at the UofA.* Red Deer County, AB: Robert Lampard, 2011.

Langley, G. Ross, and Joanne M. Langley. "A Tense and Courageous Performance: The Role of the Honourable Allan J. MacEachen in the Creation, Passage and Implementation of Legislation for Medicare (Medical Care Act 1966, Bill C-227)." *Journal of the Royal Nova Scotia Historical Society* 18 (2015): 1–29.

Large, R.G. *Prince Rupert: Gateway to Alaska and the Pacific.* Prince Rupert, BC: Mitchell Press, Ltd., 1960.

Laskier, Michael M. *The Jews of Egypt, 1920–1970: In the Midst of Zionism, Anti-Semitism, and the Middle East Conflict.* New York: New York University Press, 1992.

Lawson, Gordon, and Andrew Noseworthy. "Newfoundland's Cottage Hospital System, 1920–1970." In *Making Medicare: New Perspectives on the History of Medicare in Canada,* edited by Gregory P. Marchildon, 229–48. Toronto: University of Toronto Press, 2012.

Leah, Vince. "A Most Extraordinary Mining Town." *Winnipeg Tribune,* 4 September 1965.

Lepnurm, Rein, and Mark Trowell. "Satisfaction of Country Doctors." *Healthcare Management Forum* 2, no. 3 (1989): 14–20.

Lewis, David. *Bangladesh: Politics, Economics, and Civil Society.* Cambridge: Cambridge University Press, 2011.

Lomas, Jonathan. *First and Foremost in Community Health Centres: the Centre in Sault Ste Marie and the CHC Alternative.* Toronto: University of Toronto Press, 1985.

Louttit, Neil. "Thompson: Mining Town that Faces Boom Time." *Winnipeg Tribune,* 3 May 1967.

Lowry, Fran. "Quebec's Hunger-Striking MDs: Do FMGs Automatically Have a Right to Practice?" *Canadian Medical Association Journal* 140, no. 11 (1989): 1341–5.

Lucas, R.A. *Minetown, Milltown, Railtown: Life in Canadian Communities of Single Industry.* Toronto: University of Toronto Press, 1971.

Lyon, E.K. "Aspects of Group Medical Practice: Basic Considerations in the Formation of a Group Practice." *Canadian Medical Association Journal* 98, no. 17 (1968): 799–803.

MacFarlane, George. "Brain Gain From Immigrants Called a Mixed Blessing." *The Globe and Mail*, 9 March 1967, 29.

MacKay, D.I. *Geographical Mobility and the Brain Drain: A Case Study of Aberdeen University Graduates, 1860–1960*. London: George Allen and Unwin Ltd, 1969.

MacLeod, Malcolm. "Crossroads Campus: Faculty Development at Memorial University of Newfoundland, 1950–1972." In *Historical Identities: The Professoriate in Canada*, edited by Euthalia Lisa Panayotidis and Paul James Stortz, 131–57. Toronto: University of Toronto Press, 2006.

MacMillan, J.A. "The Impact of Hospital Insurance on Medical Prepayment Plans." *Canadian Medical Association Journal* 78, no. 10 (1958): 766–7.

MacMillan, J.B. "Letter to the Editor." *Canadian Medical Association Journal* 84, no. 4 (1961): 800.

Madison, Donald L. "Notes on the History of Group Practice; the Tradition of the Dispensary." *Medical Group Management Journal* 37, no. 5 (1990): 52–4, 56–60, 86–93.

Madison, Donald L. "Preserving Individualism in the Organizational Society: 'Cooperation' and American Medical Practice, 1900–1920." *Bulletin of the History of Medicine* 70, no. 3 (1996): 442–83.

Madokoro, Laura. *Elusive Refuge: Chinese Migrants During the Cold War*. Cambridge, MA: Harvard University Press, 2016.

– "Good Material: Canada and the Prague Spring Refugees." *Refuge: Canada's Journal on Refugees* 26, no. 1 (2010): 161–71.

Maioni, Antonia. *Health Care in Canada*. Toronto: Oxford University Press, 2015.

– *Parting at the Crossroads: The Emergence of Health Insurance in the United States and Canada*. Princeton, NJ: Princeton University Press, 1998.

Mair, Alex, and Gordon H.M. Hatcher. "The Pattern of Health Organization in Canada." *The British Medical Journal* 2, no. 5044 (1957): 539–44.

Manfredi, Christopher, and Antonia Maioni. "Courts and Health Policy: Judicial Policy Making and Publicly Funded Health Care in Canada." *Journal of Health Politics, Policy and Law* 27, no. 2 (2002): 213–40.

Manga, Pran. "Arbitration and the Medical Profession: A Comment on the Hall Report." *Canadian Public Policy* 6, no. 4 (1980): 670–7.

Manitoba Association of Registered Nurses. "Exhibit No. 65: Submission of the Manitoba Association of Registered Nurses." In *Hearings of the Royal Commission on Health Services, 1961–1962*. Vol. 14: Hearings Held at Winnipeg, Manitoba. 3589-3614. Handbound at the University of Toronto Press [1964].

Manitoba Health Survey Committee. *An Abridgement of the Manitoba Health Sur-vey Report Made by the Manitoba Advisory Health Survey Committee to the Gov-ernment of Manitoba (under the terms of the Federal Health Survey Grant).* Winnipeg: CE Leech Queen's Printer for the Province of Manitoba, 1953.

Manitoba Hospital Survey Board. *Manitoba Hospital Survey Board Report: Hospital Personnel.* Vol. 2. [Manitoba: Queen's Printer], 1961. [Handbound at the Univer-sity of Toronto Press, 1965].

Manitoba Medical Association. "Exhibit No. 55: Submission of the Manitoba Medi-cal Association." In *Hearings of the Royal Commission on Health Services.* Vol. 13: Hearings Held at Winnipeg, Manitoba. 3270-3381. Handbound at the University of Toronto Press [1964].

Manning, Morris. "Canada Health Act: Unpalatable Carrot, Unconstitutional Stick." *Canadian Medical Association Journal* 134, no. 10 (15 May 1986): 1166–7.

Marble, Allan. *Surgeons, Smallpox, and the Poor: A History of Medicine and Social Conditions in Nova Scotia, 1749–1799.* Montreal and Kingston: McGill-Queen's University Press, 1993.

Marchildon, Gregory P., ed. *Making Medicare: New Perspectives on the History of Medicare in Canada.* Toronto: University of Toronto Press, 2012.

– "The Three Dimensions of Universal Medicare in Canada." *Canadian Public Administration* 57, no. 3 (2014): 362–82.

Marchildon, Gregory P., and Nicole O'Byrne. "From Bennett Care to Medicare: The Morphing of Medical Care Insurance in British Columbia." In *Making Medicare: New Perspectives on the History of Medicare in Canada*, edited by Gregory P. Marchildon, 207–28. Toronto: University of Toronto Press, 2012.

– "Last Province Aboard: New Brunswick and National Medicare." *Acadiensis: Journal of the History of the Atlantic Region* 42, no. 1 (Winter/Spring, 2013): 150–67.

Marchildon, Gregory P., and K. Schrijvers. "Physician Resistance and the Forging of Public Healthcare: A Comparative Analysis of the Doctors' Strikes in Canada and Belgium in the 1960s." *Medical History* 55, no. 2 (2011): 203–22.

Marcus, Abraham. "Think Before Moving, British Doctors Told." *The Globe and Mail*, 4 June 1962, 11.

Margulies, H., and L.S. Bloch. *Foreign Medical Graduates in the United States.* Cambridge: Harvard University Press, 1969.

Marks, Shula. *Divided Sisterhood: Race, Class and Gender in the South African Nursing Profession.* New York: St Martin's Press, 1994.

Marks, Shula, and Neil Andersson. "Diseases of Apartheid." In *South Africa in Question*, edited by John Lonsdale, 172–99. Cambridge: University of Cambridge African Studies Centre, 1988.

Martin, Paul. "An Address to the British and Canadian Medical Associations." *Canadian Medical Association Journal* 73, no. 2 (July 1955): 139–43.

McAlister, C., and P. Twohig. "The Check Off a Precursor to Medicare in Canada?" *Canadian Medical Association Journal* 173, no. 12 (December 2005): 1504–6.

McKellar, Don, dir. *The Grand Seduction*. Toronto: Entertainment One (distributor), 2013.

McKenzie, Robert. "Canada Found Stopover Point for Brain Drain from Europe." *The Toronto Star*, 19 January 1968, B21.

McLaren, Christie. "OMA Rejects Compromise." *The Globe and Mail*, 28 April 1986, A1.

McPhedran, N. Tait. *Canadian Medical Schools: Two Centuries of Medical History, 1822 to 1992*. Montreal: Harvest House, 1993.

McPherson, T.A. "The Canada Health Act 'Illegal'?" *Canadian Medical Association Journal* 133, no. 1 (1985): 78.1.

Medical Society of Prince Edward Island. "Exhibit No. 28: Submission of the Medical Society of Prince Edward Island." In *Hearings of the Royal Commission on Health Services, 1961–1962*. Vol. 8: Hearings Held at Charlottetown, PEI. 1737–1928. Handbound at the University of Toronto Press [1964].

Medical Society of Prince Edward Island and Canadian Medical Association Prince Edward Island Division. *The Submission of the Medical Society of Prince Edward Island and CMA PEI Division to the Royal Commission on Health Services*. Charlottetown: 14 October 1961.

Mejía, Alfonso. "Health Manpower Migration in the Americas." *Health Policy and Education* 2, no. 1 (1981): 1–31.

– "Migration of Physicians and Nurses: A Wide World Picture." *International Journal of Epidemiology* 7, no. 3 (1978): 207–15.

Mejía, Alfonso, Helena Pizurki, and Erica Royston. *Physician and Nurse Migration: Analysis and Policy Implications – Report of a WHO Study*. Geneva: World Health Organization, 1979. .

– *World Health Organization Multinational Study of the International Migration of Physicians and Nurses*. Geneva: World Health Organization, 1981.

Mercer, Walter. "Edinburgh and Canadian Medicine." *Canadian Medical Association Journal* 84, no. 23 (10 June 1961): 1313–17.

Merry, Robert. "Doctors Sign in Britain to Aid Canadians." *Chicago Daily Tribune*, 7 July 1962.

– "More British Medics Fly to Help Canada." *Chicago Daily Tribune*, 10 July 1962, A4.

Meslin, Eric M. "The Moral Costs of the Ontario Physicians' Strike." *The Hastings Center Report* 17, no. 4 (August–September 1987): 11–14.

Micay, Jack. "The Strike That Backfired." *The Globe and Mail*, 12 June 1989, A7.

Millar, W.P.J. "'We Wanted Our Children Should Have it Better': Jewish Medical Students at the University of Toronto, 1910–51." *Journal of the Canadian Historical Association* 11, no. 1 (2000): 109–24.

Miller, Leonard. "Public Health and Medical Care in Newfoundland." *Canadian Medical Association Journal* 64, no. 1 (1951): 52–5.

Mills, Sean. *A Place in the Sun: Haiti, Haitians, and the Remaking of Quebec*. Montreal and Kingston: McGill-Queen's University Press, 2016.

Ministry of Health [Great Britain] and Department of Health for Scotland. *Report of the Committee to Consider the Future Numbers of Medical Practitioners and the Appropriate Intake of Medical Students*. London: HMSO, 1957.

Minn, Pierre. "Where They Need Me: The Moral Economy of International Medical Aid in Haiti." PhD diss., McGill University, 2011.

Mitchinson, Wendy. *Giving Birth in Canada, 1900–1950*. Toronto: University of Toronto, 2002.

Mody, Fallon. "'The Intellectual Boys are the Ones in a Mess': The Unregistered Doctors Association in Victoria, 1951–56." *Health & History* 17, no. 1 (2015): 17–36.

– "Migrant Medical Women: A Case Study of British Medical Graduates in Twentieth-Century Australia." *Women's History Review* (September 2018): 1–23. https://doi.org/10.1080/09612025.2018.1513828.

– "Revisiting Post-war British Medical Immigration: A Case Study of Bristol Medical Graduates in Australia." *Social History of Medicine* 31, no. 3 (2018): 485–509.

Montgomery, Charlotte. "Doctors' Strike – Day 10." *The Globe and Mail*, 22 June 1986, A16.

Monnais, Laurence, and David Wright. *Doctors Beyond Borders: The Transnational Migration of Physicians in the Twentieth Century*. Toronto: University of Toronto Press, 2016.

Mooney, Magarita. *Faith Makes Us Live: Surviving and Thriving in the Haitian Diaspora*. Berkeley: University of California Press, 2009.

Morgan, H.V. "The Impact of Hospital Insurance on Medical Practice in Alberta." *Canadian Medical Association Journal* 78, no. 10 (15 May 1958): 747–8.

Mott, Frederick. "A Pattern of Local Services in the Saskatchewan Health Program." *American Journal of Public Health and the Nations Health* 39, no. 2 (February 1949): 216–20.

Mukharji, Projit. *Doctoring Traditions: Ayurveda, Small Technologies, and Braided Sciences.* Chicago: University of Chicago Press, 2016.

Mullally, Sasha. "Policing Practitioners on the Periphery: Elite Physicians and Profession-Building in a Bicultural Province, 1920–1939." In *Medicine in the Remote and Rural North, 1600–2000*, edited by Jim Connor and Stephan Curtis, 153–68. London: Chatto and Pickering Press, 2011.

Mullally, Sasha, and David Wright. "Connecting to Canada: Experiences of the South Asian Medical Diaspora during the 1960s and 1970s." In *Doctors Beyond Borders: The Transnational Migration of Physicians in the Twentieth Century*, edited by Laurence Monnais and David Wright, 230–56. Toronto: University of Toronto Press, 2016.

– "La Grande Séduction? The Immigration of Foreign-Trained Physicians to Canada c. 1954–76." *Journal of Canadian Studies* 41, no. 3 (2007), 67–89.

Mullally, Sasha, and Katherine MacDonald. "Call the Doctor? Health Service Trends in New Brunswick, Part I, 1918–1950." *Journal of New Brunswick Studies* 8 (Fall 2017): 41–68.

Mullan, F. "Doctors and Soccer Players – African Professionals on the Move." *New England Journal of Medicine* 356, no. 5 (2007): 440–3.

– "The Metrics of the Physician Brain Drain." *New England Journal of Medicine* 353, no. 17 (2005): 1810–18.

Mustard, J.F. "The Choice – Excellence or Mediocrity in Health Care." In *The Empire Club of Canada Addresses*, 43–53. Toronto, 27 October 1966. http://speeches.empireclub.org/60255/data.

Myers, Reginald. "Doctor-Draft Law." *New England Journal of Medicine* 247, no. 19 (1952): 743.

Nayar, D.P. "Undergraduate Medical Education in India." *British Journal of Medical Education* 5, no. 3 (1971): 172–80.

Naylor, C. David, ed. *Canadian Health Care and the State: A Century of Evolution.* Montreal and Kingston: McGill-Queen's University Press, 1992.

– *Private Practice, Public Payment: Canadian Medicine and the Politics of Health Insurance, 1911–1966.* Montreal and Kingston: McGill-Queen's University Press, 1986.

Neary, Peter F. *Newfoundland in the North Atlantic World, 1929-1949.* Montreal and Kingston: McGill-Queen's University Press, 1996.

Nelson-Jones, Richard and David G. Fish. "Canadian and Landed Immigrant Applicants to Canadian Medical Schools for 1968-69." *Canadian Medical Association Journal* 102, no. 2 (1970): 186–91.

– "Medical Student Enrolment in Canada: Report Of Statistics, 1968–69." *Canadian Medical Association Journal* 100, no. 14 (1969): 646–52.

– "Projections of Graduates From Canadian Medical Schools, 1970–81." *Canadian Medical Association Journal* 102, no. 8 (1970): 850–3.

Newell, R.L. and G.A. Mahon. "Medical Group Income Distribution Accounting." *Canadian Medical Association Journal* 80, no. 3 (1959): 224–5.

Noble, Vanessa. *A School of Struggle: Durban's Medical School and the Education of Black Doctors in South Africa*. Scottsville: University of KwaZulu-natal Press, 2013.

Noether, M. "The Growing Supply of Physicians: Has the Market Become More Competitive?" *Journal of Labour Economics* 4, no. 4 (1986): 503-37.

Numbers, Ronald L. *Almost Persuaded: American Physicians and Compulsory Health Insurance, 1912–1920*. Baltimore: Johns Hopkins University Press, 1978.

Ontario Medical Association. "Exhibit No. 238: Submission of the Ontario Medical Association." In *Hearings of the Royal Commission on Health Services 1961–1962*. Vol. 47: Hearings Held at Toronto Ont. 8828–9. Handbound at the University of Toronto Press [1964].

– *The Submission of the Ontario Medical Association (Appendices) to the Royal Commission on Health Services*. Toronto: May 1962.

Ontario Public Health Association, "Exhibit No. 344: Submission of the Ontario Public Health Association." In *Hearings of the Royal Commission on Health Services 1961–1962*. Vol. 63: Hearings Held at Toronto Ont. 11875–908 Handbound at the University of Toronto Press [1964].

Ostry, Aleck. *Change and Continuity in Canada's Health Care System*. Ottawa: CHA Press, 2006.

Palmer, Howard. "Anglo-Canadian Views of Multiculturalism." In *Immigration in Canada: Historical Perspectives*, edited by Gerald Tulchinsky, 297–333. Mississauga, ON: Copp Clark, 1994.

Panayotidis, Euthalia Lisa and Paul James Stortz, eds. *Historical Identities: The Professoriate in Canada*. Toronto: University of Toronto Press, 2006.

Paul, Kathleen. *Whitewashing Britain: Race and Citizenship in the Postwar Era*. Ithaca, NY: Cornell University Press, 1997.

Paulick, Janice M. and Noralou P. Roos. "The Young Physician: Types of Practice." *Canadian Medical Association Journal* 118, no. 3 (1978): 276–8.

Pegram, Scooter. *Choosing Their Own Style: Identity Emergence Among Haitian Youth in Quebec*. Peter Lang, 2005.

Penfield, Wilder. "Health Insurance and Medical Education." *Canadian Medical Association Journal* 47, no. 6 (December 1942): 523–8.

Peterson, David. "Doctors' Strike Day 10: Excerpts from Final Debate on Extra-Billing Ban." *The Globe and Mail*, 21 June 1986, A16.

Philipp, Thomas. "Copts and Other Minorities in the Development of the Egyptian Nation-State." In *Egypt from Monarchy To Republic: A Reassessment of Revolution and Change*, edited by Shimon Shamir, 131–50. Boulder: Westview Press, 1995.

Polyné, Millery. *From Douglass to Duvalier: U.S. African Americans, Haiti, and Pan Americanism, 1870–1964*. Gainesville: University Press of Florida, 2010.

Pouliot, Jean-Francois, dir. *La Grande Séduction*. Distributed by Alliance Atlantis, Toronto. 2003.

President's Materials Policy Commission. *The Outlook for Key Commodities*. Vol. 2 of *Resources for Freedom; A Report to the President* [Paley Report]. Washington, DC: US Government Printing Office, 1952.

Qadeer, Mohammad. *Pakistan – Social and Cultural Transformations in a Muslim Nation*. London: Routledge, 2006.

Quiñonez, Carlos. "Why Was Dental Care Excluded From Canadian Medicare?" *Network for Canadian Oral Health Research Working Papers Series* 1, no. 1 (2013): 1–5.

Raghavan, Srinath. *1971: A Global History of the Creation of Bangladesh*. Cambridge, MA: Harvard University Press, 2013.

Randall, James E., and R. Geoff Ironside. "Communities on the Edge: An Economic Geography of Resource-Dependent Communities in Canada." *Canadian Geographer/Le Géographe canadien* 40, no. 1 (1996): 17–35.

Raska, Jan. "Freedom Voices: Czech and Slovak Immigration to Canada during the Cold War." PhD diss., University of Waterloo, 2013.

– "Welcoming the Sick and Afflicted: Canada's Tubercular Admissions Program, 1959–1960." *Social History/Histoire Sociale* (May 2019): 171–92.

Richards, John and Larry Pratt. *Prairie Capitalism: Power and Influence in the New West*. Toronto: McClelland and Stewart, 1979.

Richmond, Anthony, and G. Lakshmana Rao. "Recent Developments in Immigration to Canada and Australia: A Comparative Analysis." *International Journal of Comparative Sociology* 17, no. 3-4 (1976): 183–205.

Robson, Robert. "Manitoba's Resource Towns." *Manitoba History* 16 (1988). https://web.archive.org/web/20180502170157/http://www.mhs.mb.ca/docs/mb_history/16/resourcetowns.shtml.

Rockett, Ian R.H., and S.L. Putnam. "Physician-Nurse Migration to the United

States: Regional and Health Status Origins in Relation to Legislation and Policy." *International Migration* 27, no. 3 (1989): 389–409.

Roemer, Ruth, and Milton Roemer. *Health Manpower Policy Under National Health Insurance: the Canadian Experience*. Hyattsville, MD: US Dept. of Health, Education, and Welfare, Public Health Service, Health Resources Administration, Bureau of Health Manpower, Division of Medicine, 1977.

Roland, Charles G. "Ontario Medical Periodicals as Mirrors of Change." *Ontario History* 72 (March 1980): 3–16.

Roman, Howaida. "Emigration Policy in Egypt." CARIM Euro-Mediterranean Consortium for Applied Research on International Migration. European University Institute Robert Schuman Centre for Advanced Studies, 2006. https://web.archive.org/web/20190507030447/http://migrationpolicycentre.eu/docs/Emigration-Policy-in-Egypt.pdf.

Romano, Terrie. "Professional Identity and the Nineteenth-Century Ontario Medical Profession." *Social History/Histoire Sociale* 28 (1995): 77–98.

Rompkey, Ronald. *Grenfell of Labrador: A Biography*. Montreal and Kingston: McGill-Queen's University Press, 2009.

Roos, Noralou P., Michel Gaumont, and John M. Horne. "The Impact of the Physician Surplus – the Distribution of Physicians across Canada." *Canadian Public Policy* 2, no. 2 (Spring, 1976): 169–91.

Rorem, C. Rufus. "Economics of Private Group Practice." *Canadian Medical Association Journal* 70, no. 4 (1954): 462–6.

Rousselot, Louis M. "Doctor Draft." *Archives of Surgery* 102, no. 1 (1971): 87–8.

Roussillon, Alain. "Republican Egypt Interpreted: Revolution and Beyond." In *Modern Egypt, from 1517 to the End of the Twentieth Century*, edited by M.W. Daly, 334–93. Vol. 2 of *The Cambridge History of Egypt*. Cambridge: Cambridge University Press, 1998.

Roy, Denny. *Taiwan: A Political History*. Ithaca: Cornell University Press, 2003.

Roy, Patricia. *The Triumph of Citizenship: The Japanese and Chinese in Canada, 1941–67*. Vancouver: University of British Columbia Press, 2007.

Royal College of Dental Surgeons of Ontario and Ontario Dental Association. "Exhibit No. 325: Submission of the Royal College of Dental Surgeons of Ontario and Ontario Dental Association." In *Hearings of the Royal Commission on Health Services 1961–1962*. Vol. 61: Hearings Held at Toronto Ont. 11486-11539. Hand-bound at the University of Toronto Press [1964].

Royal Commission on Doctors' and Dentists' Remuneration. *Royal Commission on Doctors' and Dentists' Remuneration, 1957–1960*. London: HMSO, 1960.

Royal Commission on Health Services. *Briefs and Submissions to the Canada Royal Commission on Health Services.* 1961–1962. [unpublished].

– *Hearings of the Royal Commission on Health Services, 1961–1962.* 66 Vols. Official Reporters: Angus, Stonehouse & Co. Ltd. Handbound at the University of Toronto Press [1964].

– *Report of the Royal Commission on Health Services.* Ottawa: Queen's Printer, 1964.

Russell, George. "Enlarge Immigration Staff to Clear Backlog." *The Globe and Mail,* 31 May 1972, 8.

Rusted, Ian E. "Faculty of Medicine Memorial University of Newfoundland." In *New Medical Schools at Home and Abroad,* edited by John Z. Bowers and Elizabeth F. Purcell, 219–59. New York: Josiah Macy Jr Foundation, 1978.

Sackley, Nicole. "Foundation in the Field: The Ford Foundation's New Delhi Office and the Construction of Development Knowledge, 1951–1970." In *American Foundations and the Coproduction of World Order in the Twentieth Century,* edited by John Krige and Helke Rausch, 232–60. Gottingen: Vandenhoeck & Ruprecht.

Saskatchewan Advisory Planning Committee on Medical Care. *Interim Report of the Advisory Planning Committee on Medical Care to the Government of Saskatchewan.* Regina: Queen's Printer, 1961.

Saskatchewan Farmer's Union. *The Submission of the Saskatchewan Farmer's Union to the Royal Commission on Health Services.* Regina: January 1962.

Saskatchewan Federation of Labour. *The First Fight for Medicare.* Regina: The Federation of Labour, 1962.

Sayyid Marsot, Afaf Lutfi. *A History of Egypt: From the Arab Conquest to the Present,* 2nd ed. Cambridge: Cambridge University Press, 2007.

Schofield, J.R. *New and Expanded Medical Schools, Mid-Century to the 1980s: An Analysis of Changes and Recommendations for Improving the Education of Physicians.* Washington, DC: Association of American Medical Colleges, 1984.

Seale, John. "Medical Emigration from Great Britain and Ireland." *British Medical Journal* 1, no. 5391 (May 1964): 1173–8.

Sehgal, Deep, and Tim Whitby, dir. and prod. *The Indian Doctor.* London: BBC, 2010–2013.

Sen, S.C. "Misdistribution and Not Shortage of Doctors." *Journal of the Indian Medical Association* 38 (1 January 1962): 46–7.

Shillington, Howard C. *The Road to Medicare in Canada.* Toronto: Del Graphics Pub. Dept., 1972.

Shivapuri, H.N. "Shortage of Doctors." *Journal of the Indian Medical Association* 36 (1 January 1961): 28.

Shkimba, Margaret, and Karen Flynn. "'In England We Did Nursing': Caribbean and British Nurses in Great Britain and Canada, 1950–70." In *New Directions in Nursing History: International Perspectives*, edited by Barbara Mortimer and Susan McGann, 141–57. London: Routledge, 2005.

Shortt, S.E.D. "Physicians, Science, and Status: issues in the Professionalization of Anglo-American Medicine in the Nineteenth Century." *Medical History* 27, no. 1 (1983): 51–68.

Shuval, J.T. and J.H. Bernstein. *Immigrant Physicians: Former Soviet Doctors in Israel, Canada, and the United States.* Westport, CT: Praeger Publishers, 1997.

Sigerist, Henry E. *Report of the Saskatchewan Health Services Survey Commission.* Regina: Thomas H. McConica, King's Printer, 1944.

Silversides, Ann. "Money is Still Central Issue, Fear of Losing Power Galvanizes MDs." *The Globe and Mail*, 29 April 1986, A17.

– "Non-participation by Many MDs Will Likely Soften the Blow of Walkout." *The Globe and Mail*, 12 June 1986, A1.

– "OMA Votes to Continue Strike Action." *The Globe and Mail*, 26 June 1986, A1.

Silversides, Ann, John Douglas, and David Todd. "Doctors Wrestle with Call to Strike." *The Globe and Mail*, 11 June 1986.

Simpson, Jeffrey. "A Losing Battle." *The Globe and Mail*, 20 June 1986, A6.

Simpson, Julian M. *Migrant Architects of the NHS: South Asian Doctors and the Reinvention of British General Practice (1940s–1980s).* Manchester: Manchester University Press, 2018.

Simpson, Julian, Aneez Esmail, Virinder Kalra, and Stephanie Snow. "Writing Migrants Back into NHS History: Addressing a 'Collective Amnesia' and Its Policy Implications." *Journal of the Royal Society of Medicine* 103, no. 10 (2010): 392–6.

Smith, John, dir. *Prairie Giant: The Tommy Douglas Story.* Miniseries aired 12 and 13 March 2006 on CBC.

Spasoff, R.A. and S. Wolfe. "Trends in the Supply and Distribution of Physicians in Saskatchewan." *Canadian Medical Association Journal* 92, no. 10 (1965): 523–8.

Spaulding, W.B., and W.O. Spitzer. "Implications of Medical Manpower Trends in Ontario, 1961–1971." *Ontario Medical Review* 39, no. 9 (September 1972): 527–33.

Spaulding, W.B., and Janet Cochran. *Revitalizing Medical Education: McMaster Medical School, the Early Years 1965–1974.* Philadelphia: BC Decker, 1991.

Spencer, Ian R.G. *British Immigration Policy Since 1939: The Making of Multi-Racial Britain.* New York: Routledge, 2002.

Spinks, J.W.T. *Decade of Change: The University of Saskatchewan 1959–70.* Saskatoon: University of Saskatchewan, 1972.

Stevens, Rosemary. *Medical Practice in Modern England: The Impact of Specialization and State Medicine.* New Haven, CT: Yale University Press, 1966.

Stevens, Rosemary and Joan Vermeulan. *Foreign Trained Physicians and American Medicine.* Washington, DC: United States National Institutes of Health, 1972.

Stevens, Rosemary, L.W. Goodman, and S.S. Mick. *The Alien Doctors: Foreign Medical Graduates in American Hospitals.* New York: John Wiley, 1978.

Stevenson, H. Michael, and A. Paul Williams. "Physicians and Medicare: Professional Ideology and Canadian Health Care Policy." *Canadian Public Policy* 11, no. 3 (September 1985): 504–21.

Stevenson, H. Michael, A. Paul Williams, and Eugene Vayda. "Medical Politics and Canadian Medicare: Professional Response to the Canada Health Act." *The Milbank Quarterly* 66, no. 1 (1988): 65–104.

Strong-Boag, Veronica. "Canada's Women Doctors: Feminism Constrained." In *Medicine in Canadian Society: Historical Perspectives*, edited by S.E.D. Shortt, 207–35. Montreal and Kingston: McGill-Queen's University Press, 1981.

Susser, M., and V.P. Cherry. "Health and Health Care under Apartheid." *Journal of Public Health Policy*, 3, no. 4 (December 1982): 455–75.

Svobodny, Petr. "The Medical Faculty." In *A History of Charles University*, edited by František Kavka and Josef Petráň, 405–38. Chicago: Karolinum & University of Chicago Press, 2001.

Swope, C.D. "Doctor Draft Regulations." *The Journal of the American Osteopathic Association* 50, no. 4 (1950): 232–4.

Talani, Leila Simona. *From Egypt to Europe: Globalisation and Migration Across the Mediterranean.* 5 vols. New York: Tauris Academic Studies, 2010.

Talbot, Ian. *Pakistan: A New History.* London: Hurst & Company, 2012.

Taylor, Kenneth Lyle. "The Pursuit of Industrial Development in New Brunswick and Saskatchewan, 1945–1970: A Comparative Study." MA Thesis, University of New Brunswick, 1995.

Taylor, Lord Stephen. "Saskatchewan Adventure: A Personal Record. I. Background to the Story." *Canadian Medical Association Journal* 110, no. 6 (1974): 720–passim [720, 723, 725, 727].

Taylor, Malcolm G. "The Canadian Health System in Transition." *Journal of Public Health Policy* 2, no. 2 (1981): 177–87.

– *Health Insurance and Canadian Public Policy.* 3rd ed. Montreal and Kingston: McGill-Queen's University Press, 2009.

– *Health Insurance and Canadian Public Policy: The Seven Decisions That Created*

The Canadian Health Insurance System. Montreal and Kingston: McGill-Queen's
   University Press, 1978.

Tesson, Geoffrey, Geoffrey Hudson, Roger Strasser, and Dan Hunt, eds. *The Making
   of the Northern Ontario School of Medicine*. Montreal and Kingston: McGill-
   Queen's University Press, 2009.

The Canadian Medical Association. "A Submission Respecting Health Insurance
   Presented to the Special Committee on Social Security of the House of Commons." *Canadian Medical Association Journal* 48, no. 5 (May 1943): 383–94.

Tignor, Robert L. *Egypt: A Short History*. Princeton, NJ: Princeton University Press,
   2011.

Todd, David. "Patient Having Miscarriage Turned Away by Hospital." *The Globe
   and Mail*, 19 June 1986, A22.

Tollefson, E.A. *Bitter Medicine: The Saskatchewan Medicare Feud*. Saskatoon, SK:
   Modern Press, 1964.

Troper, Harold. "Canada's Immigration Policy since 1945." *International Journal* 48,
   no. 2 (1993): 255–81.

Tudiver, Neil. *Universities for Sale: Resisting Corporate Control Over Canadian
   Higher Education*. Toronto: Lorimer, 1999.

Twohig, Peter L. "'Everything Possible Is Being Done': Labour, Mobility, and the
   Organization of Health Services in Mid-Twentieth Century Newfoundland."
   Canadian Bulletin of Medical History 36, no. 1 (2019): 1–26.

United States Congress, Senate Committee on Armed Services. *Armed Services
   Security Cases: Hearing Before the Committee on Armed Services, United States Se-
   nate, Eighty-third Congress, Second Session, on Report on Progress in Implementing
   Defense Department Directive on Armed Services Security Cases Having a Loyalty
   Connotation, as Requested in Hearings on S. 3096, Doctor Draft Act Amendments.
   July 15, 1954*. Washington, DC: United States Government Printing Office, 1954.

– *Doctor Draft Substitute: Amending the Universal Military Training and Service Act,
   as Amended, as Regards Persons in the Medical, Dental, and Allied Specialist Categories. June 6, 1957. Hearing Before the Committee on Armed Services, United
   States Senate, Eighty-fifth Congress, First Session, on HR 6548*. Washington, DC:
   United States Government Printing Office, 1957.

University of Sherbrooke. *Université de Sherbrooke Annuaire General 1970–71*.
   Sherbrooke, QC: 1971.

University of Western Ontario. UWO *Composite Calendar 1970–71*. London, ON:
   University of Western Ontario.

Van Hoek, F.J. *The Migration of High Level Manpower from Developing to Developed Countries*. The Hague: Mouton, 1970.

Van Schendel, Willem. *A History of Bangladesh*. Cambridge: Cambridge University Press, 2009.

– "The Pakistan Experiment and the Language Issue." In *The Bangladesh Reader: History, Culture, Politics*, edited by Meghna Guhathakurta and Willem van Schendel, 177–83. Durham, NC: Duke University Press, 2013

Vaněk, Miroslav and Pavel Mücke. *Velvet Revolutions: An Oral History of Czech Society*. New York: Oxford University Press, 2016.

Vayda, Eugene. "Prepaid Group Practice Combines Personal Health Care Services, Good Organization." *Canadian Medical Association Journal* 109, no. 1 (1973): 72–3, 75, 77.

Walsh, Jeanette and Marilyn Beaton. *Come From Away: Nurses Who Immigrated to Newfoundland and Labrador*. St John's, NL: Breakwater Books, 2011.

Wang, Ru-jer. "From Elitism to Mass Higher Education in Taiwan: The Problems Faced." *Higher Education* 46, no. 3 (2003): 261–87.

Waring, Gerald. "Report from Ottawa." *Canadian Medical Association Journal* 95, no. 1 (2 July 1966): 36.

Webster, Charles. *The National Health Service: A Political History*. Oxford: Oxford University Press, 2002.

Weindling, Paul. "Medical Refugees and the Modernisation of British Medicine, 1930–1960." *Social History of Medicine* 22, no. 3 (2009): 489–511.

Weinerman, Edwin Richard, and Shirley B. Weinerman. *Social Medicine in Eastern Europe: The Organization of Health Services and the Education of Medical Personnel in Czechoslovakia, Hungary, and Poland*. Boston: Harvard University Press, 1969.

Weisz, George. "The Geographical Origins and Destinations of Medical Graduates in Quebec, 1834–1939." *Histoire Sociale/Social History* 19, no. 37 (1986): 93–119.

Westell, Anthony. "$500 Million Is Allocated for Hospitals, Medical Schools, Research." *The Globe and Mail*, 23 September 1965, 1.

– "Ontario to Get $100,000,000 in Health Aid." *The Globe and Mail*, 1 February 1966, 1.

Wilbur, Richard. "From Family History to Local History: Doris Calder and the Kingston Peninsula." In *The Maritimes: Tradition, Challenge and Change*, edited by George Peabody, Carolyn Macgregor, and Richard Thorne, 195–8. Toronto: James Lorimer and Company, 1987. Reprinted from Doris Calder, *All Our Born*

Days: A Lively History of New Brunswick's Kingston Peninsula, New York: Percheron Press, 1984.

Winnipeg Chamber of Commerce. "Exhibit No. 66: Submission of the Winnipeg Chamber of Commerce." In *Hearings of the Royal Commission on Health Services, 1961–1962*, vol. 15, *Hearings Held at Winnipeg, Manitoba*, 3615–61. Handbound at the University of Toronto Press [1964].

Woods, David. "The Alleged MD Surplus: A Need for Superb Data, National Policy." *Canadian Medical Association Journal* 129, no. 11 (1983): 1171.

World Health Organization. *Multinational Study of the International Migration of Physicians and Nurses*. Geneva: World Health Organization, 1973.

– *Multinational Study of the International Migration of Physicians and Nurses: An Analytical Review of the Literature*. Geneva: World Health Organization, 1976.

– "World Health Assembly Concludes: Adopts Key Resolutions Affecting Global Public Health." World Health Organization News. 25 May 2005. https://web.archive.org/web/20050527220627/https://www.who.int/mediacentre/news/releases/2005/pr_wha06/en/ [Archived 27 May 2005].

Wright, David Stuart. "Factors Influencing the Location of Practice of Residents and Interns in BC: Implications for Policy Making." MSc thesis, University of British Columbia Department of Health Care and Epidemiology, 1985.

Wright, David. *SickKids: The History of the Hospital for Sick Children*. Toronto: University of Toronto Press, 2016.

Wright, David, Nathan Flis, and Mona Gupta. "The 'Brain Drain' of Physicians: Historical Antecedents to an Ethical Debate, c. 1960–79." *Philosophy, Ethics and Humanities in Medicine* 3, no. 24 (November 2008).

Wright, David, Sasha Mullally, and Colleen Cordukes. "'Worse than Being Married': The Exodus of British Doctors from the National Health Service to Canada, c. 1955–1975." *Journal of the History of Medicine and Allied Sciences* 65, no. 4 (2010): 546–75.

Wu, Wen-Hsing, Shun-Fen Chen, and Chen-Tsou Wu. "The Development of Higher Education in Taiwan." *Higher Education* 18, no. 1 (1989): 117–36.

Xierali, Imam M. "The Characteristics and Distribution of International Medical Graduates From Mainland China, Taiwan, and Hong Kong in the US." *GeoJournal* 78, no. 1 (2013): 139–50.

Young, Morley A.R. "The Impact of Hospital Insurance on the Practice of Medicine: Bill 320 et Sequentia." *Canadian Medical Association Journal* 78, no. 10 (May 1958): 754–8.

Zarecor, Kimberly Elman. *Manufacturing a Socialist Modernity: Housing in Czechoslovakia, 1945–1960*. Pittsburgh: University of Pittsburgh Press, 2011.

Zohry, Ayman. "Migration and Development in Egypt." In *Migration from the Middle East and North Africa to Europe: Past Developments, Current Status and Future Potentials*, edited by Michael Bommes, Heinz Fassman, and Wiebke Sievers, 75–98. Amsterdam: Amsterdam University Press, 2014.

Index

cil of Canada (LMCC), 32, 40, 187, 188; in
Ontario, 132; prearranged job contracts/
provincial approval and, 231; protectionism in, 39–40; provincial governments
and, 31–2; provincial variations, 32;
provisional/conditional, 231; of refugee
doctors, 38; and underserviced areas, 32;
in US, 295n49. *See also* accreditation;
reciprocity
Lomas, Jonathan, 210

MacDonald, Iain, 71–2
McEachern, Justice, 235–6
McGeachy, James Burns, 39 40
McGill University: and Jewish students, 29;
medical school, 26, 27f, 28, 29, 30, 120
McIntosh, Lachlan, 216–21
Mackasey, Bryce, 97
Maclean's, on foreign-trained doctors in
Ontario, 132, 133f
McMaster University: Faculty of Health
Sciences, 113, 115–16; medical school, 91,
92, 96
MacMillan, J.A., 76
McNair, David, 209–12
McPherson, T.A., 241
Madison, Donald, 201
Maioni, Antonia, 8, 94–5
Makerere University (Uganda), 168
Malaysian American Commission, Educa-
tion Council for Medical Graduate Exam-
inations, 164
maldistribution of doctors: declining/
converging physician–population ratios
vs, 230–1; and entitlement to services, 254;
foreign-trained doctors and, 251; Hall
Commission and, 93–4, 180; interprovincial, 82, 196; local solutions, 197; national
health insurance and, 195; in Ontario, 184–
5, 196; recruitment of medical migrants
and, 177; and rural/remote areas, 193–4,
248–9; in rural/remote vs urban areas, 21,
80; shortage vs, 23, 184–5, 198, 225; in
South Africa, 168–9; supply/demand economic model and, 232; supply vs, 149, 184–5,
194, 256; between urban vs rural/remote
areas, 82
Mandela, Nelson, 174
Manitoba: credentialing in, 187; extra billing
in, 245; foreign-trained doctors in, 195,
208; medical education in, 28; medical
graduating class remaining in, 80; physician–population ratio, 82; and Quebec

hunger strike, 247; reciprocity of foreign-
trained doctors with GMC qualifications,
187; resource/industrial towns in, 208,
212–16 (*see also* Thompson, Manitoba);
retention of recruited doctors in, 225;
rural/remote areas in, 47, 195; Taiwanese-
trained doctors in, 139–40
Manitoba, University of: Faculty of Medicine regarding doctor shortage, 193; and
Jewish students, 29
Manitoba College of Physicians and Sur-
geons, 80
Manitoba Medical College, 28
Manpower and Immigration Act, 194
Marchand, Jean, 101–2
Marchildon, Greg, 8
Margulies, H., 154–5, 156–7, 160
Maritime Hospital Service Association, 76
Maritime provinces: British Isles-trained
medical graduates in, 30; foreign-trained
doctors in, 196; Irish-trained doctors in,
30; Pakistan-trained doctors in, 144;
physician–population ratios, 82. *See also*
New Brunswick; Nova Scotia; Prince
Edward Island
Martin, Paul Sr, 73
Mayo Clinic, 202
medical associations. *See* medical societies
Medical Care Act (1966), 7, 128; about, 106–7;
and Albertan for-profit health insurance
companies, 108; Canada Health Act (1984)
and, 10, 238; and cost sharing, 237; and
extra billing, 109; and nation building, 120;
and numbers of foreign-trained doctors
in Canada, 127; and opting-out of Medicare, 95; and points system, 20; royal assent, 104; as taking effect in 1968, 270n41;
White Paper on Immigration and, 104.
See also Medicare
Medical Care Insurance Act (Saskatchewan),
84–5
Medical Care Insurance Commission
(MCIC), 84, 86
Medical Council of Canada (MCC), 32, 40,
131, 132; Licentiate (LMCC), 32, 40, 187, 188
medical doctorate (MD), 26, 32, 48
medical draft (US). *See* doctor draft (US)
medical education: about, 26–34; Association of Medical Students of South Africa,
170f; baby boom and, 26; within British
Empire, 54; British-/Irish-trained doctors
and, 26; changes in, 48; completion in
Britain, 54; federal funding for, 20; and

medical doctorate (MD), 26, 32; medical
research vs, 113, 115; numbers of Canadian-
trained graduates, 30; in Ontario, 28;
population growth and, 78, 79; postwar
economic growth and, 26; in South Africa,
224–5; South Asian, 133; and supply of
doctors, 250; and urban vs rural practice,
48; in US, 115. *See also* medical schools
medical migration: from African countries,
157; bilateral programs, 161–2; Canada as
crossroads of, 264; and compulsory national service, 163–4; cost, in Ontario, 226;
countries encouraging training for export,
173–4; and developed countries as both
donor and recipient, 173; domino effect,
163; donor countries, 160–4; economic impact on poorer countries, 157–8; geopolitical events and, 152, 264; and global health
care ethics, 6, 23, 152–3, 154, 162, 260–1;
immigration regulation/policies and, 6;
from India, 157; individual loss/regret/
self-questioning regarding, 175–7; "international" doctors and, 174; interprovincial,
226–7; for knowledge transfer vs permanent resettlement, 161; Medicare and, 6–9,
177; oral history of, 8–9; peak of, 20; and
permanent resettlement vs returning to
home countries, 173; as physician's personal choice, 174; points system and, 177;
polarizing debate over, 20–1; for postgraduate education, 9; and prearranged
contracts/ provincial approval, 227; pro-
hibition/ethical regulation of, 261; and return to native countries, 154–5; subsidence
of interest in, 260; towards economically
advantages vs disadvantaged countries,
159; unpredictable movement of physicians, 172–3; volume of, 263–4; who reports on, 159–60. *See also* immigration;
international medical graduates (IMGs)
medical profession: attitudes toward foreign-
trained medical residents, 155–6; CMA and,
43; and federal vs provincial responsibilities for medical practice, 31–2; federal vs
provincial responsibilities for regulation
of, 31–2; and medical journals, 26; and
professionalization of medicine, 26, 30; in
Saskatchewan community care clinic system, 43; vs state regarding medical insurance systems, 7; and universal health
insurance, 8. *See also* medical societies
medical schools: and bilateral agreements,
177–8; in Caribbean, 174; closures, 235;

Commonwealth doctors as faculty in, 115–
16; development of, 26–30; discrimina-
tory/restrictive admission to, 29–30;
in Egypt, 131; enrolment, 78–9, 120, 249;
faculty, 113, 115–18; foreign students in, 119–
20; global diversity of, 128; Hall Commission and, 91–2, 93f, 96; in Ireland, 127;
location in urban areas, 80, 82, 256; location outside principal cities urban areas,
249; Medicare and, 106, 111; new, 11, 22, 96,
106, 111, 112, 113, 115–18, 227, 254, 257; New
Brunswick and, 187; numbers of, 28, 33f,
250; numbers of IMGs vs numbers of
graduates from, 56; and oversupply of
doctors, 55; in Quebec, 246, 271n12; and
rural areas practice, 249; and self-
sufficiency of doctor supply, 227–8; in
South Africa, 169, 223, 224; South Asian,
133–4; and supply of doctors, 250; in US,
30; women students, 29–30, 120. *See also*
medical education; *names of universities
and places*
Medical Service Amendment Act (1985)
(BC), 236
medical societies: on extra billing, 243; and
group practice, 202; and health policy, 47;
and HIDS, 76; tensions with provincial
governments over credentialing, 187; universal health insurance and, 47. *See also*
British Medical Association; Canadian
Medical Association (CMA)
Medicare: accessibility under, 242; and access to physicians/services, 254; Canada
Health Act (1984) as consolidation of rules
governing, 244–5; and Canadian self-
identity, 6; as centennial project, 111; comparative developmental perspective, 8;
comprehensiveness of, 107, 108; copayments, 237; as creation of Medical Care
Act, 106; and distribution of doctors, 259;
doctor opting-out of, 108–9; and doctor
shortage, 185; Douglas and, 6–7; extra billing under, 109–10, 237–8, 240; and federal
health transfers to provinces, 95–6; fee-
for-service remuneration, 109; fee schedules, 109; foreign-trained doctors and, 11,
96; and for-profit/not-for-profit insurance
companies, 108; four principles of, 107–11;
global diversity of foreign-trained doctors,
and impact on, 128; and group practices,
22, 202; Hall Commission on implementation challenges, 95–6; and health care as
provincial responsibility, 7; launch date,

225; for rural/remote areas, 46–7, 180; in
South Africa from other African countries, 260; of South African doctors, 260;
for underserviced areas, 258–9
Red Deer, numbers of physicians/foreign-
trained physicians in, 207–8
refugee doctors: licensing of, 38; in NHS, 55;
and underserviced areas, 38
refugees: after Indian Partition, 141; Chinese,
283n12; Hungarian Revolution (1956) and,
36, 283n12; under Immigration Act (1976),
228–9; as medical students, 120; postwar,
35; Prague Spring and, 283n12; Syrian,
264–5
registration: in Alberta, 187; foreign-trained
doctors and, 64; of foreign-trained doctors in Ontario, 131–4; between GMC and
Commonwealth, 30–1; GMC responsibility
for, 278n50; in Ontario, 131–2, 134. See also
licensing; reciprocity
remigration, 173; within British Empire, 53–
4; foreign-trained doctors and, 256; from
New Brunswick, 39; and oversupply of
doctors, 22; of Pakistan doctors after
advanced training in Britain, 144; from
rural/remote areas, 47; and rural vs urban
areas, 257; of skilled professionals, 156; of
South African doctors, 172; of South Asian
doctors from Britain to US, 154; from
underserviced areas, 225–6
remuneration: British-trained doctors and,
203–4; in Canada vs UK, 193, 217; Canadian vs British, 59; caps on earnings, 241;
in community hospitals, 46; doctor attitudes toward salaries, 204; doctor-initiated
demand for services and, 233; extra billing,
95, 109–10, 234, 237–8, 240–5, 251; fee-for-
service, 109; fee schedules and, 109, 234,
236, 237, 243, 245; for foreign doctors as
Saskatchewan strikebreakers, 86–7;
foreign-trained doctors in Canada vs NHS,
64; licensing restrictions and, 39; of NHS
vs foreign physicians, 59; in Nova Scotia
vs NHS, 62; payment model of health
care system and, 258–9; prescription of
more/more expensive services for, 234; in
rural vs urban areas, 258; salaries in niche
sectors, 109; in urban vs rural/remote
areas, 82; in US vs Canada, 186–7. See also
fee-for-service system
Requirements Committee on Physician
Manpower (ON), 226
research, medical: clinical training vs, 119;

facilities, 119; federal government and, 119;
general practice vs, 256; Hall Commission
studies, 78; Health Research Infrastructure
Grant, 96; medical education vs, 113, 115
Research Ethics Board, 17
residencies. See internships/residencies
resource/industrial towns: about, 200; about
resource towns, 204–5; in Alberta, 207–8;
in British Columbia, 208; British-trained
doctors in, 199–200; in Cape Breton, 205,
207; defined, 204; expansion of physician
population in, 205–6; foreign-trained doctors in, 22, 200–1, 204, 205–9, 206t, 209–12,
221–2; group practices in, 256; managing
doctor supply in, 221–2; in Manitoba, 208,
212–16; in New Brunswick, 207; in Newfoundland, 207; in Ontario, 205, 209–12;
and resource development and economic
growth, 213–14; in Saskatchewan, 208–9.
See also Sault Ste Marie; Thompson,
Manitoba; and names of other towns
Resources for Freedom program (US),
213–14
retention: democratization of group practices and, 220–1; of foreign-trained doctors in Canada, 149–50; of medical
practitioners, 47; mobility restraints and,
231; of recruited doctors, 38, 225; in
rural/remote areas, 180; turnover vs, 44, 46
Roberts, Harry, 227–8
Rockefeller Foundation, 157
Roddick, Sir Thomas, 27f
Roos, Noralou, 257–8
Rorem, C. Rufus, 201–2
Roy, Patricia, 35
Royal Canadian Mounted Police, 151–2
Royal Commission on Doctors' and Dentists' Pay (UK, 1960), 55
Royal Commission on Health Services (Hall
Commission), 16, 21, 56, 82, 84, 90–1, 103;
and challenges in Medicare implementation, 95–6, 104, 106; CMA and, 94; commissioners, 78; Fairclough Directive and
conclusion of, 104; final report, 94; and
foreign-trained doctors in Ontario, 132;
hearings, 78; and loss of medical graduates
to US, 149; and maldistribution of doctors, 93–4, 180; mandate, 77–8; and medical manpower, 78; and medical schools,
91–2, 93f, 96; on numbers of Canadians
without health care for medical services,
76; and nursing shortage, 92; and physician access/supply, 171; and reliance on

foreign-trained doctors, 91, 93; research studies, 78; on staffing, 104, 106, 111; tabling of report, 91; and universal health insurance, 91. *See also* Medical Care Act (1966); Medicare

Royal Society (British), and out-migration of scientists, 54

Royal Victoria Hospital, 26

rural/remote areas: access to physicians in, 185, 233; alternatives to physicians for, 248–9; in British Columbia, 236–7; British-trained doctors in, 47, 191–3; dentistry services in, 184; diversity of life in, 180; federal government and, 194; foreign-trained doctors in, 45, 82, 149, 190–3, 208, 248–9, 260; health insurance and physician recruitment for, 46–7; incentives for moving into, 43, 196, 197; local solutions to influence physicians to move into, 197; maldistribution of doctors and, 21, 80, 82, 193–4, 248–9; in Manitoba, 195; medical care in, 11; medical education in urban areas, and doctor supply for, 48; medical schools, and practice in, 249; in New Brunswick, 187–91; in Ontario, 46–7, 184–5; and physician mobility, 185–6; physicians choosing, 179–80; physician workload in, 182, 185; in Prince Edward Island, 181, 182–3; private practice in, 46, 182, 184, 185; provincial government incentives for service in, 180; provincial governments and, 38–9; public health problems in, 184; reaction of physicians to HIDS, 75–6; reasons for medical graduates settling in urban areas, vs, 80, 82; recruitment for, 180; remigration from, 47; retention in, 180; in Saskatchewan, 181, 183–4; shortages of doctors in, 198; social norms and expectations of access/physicians, 181–2; staff shortages in, 69; subsidies for practice in, 184–5; supply in, 38–9; in UK vs Canada, 191–2; variations among, 181

rural vs urban areas: amenities for rural practitioners, 183–4; foreign-trained doctors in, 251; hospitals and, 190–1; in New Brunswick, 190–1; over- vs underdoctored populations in, 180–1; physician–population ratio(s) in, 195; remigration and, 257; remuneration in, 258; in South African primary care, 168–9; types of professions and, 159; young doctors and practice in, 256. *See also* rural/remote areas; urban areas

Rusted, Ian, 117–18

Sadat, Anwar, 131

St John's, Newfoundland, 45–6

St Laurent, Louis, 73, 74

salaries. *See* remuneration

Sappier, Michael, 262–3

Saskatchewan: anti-Medicare protest, 89f; British-trained doctors in, 48, 68; community care clinics in, 42–4, 273n49; credentialing in, 187; as crucible of experimentation, 77; Depression in, 41, 42; doctors' strike (1962), 7, 19, 48, 78, 83, 85–90, 94; experimentation with programs, 41; extra billing in, 245; foreign-trained doctors in, 7, 45, 68, 90, 149, 208–9; free, state-funded health care in, 7; Health Services Planning Commission, 42; hospital care insurance in, 42, 73, 75; medical education in, 28, 44–5; Medicare in, 77, 84–5; numbers of practitioners, 43–4; personnel shortages, 43; physician–population ratio, 44, 90, 183; prepaid universal health insurance, 44; reciprocity with GMC qualifications, 187; resource/industrial towns in, 208–9; retention of doctors in, 44, 225; rural/remote areas in, 40–5, 181, 183–4; rural vs urban divide in, 183–4; Sigerist and, 41; Social Assistance Plan, 41–2; state-run hospital systems/community care in, 26; Taiwanese-trained doctors in, 140; underserviced areas in, 197; universal health insurance in, 40–5, 77; Wheat Pool farmers' union, 184. *See also* Co-operative Commonwealth Federation (CCF)

Saskatchewan, University of (Saskatoon): faculty obtaining first degrees in Canada, 116; medical school, 28, 44–5; medical sciences/dental sciences buildings, 119

Saskatchewan College of Physicians and Surgeons (SCPS), 280–1n31; conflict with CCF, 83, 84–5; and doctors' strike, 83–5, 88; health plan for indigence/social assistance, 41; and Medical Care Insurance Act, 84–5; opposition to universal medical care program, 84; and private insurance plans, 85

Saskatchewan Federation of Labour, 86

Saskatchewan Hospitalization Act (1946), 19

Saskatchewan Medical Care Insurance Act (1961), 84–5, 89f

Saskatoon Agreement, 88, 90

Sault Ste Marie: advancement in, vs Ottawa, 211–12; Algoma Steel, 205; Community Health Centre, 22; Community Health Centre (CHC), 209, 212; foreign-trained physicians in, 205, 209, 210–12; General

Hospital, 210; group practices in, 211; labour unions and prepaid health care schemes, 209; number of physicians in, 205; Plummer Hospital, 210

Scotland: community/cottage hospitals in, 46; medical migrants in Nova Scotia, 30; South Africa, 50–1

Scottish-trained doctors, 71–2; in Thompson, 216, 217–20, 221

Scott's Medical Database, 16, 17

Seale, John, 56

Sherbrooke, University of: Egyptian-trained doctors at, 131; medical school, 91, 96, 113, 115, 246

shortage(s) of doctors: during 2000s, 249; discussion as coming full circle, 258; and expansion of domestic capacity, 111–12; group practices and, 203; growing discourse regarding, 83; hospitalization insurance and, 19; IMGs and, 254; maldistribution and, 23, 80, 184–5, 198, 225; Medicare and, 185–6, 254; in Newfoundland, 46; and new training facilities, 111–12; oversupply vs, 193; in parts of Ontario, 39; as persistent problem, 254; in Prince Edward Island, 182; protectionism and, 40; reasons for regional, 256; in rural/remote areas, 198. See also supply of doctors

shortage(s) of nurses. See under nurses

Shuval, J.T., 250

Sigerist, Henry, 41, 42

Silversides, Ann, 244

Simpson, Jeffrey, 244

Simpson, Julian, 9

single-payer systems: and doctors as civil servants, 240–1; and group practice, 202; microeconomic models and, 251–2

Six-Day War, 128–9

Skála, Josef, 124f

skilled labour, 25; free movement of, 261; immigration of, 20; incentives to return home, 164; Indian loss of, 162–3; loss of poorer to wealthier nations, 162; migration of, 158–9; points system and, 156; recruiting of, 156; transnational migration of, 156–7; US reconstruction programs for, 161

small towns: foreign-trained doctors in, 149; numbers of physicians/surgeons in, 84t; in Ontario, 186; practice in Prince Edward Island, 182; in Quebec, 247

Smallwood, Joey, 179

Smith-Mundt Act (1948) (US), 161

Snow, Stephanie, Against the Odds, 9

Social Credit Party, 225

socialist/socialized medicine, 7, 8, 19, 41, 42, 48, 76, 94, 108

South Africa: aids epidemic, 175–6; Apartheid and medical care in, 168–70, 175–6; Apartheid in, 223; Association of Medical Students of South Africa, 170f; Bantustans, 168–9, 170; black medical students/ doctors in, 169–70; exodus of doctors, 260; hospitals in, 169, 223–4; Indian medical students in, 223; maldistribution of doctors in, 168–9; medical education in, 224–5; medical schools, 169, 223, 224; Polish doctors in, 50–1; post-Apartheid rebuilding, 260; recruitment from other African countries, 260; Sharpeville massacre, 172

South African doctors: in British Columbia, 225; in Canada, 146f, 171f, 260; global migration of, 168; feelings regarding migration, 175–6; remigration of, 172; in US, 171; Vietnam War, and choice of Canada vs US, 147–8

South African Medical Association, 260

South African medical graduates: in Britain, 171; emigration during internship year, 224–5; postgraduate education abroad, 170–1

South African Medical Journal, 260

Southam Medical Database, 13. See also Canadian Medical Directory (CMD)

South Asia: circulation of ideas/practitioners between East Africa and, 9; and Colombo Plan, 161–2; emigrants in UK, 65–7; emigrants in US, 139; immigrants from, 35; immigration liberalization and emigration from, 139. See also Bangladesh; Ceylon/Sri Lanka; India; Pakistan

South Asian–trained doctors: barring in Ontario, 132, 133–4; in British training courses, 66; in NHS, 53, 55, 69, 154; on permanent settlement vs returning home, 176–7; place of undergraduate training, 141t; remigration from Britain to Canada/US, 154; in Sydney, NS, 3–6. See also Indian-trained doctors; Pakistan-trained doctors

Soweto, 223, 224

Spaulding, William, 196

specialization, 32–4; consultants and, 57, 58; diploma courses, 32; foreign-trained doctors and, 195, 209–12, 226; graduate medical training and, 32–4; as growing trend, 256; medical education in Britain for, 54; in Ontario, 226; Quebec strike, 94;

health insurance and, 195; nurse practi-tioners/nursing assistants and, 196–7; in Ontario, 186; oversupply of doctors and, 193, 258; recruitment for, 258–9; refugee doctors and, 38; reimbursement for service, vs in overserviced areas, 236–7; remigration from, 225–6; in Saskatchewan, 197. *See also* rural/remote areas
Union Public Service Commission, 164
United Kingdom. *See* Britain
United Nations Convention on Refugees, 98
United States: brain drain to, 173, 249; British-trained doctors' attitudes toward, 60; Canadian restriction of access for doctors trained in, 30; Canadian-trained American graduates returning to, 30; Canadian-trained doctors in, 79–80, 81t, 149; Canadian-trained medical graduates in, 82; and Colombo Plan, 161–2; compensation for physicians, vs Canada, 186–7; Czech refugees in, 125; doctor draft, 145–9, 152; East Asian emigrants in, 139; expansion of medical education, 115; foreign medical graduate immigration for advanced training, 154–5; foreign-trained doctors in, 21, 154; group practice in, 201–2; health insurance tied to employment in, 313n24; Indian doctors in, 162, 295n49; Indian scientists in, 162–3; Irish-trained American doctors, 151–2; and Korean War, 136, 137; licensing in, 295n49; loss of graduates to, 186–7; medical school enrolment in, 120; medical schools in, 30; medical students from, 120; Military Selective Service Act, 144, 146–7; NHS doctor migration to, 54–6; numbers of foreign-trained doctors in, 153; reconstruction programs in Europe, 161; remigration of South Asian doctors from Britain to, 154; Resources for Freedom program, 213–14; rural health care in, 41; South African-trained doctors in, 171; South Asian emigrants in, 139; state-subsidized health care in, 94–5; stockpiling of strategic minerals, 213–14; and Taiwan, 135–7; Taiwanese emigrants in, 139; and Vietnam War, 136; Vietnam War and, 144–9. *See also* Vietnam War
universal health insurance: and access to physicians, 91; Beveridge Report and, 41; Canadian vs US paths, 8; and demand for services, 91; and fee-for-service remuneration, 234; foreign-trained doctors and, 254–5; globalization and, 12; Hall Com-

mission and, 91; and immigration regulation/policy changes, 104; and medical personnel supply, 47, 78; medical practitioners and, 8; and medical schools, 91; in nursing history, 8; political science perspectives, 8; prepayment schemes and, 26; in Saskatchewan, 40–5, 77; social history perspectives, 8; and supply/demand economic model, 232. *See also* Medicare
Université de Montréal, 28
Université du Québec network, 112
Université Laval medical school, 28, 119
universities: and Health Resources Fund (HRF), 112; health sciences centres, 111, 112, 119; nursing education in, 92, 113; outreach training projects, 177
Uranium City, immigrant physicians in, 208–9
urban areas: foreign-trained doctors in, 149; maldistribution of doctors and, 80, 82; medical education and, 48; medical schools located in, 80, 82, 256; physician–population ratio in smaller, 84t; practice in British Columbia, 235; reasons for medical graduates settling in, vs rural/remote areas, 80, 82. *See also* rural vs urban areas
Urovitz, Edwin, 241

Verma, Prem, 182–3
Verma, Terrance, 182–3
Victoria, University of: medical school, 91, 92
Vietnam War, 60, 136, 144–9; Canadian neutrality in, 151; doctor draft, 145–8, 151–2; draft, 144–5
Virick, Mohan, 5, 261–3, 263f, 264

Warsaw Pact, 125, 147, 264
Western Ontario, University of (London): as coeducational, 29; dental school, 116; health sciences centre, 116–17; medical school, 28
West Indies. *See* Caribbean
Wheelan, Thomas J. Jr, 145
White Paper on Immigration (1966), 96, 102, 104
Willink Committee, 54–5
Wilson v. Medical Services Commission (British Columbia), 236
Witwatersrand University (Johannesburg), 169, 223, 224
Wolfe, Samuel, 87, 89–90
Wolfville (NS), 51–2

women: enrolment in medical schools, 120;
  medical students, 29–30; in South African
  medical schools, 169, 223
women doctors: choice of destination as
  emigrants, 65; as percentage of physician
  workforce, 29–30; types of practice, 30
Women's College Hospital (Toronto), 29
Women's Medical College (Toronto), 29
Woods, Gordon & Co., 119
workforce, physician: expansion of, vs population growth, 127, 149; foreign-trained
  doctors as proportion of, 10, 127, 254;
  women doctors as percentage of, 29–30
World Congress on Group Practice, 203
World Health Organization (who): brain
  drain chart, 158f; decade of global health
  human resources, 261; on migrant
  physicians/nurses, 153, 159–60, 172; on
  physician–population ratio, 82; and Sault
  Ste Marie Community Health Centre, 209;
  and transnational migration of health care
  personnel, 21
*World Health Organization: Multinational
  Study of the International Migration of
  Physicians and Nurses* (Mejía), 21, 313n24

York University, proposed medical school,
  91, 113, 118, 282n81
Young, Morley, 75–6